Notice to users:

1. User agrees not to redistribute any electronic artifacts of this resource without prior written permission from Free Radical Publishing Co.

2. Except as permitted under the United States Copyright Act of 1976, no part of this publication may be reproduced or distributed in any form or by any means, or stored in a data base or retrieval system, without prior written permission of the publisher.

It is understood that medicine is an ever-changing science. As new research and clinical experience broaden our knowledge, changes in treatment and drug therapy are required. The author and the publisher of this work have checked with sources believed to be reliable in their efforts to provide information that is complete and generally in accord with the standards accepted at the time of publication. However, in view of the possibility of human error or changes in the medical sciences, neither the authors nor the publisher nor any other party who has been involved in the preparation of publication of this work warrants that the information contained herein is in every respect accurate or complete, and they disclaim all responsibility to any errors or omissions or for the results obtained from use of the information contained in the work. Readers should confirm the information contained herein with other sources. For example and in particular, readers are advised to check the product information sheets (or labels) included in the package of each drug they plan to administer to be certain that the information contained in this work is accurate and that changes have not been made in the recommended dose or in the contraindications for administration. This recommendation is of particular importance in connection with new or infrequently used drugs, additives or supplements.

Disclaimers:

Please note: only your personal physician or other health professional you consult can best advise you on matters of your health based on your medical history, your family medical history, your medication history, and how information from any of these databases may apply to you. Neither Dr. Howes nor any party involved in creating, producing or delivering this web site shall be liable for any damages arising out of access to or use of this material or web site, or any errors or omissions in the content thereof.

The information given herein is not intended as medical advice. Always consult with your doctor for underlying illness. Before beginning dietary investigation, consult a dietician or a physician with an interest in nutrition. Information is drawn from the scientific literature, web research, and personal enquiry; while all care is taken, information is not warranted as accurate and the author cannot be held liable for any errors and omissions.

Financial disclosure:

Dr. Howes has no financial conflicts of interest and is not involved in the sale of dietary supplements or fitness equipment. The author holds no stocks or interests in companies in the food additive or antioxidant supplement business.

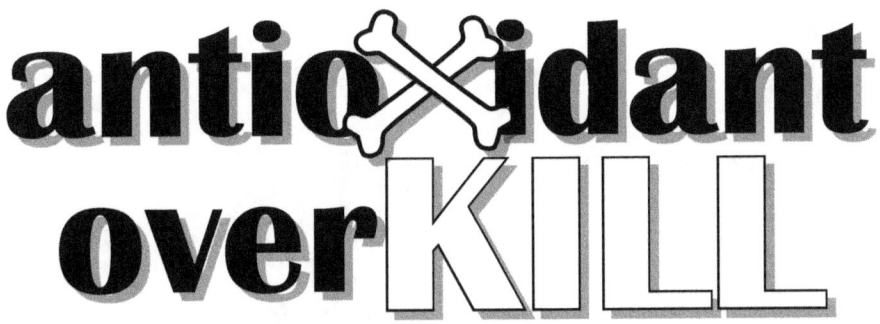

antioxidant overKILL

CRUCIAL PROOXIDANT PATHOGEN AND NEOPLASIA PROTECTION

$$^3\Sigma_g O_2 \; O_2{\cdot}^- \; ^1\Delta_g O_2 \; H_2O_2 \; {\cdot}OH \; HOCl \; NO{\cdot}$$

A SELECTIVE REVIEW
An Antioxidant Guide for the
Educated Consumer

Prof Randolph M. Howes M.D., Ph.D.
Physician, Surgeon, Scientist (Biochemist)

Adjunct Assistant Professor of Plastic Surgery,
The Johns Hopkins Hospital, Baltimore, MD USA

Espaldon Professor of Plastic and Reconstructive Surgery,
University of Santo Tomas, Manila, Philippines

Adjunct Professor of Biological Sciences,
Southeastern Louisiana University
Hammond, LA USA

Founder, Director and Chairman of the Scientific Advisory
Board;
U.S. Medical Scientific Research Foundation, Inc.

Acknowledgements:

Special thanks to Don Neale Piatt, Sr. for expert proofreading. Also special thanks to Michael R. Root, M.S. for his technical expertise.

Extraordinary theories necessitate extraordinary proof. I have amassed epic support for my innovative prooxidant theories to conquer cancer, heart disease, HIV/AIDS and malaria, the biggest global killers of mankind.

R. M. Howes, M.D., Ph.D.

11/7/10

ABOUT THE AUTHOR
RMH Biographical sketch:

Professor Randolph M. Howes M.D., Ph.D. was born on August 17, 1943 in a small rural hospital in Madisonville, Louisiana. While at the hospital, an accidental hip burn from a heating pad introduced Dr. Howes to the harsh realities of life.

Raised on a small bucolic strawberry farm in Ponchatoula, Louisiana, Dr. Howes learned ethics, morality, hard work and respect for his fellow man at a young age. Humble beginnings launched his lifetime trek of achievement as a scientist, surgeon, writer, visionary, philanthropist, international lecturer, singer, songwriter, business entrepreneur, broadcaster, inventor, author, newspaper columnist, corporate executive and rancher.

He attended St. Joseph's elementary school for eight years, served as an altar boy and sang in the choir. Next, he attended Ponchatoula High School where he finished as President of the Student Council by winning an election over the school's quarterback of the football team. He attributes this hard-fought win to his guitar playing and singing abilities. Dr. Howes began playing self-taught guitar professionally at 13 years of age.

In 1961, Dr. Howes entered Southeastern Louisiana College (now Southeastern Louisiana University, SLU), where he took premed courses, made the Dean's list, made the honors chemistry class, worked 40 hours/week at the Psychology Research Laboratory under Dr. John R. Nichols, played music in his 3 piece combo, named The Three Blind Mice, and was elected as president of the Catholic Youth Organization, the Inter-fraternity Council and the Junior class.

He was featured in his college newspaper for his versatility and industriousness and he presented his first scientific paper to the Southwestern Psychological Association on interspecies intelligence, while still in his junior year. He has since been honored as an Outstanding SLU Alumnus, along with Robin Roberts of ABC's Good Morning America. Later SLU articles would refer to him as "a da Vinci in cowboy boots" and the sobriquet stuck.

He has served as an Adjunct Professor of Biological Sciences for many years at SLU. His Southeastern Louisiana University education opened the doors of academia for him and he next matriculated to Tulane School of Medicine in New Orleans, Louisiana.

While working on double doctorate degrees, Dr. Howes worked as a technician on the isolation of thyrotropin releasing factor with Nobel Laureate, Dr. Andrew V. Schalley, studied under Dr. Richard Steele, whose mentor was Nobel Laureate, Dr. Albert Szent Gyorgii, met Nobel Laureates, George Wald and Dr. Linus Pauling, who felt that Dr. Howes could help bridge the gap between physicians and scientists, served as president of the Biochemistry graduate students, graduated in the top 10, received the 1971 Pathology Association Award, was elected to Sigma Xi honor fraternity and was the first in the history of Tulane School of Medicine to receive double doctorate degrees in medicine and biochemistry simultaneously.

He was the first to be designated by the late Dr. Theodore Drapanas as a trained "surgical scientist" at Tulane Medical School.

He matched with his first choice at the prestigious Johns Hopkins Hospital for his surgical internship and residency training. He chose it over other top notch programs because Dr. George Zuidema, Chief and Blalock Professor of Surgery, gave him permission to conduct research studies concurrent with his surgical training in the highly sought after William Stewart Halstead surgical training program.

Even during his internship year, he was permitted lab space by Dr. John Cameron, past president of the American Surgical Association, and he secured his own grants, trained his own lab technicians, slept on the lab floor and later wrote many papers on surgical and oxygen free radical subjects during his residency training.

At the end of his second year of training, he was selected (as only the second resident to do so) to enter a double training surgical program in general and plastic surgery, to be completed in a six year interval.

He played music and sang for many of the surgery resident's functions and broke an ankle in a resident's football game and sustained significant trauma from a motorcycle accident, neither of which caused him to miss a single minute of work.

He was the first to complete board eligibility in both general and plastic surgery at The Johns Hopkins Hospital, while doing basic research on oxygen metabolism, all in a six-year period.

He had the opportunity to work with the pioneer of mitochondrial biochemical function, Dr. Albert L. Lehninger, and rubbed elbows with many of the greats of science, surgery and medicine. He trained with Dr. Edward Luce and Dr. James Wells, both of whom have served as president of the American Society of Plastic and Reconstructive Surgeons. He trained under Dr. John E. Hoopes, past president of the American Association of Plastic Surgeons.

He received many grants, honors and awards from 1971-1977 during his years at Johns Hopkins, which are detailed in his full curriculum vitae. He was Dr. Paul Manson's chief resident, who just retired as Chief of Plastic Surgery at Johns Hopkins Hospital. Also, he was granted a position as Adjunct Assistant Professor of Plastic Surgery at Johns Hopkins Hospital, which was another first at Johns Hopkins.

His musical interests have carried him to perform at the New Orleans World's Fair, on many televised shows, appearing with numerous country superstars and ultimately to center stage at the famed Grand Ole Opry Gospel Hour in Nashville, Tennessee. He has composed over 500 songs and his original "Fantasies of You" recording went to the # 1 chart spot on Nashville's Panel Report for nationwide independent air play.

He was honored by the Country Music Associations of America with a Lifetime Achievement Award, Inducted into the Tracker Hall of Fame, received the King Eagle Humanitarian Award for "Your Devotion To the Betterment of Mankind", received the 1999 Golden Music Award, Lifetime Achievement Award for Songwriter/Artist/Humanitarian and many other such honors.

In 1994, he received Dr. Norman Vincent Peale's America's Awards honoring Unsung Heroes, known as "The Nobel Prize for Goodness," and in 1995, he was awarded an Honorary Doctorate of Humanities Degree by SLU. That same year he was sworn in by Rudolph W. Giuliani, Mayor of New York City, as the Community Mayor for the State of Louisiana, International Council of Mayors and was an awardee, along with the late Dr. Stephen Ambrose, for the George Washington Honor Medal.

Even though he had been told that he could not go directly into solo practice, he boldly returned to New Orleans in 1977 and opened his private practice at the Institute of Cosmetic Plastic Surgery, which became a bona fide success story.

He has served as president of the Metropolitan Cosmetic Surgery Society and the Louisiana Cosmetic Surgery Society, and has served the American Academy of Cosmetic Surgeons in numerous national offices and in many capacities, including national First Vice President of the American Board of Cosmetic Surgery and chairman of the Board of Advisors for the American Society of Liposuction Surgery.

He was awarded a patent certificate for inventing the triple lumen venous catheter in 1977, licensed it to Arrow International, Inc. in 1981, successfully defended it is a multimillion dollar six year patent infringement suit and watched it become recognized as the number one venous catheter in the world. His multilumen catheter has been credited with helping save the lives of over 20 million critically ill patients worldwide and the name of Howes is well-known in over 100 countries.

In the 1980s he became friends with Nobel laureate, Fritz Lipmann, through their work with the Institute of All Nations and the Louisiana University of Medical Science.

He performed pro bono surgery, since 1982 throughout the Philippines, was honored by the Philippine Ministry of Health in 1985 and since 2004, he holds the Espaldon Professorial Chair in Plastic and Reconstructive Surgery at the University of Santo Tomas in Manila.

He was the recipient of the Humanitarian of the Year Award from the Community Mayors of New York, New Jersey and Connecticut in 1996. His philanthropic and humanitarian efforts have been acknowledged by Presidents Ronald Reagan and George H. Bush and he has received a letter of appreciation from past USA President, George W. Bush.

He retired from his private practice to pursue his dream of contributing to a better understanding of oxygen biochemistry and of conducting an arduous in depth review of the world's scientific literature on oxygen metabolism. In 2004, he published his first in a series of e-books on oxygen metabolism, which was a 767-page tome entitled, "U.T.O.P.I.A.: Unified Theory of Oxygen Participation In Aerobiosis."

Also in 2004, in an unprecedented move, The Johns Hopkins Hospital gave him an appointment as an Adjunct Assistant Professor of Plastic Surgery.

In 2005, he published his second e-book, a 931-page tome, entitled, "The Medical and Scientific Significance of Oxygen Free Radical Metabolism." In 2006, he published a third companion e-book, 274-pages, entitled, "Hydrogen Peroxide: Monograph 1: Scientific, Medical and Biochemical Overview and Antioxidant Vitamins: A, C & E: Monograph 2: Equivocal Scientific Studies."

Also in 2006, he published "Cardiovascular Disease and Oxygen Free Radical Mythology, © 2006, 308 pages"; "Diabetes and Oxygen Free Radical Sophistry, © 2006, 366 pages."

After 3 years of work he published the "Reactive Oxygen Species Insufficiency (ROSI) as the Basis for Disease Allowance and Coexistence: Extraordinary Support for an Extraordinary Theory" Volumes 1-3 © 2008; 1564 pages. In 2009, he finished "Reactive Oxygen Species vs. Antioxidants: 'The Oxypocalypse': or The war that never happened" which is a 574 page tome.

He also published "Coffee table musings of the Da Vinci in cowboy boots" © 2009; 104 pages and "The Pundit Speaks: an anthology of neoclassical poetic philosophy" © 2009; 140 pages. In 2009, he also completed, "Antioxidant Vitamins: Vitamins A, C and E, Negligible results, half truths and potential harm as demonstrated by failed intervention trials" © 2009; 130 pages.

In 2010, he published, Death in Small Doses: Antioxidant Vitamins A, C & E in the 21st Century. Book One: A Health Impact Statement For The Layman © 2010; 90 pages and Antioxidant Vitamins are Making A Killing; Antioxidant Vitamins A, C & E in the 21st Century Book Two: A Health Impact Statement For The Medical Scientist© 2010; 184 pages.

In 2011, he is publishing *Killer Antioxidants?* and has an article, *Mythology of the Antioxidant Vitamins,* appearing in the inaugural issue of the Journal of Evidence Based Complementary and Alternative Medicine.

These books contain about 6,000 pages of material and tens of thousands of peer-reviewed references, which represents the most comprehensive selective overview of oxygen metabolism available today. His belief is that the free radical theory is unfounded and that electronically modified oxygen derivatives (EMODs) are of low toxicity and are essential for energy production, for pathogen protection, as secondary cell messengers and as tumoricidal agents.

His Unified Theory states that EMOD insufficiency levels "allow" for the manifestation of diseases, including neoplasia and is a contributing factor in the aging phenomenon. He also postulates that an EMOD insufficiency is the basis for coexistence of diseases.

Dr. Howes, who is both an experimentalist and a theoretician, is an international lecturer on plastic surgery and a world expert on the biochemistry of oxygen free radicals. His passionate goal is to have cures at the bedside, based on his innovative theories involving electronically modified oxygen derivatives, within his lifetime.

THE HOWES SELECTIVE WORLD LIBRARY OF OXYGEN METABOLISM

Dr. R.M. Howes' magnum opus of electronically modified oxygen derivatives (EMODs) in obligate aerobic systems

My series and companion books are the following:

#1. U.T.O.P.I.A. © 2004 Unified Theory of Oxygen Participation In Aerobiosis; 767 pages

#2. The Medical and Scientific Significance of Oxygen Free Radical Metabolism © 2005; 934 pages

#3. Hydrogen Peroxide Monograph 1: Scientific, Medical and Bio-chemical Overview. © 2006; 200 pages

#4. Monograph 2: Antioxidant vitamins A, C & E: Equivocal Scientific Studies, © 2006; 171 pages

#5. Cardiovascular Disease and Oxygen Free Radical Mythology, © 2006; 308 pages

#6. Diabetes and Oxygen Free Radical Sophistry, © 2006; 366 pages

#7, 8, 9. Reactive Oxygen Species Insufficiency (ROSI) as the Basis for Disease Allowance and Coexistence:

Extraordinary Support for an Extraordinary Theory

Vol I, II & III. © 2008; 1564 pages

Volume I 501 pages #7 © 2008

Volume II 505 pages #8 © 2008

Volume III 562 pages #9 © 2008

#10 THE HOWES PAPERS © 2009; 211 pages

#11. Reactive Oxygen Species vs. Antioxidants: "The Oxypoca-lypse" or "The war that never was" © 2010; 550 pages

#12. Death in Small Doses: Antioxidant Vitamins A, C & E in the 21st Century Book One: A Health Impact Statement For The Layman©

Prof Randolph M. Howes MD, PhD

2010; 90 pages

#13. Antioxidant Vitamins are Making A Killing; Antioxidant Vitamins A, C & E in the 21st Century Book Two: A Health Impact Statement For The Medical Scientist © 2010; 184 pages

#14. "COFFEE TABLE MUSINGS of the Da Vinci in COWBOY BOOTS" Pithy Prose and Perspicacious Aphorisms. © 2009; 103 pages

Total pages over 5,700
Over 3,000 pages of my opus are available online
in a searchable format
www.iwillfindthecure.org

Companion Papers:

Citation: R. Howes : Cancer Therapy: A Review with Scientific Validation for the Role of Electronically Modified Oxygen Derivatives in Oncologic Treatment Modalities. *The Internet Journal of Alternative Medicine.* 2010 Volume 8 Number 1.

Citation: R. Howes : Hydrogen Peroxide: A review of a scientifically verifiable omnipresent ubiquitous essentiality of obligate, aerobic, carbon-based life forms. *The Internet Journal of Plastic Surgery.* 2010 Volume 7 Number 1.

Howes M.D., PhD., R. (2009). Dangers of Antioxidants in Cancer Patients: A Review. *PHILICA.COM Article number 153.* Published 7th February, 2009. (20 pages)

Howes M.D., PhD., R. (2008). Aging and anti-aging claims: a review on antioxidant vitamins A, C & E. *PHILICA.COM Article number 116.* Published on 12th January, 2008. (16 pages)

Howes M.D., PhD., R. (2007). Sleep: An original "radical" proposal. *PHILICA.COM Observation number 42.* Published on 5th October, 2007. (1 page)

Howes M.D., PhD., R. (2007). Antioxidant Vitamins A, C & E; Death in Small Doses and Legal Liability? PHILICA.COM Article number 89. Published on 5th April, 2007. (23 pages)

Howes M.D., PhD., R. (2007). Cancer, Apoptosis and Reactive Oxygen Species: A New Paradigm. PHILICA.COM Article number 86. Published on 26th February, 2007. (11 pages)

Howes M.D., PhD., R. (2007). Antioxidant Vitamins A, C and E: Assessing Potential for Harm PHILICA.COM Article number 83. Published on 15th February, 2007. (14 pages)

Howes M.D., PhD., R. (2007). The Consequent Downfall of the Free Radical Theory. PHILICA.COM Article number 75. Published on 22nd January, 2007. (9 pages)

Howes, R.M.: "The Free Radical Fantasy," The Annals of New York Academy of Sciences, 2006, Vol. 1067, pp. 22-26.

Available at www.philica.com
www.medi.philica.com
www.iwillfindthecure.org

OTHER BOOKS PUBLISHED:

The Fire Eaters, Molding your own destiny more easily, Carnivore Press, © 1982

Uplift, The Answer Book to your plastic and cosmetic surgery questions, Carnivore Press, © 1986

The Pundit Speaks, An Anthology of Neoclassical Poetic Philosophy, Carnivore Press, © 1990

The Pundit Speaks, Volume II, An Anthology of Neoclassical Poetic Philosophy, Free Radical Press, © 1994

The Pundit Speaks, Volume III, An Anthology of Neoclassical Poetic Philosophy, Free Radical Press, © 1996

The Fable of the Chocolate Covered Strawberry Coloring Book, Free Radical Press, © 2001

Prof Randolph M. Howes MD, PhD

The Pundit Speaks, Volume IV, An Anthology of Neoclassical Poetic Philosophy, Free Radical Press, © 2003

The Pundit Speaks, Volume V, An Anthology of Neoclassical Poetic Philosophy, Trafford Publishing, © 2009

DEDICATION

To the pantheistic presence
that has persistently enabled my efforts,
maintained my bliss and
provided personal scientific solace
throughout this journey of discovery.

TABLE OF CONTENTS:
(if ever I cease to dream)

"Future's shape is sculpted by the
persistent kneading hands of
the impossible dreamer."

R. M. Howes, M.D., Ph.D.
5/2/04

Book summary: 69 new studies in section one from 2011 plus 181 from 2010 studies from section three, for a total of 250 studies, with 80 of these studies showing harmful effects

EMODs (electronically modified oxygen derivatives) are not as harmful as you might've imagined, not as destructive as you might've thought and not the "inner enemy" you might've feared. In fact, your life depends on them.

R. M. Howes, M.D., Ph.D.
5/28/10

SECTION ONE
DISCUSSIONS FOR THE EDUCATED CONSUMER

American psychologist, the late Anne Roe Simpson, said, "Nothing in science has any value to society if it is not communicated, and scientists are beginning to learn their social obligations." My books are my attempts to communicate the potential dangers of antioxidants to the medical community and to the overall populous. Also, they are my way of introducing people to my attempts at revolutionizing cancer and heart disease prevention and cure, based on oxygen metabolism.

News flash: An apple a day....is highly over rated....and can not guarantee to keep the doctor away. If only it was that simple!

Antioxidant Supplement Guide — Informing the Public

It is mandatory that the public have information about the adverse reactions to antioxidant supplements. The public must know the reasons for avoiding excessive antioxidant supplement intake and when and how to react to protect themselves at the first sign of an adverse drug reaction. Serious medical damage, and potentially death, may be averted only if the patients taking excessive antioxidant supplements stop the drugs at the first sign of untoward effects. Likely, the first sign will be lethargy or unexplained tiredness, as was described by Dr. Denham Harman in a discussion with Jack Challem. Even early stoppage may not guarantee avoidance of long term unintended consequences.

In its announcement proposing Medication Guides (patient package inserts) to provide prescription drug customers with comprehensive and reliable drug information, the FDA stated, "FDA believes that improved dissemination of information about prescription drug products is necessary to fulfill patients' need and right to be informed." Medication Guides are intended to be used in products "that pose a serious and significant public health concern" requiring immediate distribution of drug information to the public." (FDA, 1995).

I am hereby making this book an "Antioxidant Supplement Guide," because, just like drugs, they can also result in significant public health concern. The public must be informed of this and the manufacturers, purveyors, vendors or sellers of these products will not inform the public due to fear of hurting sales and incurring legal liabilities.

Logically, wide ranging antioxidant agents which block oxidation (**food industry** (preservatives, rancidity, spoilage, browning); the **rubber and plastics industry; pharmaceutical industry**; antioxidants in **beverages and herbal products**; antioxidants in all processed foods; etc.) outside of the body have the capability to block oxidation inside of the body, if ingested and absorbed. There may be as many as 25,000 phytochemicals in the human diet, many having direct antioxidant effects. That is where the potential harm and problems start with antioxidant use and overload in humans.

Specifically, the accumulating evidence presented in my books clearly identifies the antioxidant supplements as agents that pose a significant public health concern. To be sure, there are some non-randomized, non-blinded studies showing that the antioxidants can be beneficial but we can not ignore the 80 studies showing adverse effects. With such large populations taking antioxidants on a daily basis, this truly is a global public health issue.

We can not simply cherry-pick the data which favors the viewpoint we are supporting. We must base our conclusions on the best overall scientifically based evidence.

There is no over-riding, monolithic, absolute conclusion, which can be supported by all of the literature. However, acceptance or rejection of view points must be swayed by the preponderance of scientifically reliable data.

Safety

I agree with the following recommendations of the Mayo Clinic. "The U.S. Food and Drug Administration does not strictly regulate herbs and supplements. There is no guarantee of strength, purity or safety of products, and effects may vary. You should always read product labels. If you have a medical condition, or are taking other drugs, herbs, or supplements, you should speak with a qualified healthcare provider before starting a new therapy. Consult a healthcare provider immediately if you experience side effects." http://www.mayoclinic.

com/health/echinacea/NS_patient-echinacea/DSECTION=safety (accessed 12-25-10).

Recommendations for the use of vitamin supplements during cancer treatment have been particularly controversial. **Although many researchers and clinicians have suggested that vitamin supplements, especially high-dose antioxidants, should not be used by patients during cancer treatment, vitamin supplement use is widespread amongst most cancer patients.**

However, theoretical insights indicate that antioxidants could block tumoricidal therapies such as chemotherapy and radiotherapy. If antioxidants protect tumor cells to any extent, they could theoretically lower the efficacy of cancer treatments and promote cancer cell growth, metastasis, recurrence and death.

My global perspective: The antioxidant chemical family originates from a variety of agricultural, industrial, and dietary factors. My review focuses on the many antioxidant products that have been promoted in cancer and heart disease prevention and that are falsely flaunted as bolstering human health without recognizable side effects. However, it appears that these antioxidant molecules, even those originating from vegetables, fruits, plant extracts, and herbs, can have serious cumulative adverse effects when taken in excess.

SECTION ONE

INTRODUCTION

Can there be "too much of a good thing?"

Currently, antioxidants are being promoted as being capable of reversing diseases and aging caused by so-called harmful oxygen free radials. Yet, hundreds of scientific studies do not back up these bold claims and antioxidants are proving to be neither a panacea nor a Fountain of Youth. Additionally, oxygen free radicals are products of normal metabolism and are crucial agents for cellular function and messaging.

Can we ingest too many antioxidants and overload on them?

Can antioxidants be harmful? If so, how harmful?

Can we block too many protective oxidative events?

Is there such a thing as antioxidant hypervitaminosis or hypersupplementation?

As an educated consumer, please follow me and I will thoroughly discuss all of these controversial issues in this book.

First, we must maintain sufficient electron-donating antioxidants in order to form adequate protective levels of electron-accepting pro-oxidants. Problems develop when antioxidant over dosing results in an electronically modified oxygen derivative (EMOD) insufficiency. I prefer to more accurately refer to oxygen free radicals as EMODs. Antioxidant overloading specifically blocks oxidative protection from pathogens and cancer and knocks down our ability to generate sufficient energy levels via the electron transport chain.

The following notes were excerpts of Jack Challem's recount of a conversation with Dr. Denham Harman, father of the nullified free radical theory:

With all the attention given to antioxidants, a lot of questions remain un-answered. How much is enough? How much is too much? Are free radicals really all that bad? Challem began asking these questions because the vita-mins Challem took should have left him feeling energized. But over the past 10 years, he had felt far more tired than he should - tired in the morning, tired in the afternoon, tired in the evening.

It wasn't easy finding answers. Challem finally tracked down the guy who would know: Denham Harman, MD, PhD. He's the fellow who invented the free radical theory of aging back in November of 1954. To Challem's surprise, he discovered that he was doing too good a job crushing those dangerous free radicals we all hear about. Challem **was taking too many antioxidants. With all the talk about the benefits of antioxidants, we forget that free radicals are there for a reason. Free radicals are essential for health.**

Even over-exercising generates extra free radicals. The biggest source of free radicals is our own bodies. (RMH Note: The air we breathe is the biggest source of free radicals, because oxygen in its ground state is a di-radical). *White blood cells use free radicals to destroy bacteria and virus infected cells. Free radicals help the liver detoxify harmful chemicals. They are also a normal by-product of breathing, in which our bodies use oxygen and generate energy. The process of creating energy is like the childhood game "hot potato." Molecules get passed around, as the cells try to keep the good ones and get rid of the bad ones.*

The sheer scale of this activity is mind blowing. Each cell in our body suffers 10,000 free radical "hits" every day.

The relationship between free radicals and antioxidants is one of balance. Challem asked Harman which supplements he took. Unlike a lot of doc-tors who don't want to go on record with this information, he was very up front: 400 IU vitamin E, 2000mg vitamin C, 100 micrograms selenium and 30mg CoQ10 each day and 25,000 IU of beta-carotene every other day. **"I'd take more," he said, "but I can't afford to get tired."** *Challem's ears perked up.* **He explained that too many antioxidants cause fatigue and muscle weakness.**

*Several years ago, in an experiment, Harman found that large amounts of BHT, a man-made antioxidant, interfered with the ability of mice to produce energy. "**Too many antioxidants can leave you feeling very weak," Harman said.** "BHT decreases ATP and mitochondria function." ATP, or adenosine-tri-phosphate, is required for energy production in the mitochondria, which is the part of the cell biologists call the energy factory. Challem asked Harman whether too many natural antioxidants could cause fatigue.*

Harman was positive, "Yes!" There's a point where the stuff turns on you. *(Jack Challem. Some Good Things to Say About Free Radicals. Reproduced from The Nutrition Reporter® newsletter).*

Too much can be too bad. Repeatedly, benefits of antioxidants have been intentionally overstated and adverse effects have been ignored or denied. This must be stopped.

Maureen Storey, Ph.D., a nutritionist with the Georgetown Center for Food and Nutrition Policy, stated, **"You can get too much of a good thing."** People who pop large amounts of vitamins or minerals—thinking that if a little is good, a lot is better—need to know that there are dangerous levels of these compounds.

Avoid over dosing on antioxidants. Excessive levels appears to lower the levels of electronically modified oxygen derivatives (EMODs), which serve as crucial signaling molecules and as protectors against pathogens and cancer. Also, excesses of antioxidant will logically interfere with energy production and lead to fatigue. Antioxidants can interfere with oxidative phosphorylation and oxidation NADH and $FADH_2$, leading to ATP synthesis.

In November 2004, the American Heart Association warned that while the small amounts of vitamin E found in multivitamins and foods were not harmful, taking 400 International Units a day or more could increase the risk of death.

Dr. Pradeep Ramulu, of Wilmer Eye Institute at Johns Hopkins University in Baltimore, wrote in an article about retinal eye diseases (macular degeneration and diabetic retinopathy) that, **"I believe that the increase (in retinal eye diseases) is due to the increased intake of antioxidants, both supplements and fortified foods."**

Further, antioxidants do not appear to prevent or cure eye diseases such as cataracts. In 2008, William G. Christen, an associate professor of medicine at Brigham and Women's Hospital, said, "Although observational data tend to suggest benefits for vitamin E, data from a more rigorous randomized 10-year trial suggests little benefit." At the end of the study, including 37,675 women, there was no difference in the number of cataracts between the groups studied and no difference in the types of cataracts they developed. Nor did those with possible risk factors like age and cigarette smoking get any benefit from vitamin E.

The Heart Outcomes Prevention Evaluation trials, which looked at nearly 10,000 patients 55 and older with vascular disease or diabetes, found no heart benefit from taking 400 IUs of vitamin E daily for an average of seven years. In fact, those taking the vitamin were more likely to develop heart failure, which prompted the heart association warning.

The Women's Health Study, of nearly 40,000 women 45 and older who were followed for an average of 10 years, showed no overall benefit in taking 600 IUs of vitamin E every other day for major cardiovascular events (heart attacks and stroke) or total mortality.

The Physicians' Health Study, 14,641 men 50 and older were followed for up to eight years, and it found that 400 IUs of vitamin E every other day had no effect on the incidence of major cardiovascular events, including cardiovascular deaths. In short, all of these reported that supplements of vitamin E could not be relied upon to protect against eye diseases, heart disease and stroke. The same pattern has been found for the other antioxidants.

If only all those glowing forecasts had turned out to be true. Just as a well-designed clinical trial disproved the notion that postmenopausal hormones could keep women heart-healthy, controlled clinical trials of vitamin E and beta carotene have found the supplements wanting, as well. The same is true of another antioxidant, vitamin C.

Even the National Cancer Institute's website now states, "Considerable laboratory evidence from chemical, cell culture, and animal studies indicates that antioxidants may slow or possibly prevent the development of cancer. However, information from recent clinical trials is less clear. **In recent years, large-scale, randomized clinical trials reached inconsistent conclusions."** (http://www.cancer. gov/cancertopics/factsheet/prevention/antioxidants accessed 1-7-11).

But, please keep in mind that these vitamins can serve in many other important cellular functions, other than in oxidation-reduction reactions (redox reactions). Thus, one should avoid vitamin deficiencies, even of the antioxidant vitamins.

Yes, there can be too much of a (supposed) claimed good thing.

Just being alive, puts you at risk to die

Reportedly, more than 11 million Americans are living with cancer or the prospect that cancer may return, and 1.5 million more may get new diagnoses of the disease this year, driving total cancer care costs above $100 billion a year. Nearly one in four Americans are projected to die from cancer. It is said that one in every two men and one in every three women will get cancer.

In misguided attempts at modernity and to protect themselves against disease, people pop pills faster than oxygen can pick up electrons. The vast majority of the people, many of whom are in the medical sector, remain totally in the dark when it comes to the subject of antioxidant vitamins.

Some say that taking antioxidant vitamins is just "a way to make expensive urine." Others say that we should keep selling and feeding them to the uninformed, because it is, in effect, "a tax on the stupid."

We even have some of our most notable athletes and super stars pushing them onto an ill informed public....and it works!

Have you heard the saying, "I used to eat a lot of natural foods until I learned that most people die of natural causes." Well, there is some truth in that. But add to that a growing list of dangers, such as tobacco product use, alcohol, x-rays, pollution, pesticides, synthetic hormones, smoke and city smog, CAT scans, herbicides, inactivity, obesity, genetic sway, etc.

So, what is one to do? Live life to its fullest each and every day and don't worry so much because even stress can kill you. There is still no substitute for a well balanced diet of fresh fruits and vegetables, some dairy products, fish and meat (in moderation) and daily exercise.

Mistrust in our govermental agencies (FDA, EPA) and distrust of the entire pharmaceutical and dietary supplement industry is also a reality and a growing problem. Legally prescribed drugs are killing more people than illegal drugs and the deep pockets of drug companies allows them to dominate television advertising.

Just consider these recent examples of harmful drug controversy: Accutane, Baycol, Vioxx, Celebrex, hormone replacement therapy, Darvon, Darvocet, Avandia, etc. The list goes on and on. Remember, these drugs were "tested" (supplements are not) and they can still have deadly consequences.

There is even growing mistrust of the medical sector, because they are seen as promoting drugs unnecessarily and making profits off of the drugs they prescribe, many of which are deadly. As Steve Covey said, "Common sense is not so common anymore."

It is clear that far from being a benign health booster, antioxidants and supplements need to be taken with extreme caution. Our bodies are designed to utilize nutrients from food and not from chemical concoctions.

Popping pills for your ills

Today, people are encouraged to run to the doctor and gulp down handfuls of all varieties of medications, many with serious side effects. However, whatever drugs doctors claim are good for you today are likely to change by tomorrow, such as Vioxx, Celebrex, Avandia, hormone replacement therapy, etc. It seems that what was good for you today, will be bad for you next week.

More and more it appears that drug companies, most of which are foreign owned, are only interested in the profit margins and returns for their stockholders. Drugs and vaccines are being recommended and sometimes required (mandated) for a younger and younger population, such as the HPV vaccine and cholesterol lowering drugs for those as young as 8 years old. Now, they are targeting babies and toddlers with unending vaccinations. But, you have got to admit that it opens up huge new drug markets for more of their profits.

Americans are the biggest group of "pill poppers" on the planet. A government report indicates that, for the first time, abuse of painkillers and other medication is sending as many people to the emergency room as the use of illegal drugs.

In 2008, emergency room visits from people abusing prescription or over-the-counter medicines, mostly painkillers and sedatives, totaled about 1 million. That equaled the number of visits from those overdosing on heroin, cocaine and other illegal drugs. The number of drug-related visits have about doubled over the past 5 years and it seems to be still increasing. The trend was clearly led by painkillers, such as oxycodone and hydocodone and sedatives, with tranquilizers bringing up the rear.

Some cases are from mixing or combining (stacking) of drugs or combining them with alcohol. Actually, the number of prescriptions for these drugs have also been increasing and many may have legally obtained their drugs. In 2009, a CDC report found that, "The rate of drug-related deaths roughly doubled from the late 1990s to 2006, and most of the increase was attributed to prescription opiates such as the painkillers methadone, Oxycontin and Vicodin."

Gil Kerlikowske, director of the Office of National Drug Control Policy, said, "The abuse of prescription drugs is our nation's fastest-growing drug problem." In recent years, drug companies have fired up the marketing of pain medications, anti-depressants, sleep aids and tranquilizers. Experts say, "People believe that legally obtained drugs are safer because they are prescribed by doctors and approved by the FDA."

Rest assured, they can still kill you.

Now, there is a startling federal report that 30 million Americans are driving drunk and another 10 million are driving drugged. Although it varies, in some states, drunk and drugged drivers are over 20 percent, according to the Substance Abuse and Mental Health Services Administration (SAMHSA). Unfortunately, younger drivers are more likely to drive while impaired.

Sadly, over ten thousand were killed by drunk drivers in 2009 and drugged drivers caused one in three car accident deaths. These injuries and deaths are PREVENTABLE and guilty parties should be prosecuted to the fullest extent of the law (no deals, no excuses).

Good advice and bad advice

Many strategies are offered for good health and to avoid cancer and heart disease but their value can be questioned. For example, some studies show:

- Avoid all red meat products - eat fish instead but watch out for mercury poisoning.
- Marinate all meat before grilling - better still, don't eat the meat after it is cooked.
- Eat only highly colored vegetables - but watch out for the pesticides and herbicides.
- Drink coffee every day or never drink coffee? It will either help you or kill you.
- Drink eight glasses of water a day - but is their any scientific proof of benefit?
- Snack on nuts - but watch out for the extra calories.
- Avoid dry cleaners because of toxic perchloroethylene - what?
- Ladies get mammograms regularly - if only doctors can come up with a uniform plan.
- Men get PSA tests - but are they reliable?
- When in doubt, get a CAT scan - and get resulting cancer from x-ray overexposure.
- Take calcium - wait, do not take calcium.
- Eat whole grain bread - but many say do not eat carbs at all.
- Take a multivitamin - unless you have read recent reports of their harmful potential.

- Load up on antioxidants - unless you read my last book, *Death In Small Doses?*

Actually, the best advice is to exercise as tolerated, avoid tobacco products, avoid alcohol excesses, eat a balanced diet with fresh fruits and vegetables, and some meats and fish and do not worry about every little thing. There is so much that we still do not know in medicine in our current state of ignorance.

The biggest component associated with disease that we can not yet escape is our genetic makeup. If we have a obvious family trend toward certain diseases, we need to remain alert to early signs of these diseases and seek medical advise immediately. This can save your life.

Do not be fooled by those who pretend to know it all! They do not.

Even multivitamins are being questioned

Scientists at the Fred Hutchinson Cancer Research Center followed 160,000 postmenopausal women for about 10 years. Marian Neuhouser, PhD., lead author, concluded: "Multivitamins failed to prevent cancer, heart disease, and all causes of death for all women. Whether the women were healthy eaters or ate very few fruits and vegetables, the results were the same."

Two massive studies agreed. The first, a review of 63 randomized, controlled trials (the gold standard research method) on multivitamins, published by the Agency for Healthcare Research and Quality found that multivitamins did nothing to prevent cancer or heart disease in most populations (the exception being developing countries where nutritional deficiencies are widespread).

Miriam Nelson, PhD, director of the John Hancock Research Center on Physical Activity, Nutrition, and Obesity at Tufts University, said, "The multivitamin as insurance policy is an old wives' tale, and we need to debunk it." This represents a complete reversal of the thinking surrounding our health care policies, because as recently as 2002, no less an authority than the Journal of the American

Medical Association recommended that "all adults take one multivitamin daily."

Shockingly, as of November 2010, Prevention magazine said that studies show that it may be "Time to kick the multivitamin habit." Studies on boosting immunity have been "equally discouraging" and a British review of eight studies found no evidence that multivitamins reduced infections in older adults.

Other studies found that the vitamins didn't improve fatigue among breast cancer patients undergoing radiation therapy and inner-city schoolchildren who took a multivitamin did not perform any better on tests or have fewer sick days than students who didn't take one.

Other studies even indicate that multivitamins may be harmful. A 2010 study of Swedish women found that those who took multivitamins were 19% more likely to be diagnosed with breast cancer over a 10-year period than those who didn't. Other studies have shown them to cause increased breast density in women, which is associated with breast cancer.

A 2007 paper, in the Journal of the National Cancer Institute, found that men who took multivitamins along with other supplements were at increased risk of prostate cancer, especially the fatal type of prostate cancer.

And other research has linked excessive folic acid intake to higher colon cancer risk in people who are predisposed. David Katz, MD, MPH, director of the Prevention Research Center at Yale University School of Medicine, said, "In terms of a risk-benefit ratio, **why would you accept even a tiny risk if you're not getting any benefit?"**

Excellent question!

Even manufactured supplements bear little resemblance to the natural vitamins and minerals found in fruit, vegetables and other foods. Many now believe that these chemically concocted vitamin supplements are dangerous. European and British authorities are clamping down on manufacturers.

Proof of the supplements industry's fallibility came last year, when hundreds of products were quietly removed from the shelves of UK shops. This under-reported event resulted from a Food Supplements Directive brought into force by the European Commission in 2002, but which only took effect at the end of 2009 because of legal challenges from the health food industry. Nina Papadoulaki, EC spokesperson for health, explained the reasoning behind this mass product cull. "Vitamins and minerals are essential nutrients, but in some cases excessive intake can lead to adverse health effects," she said. "Therefore the Food Supplements Directive foresees the setting of maximum amounts of vitamins and minerals present in these supplements."

In addition to capping the dosage levels of supplements, the European Food Safety Authority drew up a "positive list" of vitamins and minerals deemed non-hazardous to health. Any nutrient not on the list is now banned from sale, including six minerals (tin, silicon, nickel, boron, cobalt, and vanadium) that had been used in food supplements on sale in the UK for many years.

This is worrying enough, but critics of pharmaceutical supplements want the EC to go further, banning the synthetically manufactured vitamins they regard as harmful.

What is the wisdom of taking supplements without a clear understanding of their potentially harmful side effects?

Unfortunately, consumers presume these supplements are safe and use them without their doctors' supervision. Of even more concern, many doctors are barely knowledgable of the harmful potential of the antioxidant vitamins. Many **practitioners argue that their remedies are effective, despite overwhelming scientific evidence to the contrary**. It can be a waste of both private and public money and can be downright dangerous, if used to treat a life-threatening condition like cancer or cardiovascular disease.

My research is very encouraging.

My first clue about our ability to naturally kill cancer was related to "spontaneous regression or remission," which is defined as cancers that shrink or disappear completely, without any conventional or alternative anticancer therapy. It is well-established in the medical literature (hundreds of descriptions) and amongst oncologists.

The most frequently cited cancers that may experience a spontaneous remission include kidney and testicular cancers as well as lymphoma and melanoma (estimated at 1 out of every 400 cases). Perhaps the best studied group is a type of lymphoma referred to as "low-grade, B-cell, Non-Hodgkin's lymphoma." It is well established that approximately 20% of patients diagnosed with this type of lymphoma will experience a spontaneous shrinkage of their disease. It is for this reason that oncologists do not treat these types of lymphoma unless they are causing bothersome symptoms for the patient.

In the *New York Times* (Oct 27, 2009), Gina Kolata wrote an article entitled, "Cancers Can Vanish Without Treatment, but How?" The impetus for her article was recent medical publications on screening tests for breast cancer and prostate cancer (mammography and PSA testing). Kolata wrote, "Besides finding tumors that would be lethal if left untreated, screening appears to be finding many small tumors that would not be a problem if they were left alone, undiscovered by screening. They were destined to stop growing on their own or shrink, or even, at least in the case of some breast cancers, disappear."

I believe that EMODs are, at least to a significant degree, the basis of this phenomenon. They are primarily responsible for EMOD-induced apoptosis (cell suicide), along with a vast complexity of biochemical entities.

Please remember that EMODs can be blocked by antioxidants, which can interact when combined in what is called a "cocktail effect." Others refer to it as a "synergism." Actually, my work shows that combining the antioxidant vitamins increases their harmful consequences, which I presented and discussed in *Death In Small Doses?*

The developed nations have the highest rates of common cancers, such as prostate, breast and lung and it appears that we are transferring this to the lesser developed nations. **Antioxidants are in hundreds of food products and manufactured goods in the industrialized nations.** Are they causal of these diseases? Are they related to the BPAs (bisphenols) used in the plastics industry and which is an antioxidant used to prevent polymerization? We now have excellent leads to answers concerning antioxidants.

Are developed nations like the wealthy Romans, who could afford lead-laden plates and pots and subsequently died of lead poisoning, because they could afford it? The poor were spared and this may be analogous to under developed nations not being able to afford the harmful products (antioxidants) of the industrialized nations (contaminated baby bottles, drink cans, water lines, fortified foods, antioxidant vitamin supplements, etc.).

There are those who say that "cancer is a pathway disease" and I believe that EMODs will lead the way to the cure and prevention of cancer. Redox (oxidation/reduction) pathways will lead us to the door of discovery and I am trying to open and go through that door.

The impotent FDA

Even though millions gulp down antioxidant supplements on a daily basis, most know very little about what they are taking or about the safety or effectiveness of these widely used and highly promoted products. Most are totally unaware that dietary supplements can lead to bad side effects or even life threatening problems or even death.

Some define dietary supplements as being any product in "pill, capsule, tablet, or liquid form containing vitamins, minerals, herbs, or other botanicals, amino acids, or other known dietary substance that is intended as a supplement to the normal diet." In short, this means anything taken "intended to supplement the diet."

Consequently, many people assume that these supplements are safe and effective for treating specific situations, like diseases or illnesses, but the FDA does not require manufacturers of dietary supplements to prove safety or efficacy and most supplements have not been carefully studied. Lack of regulation and government monitoring also means that supplements are not monitored to ensure that they contain the ingredients or amount of active ingredient the manufacturer claims they contain.

Most supplements, like foods, can immediately enter the market, and only after repeated instances of adverse reactions can the Food and Drug Administration (FDA) remove them. The Dietary Supplement

Health and Education Act of 1994 (DSHEA) places dietary supplements in a special category under the general umbrella of "foods," not drugs.

But, please keep in mind that the FDA (and Congress) is dominated by large pharmaceutical interests and that about half of the supplement industry is owned by drug companies. Ergo, you are not going to be successful at changing any of the laws regulating supplements or antioxidant vitamins. Also, if the FDA were to control supplements, prices would go up, just as happens with omega-3 fish oil. It costs about seven times more than the same amount of EPA/DHA fish oil you can buy as a dietary supplement.

People are still shocked that the FDA doesn't regulate supplements, including vitamins, minerals, and herbs, the same way it does for drugs. Supplements don't have to go through any safety testing before they hit stores. Despite 2007 legislation that marginally increased the FDA's authority, health and safety critics say the FDA doesn't have enough resources to oversee the industry.

And the Dietary Supplement Safety Act of 2010 was shot down within months of being introduced.

Please remember that industry can markedly influence the outcome of studies because "money talks." A documentary called, Our Daily Poison, exposes the corruption in both the pharmaceutical industry and the medical profession. Studies can be biased and dishonesty can be commonplace.

It is said that the driving force behind pharmaceutical and supplement companies is "profit at any cost." You decide.

Food for thought

We have all been told that consuming antioxidants will make us look younger, feel younger, boost our immunity, fight diseases (i.e., cancer, heart disease, strokes, diabetes, arthritis), and increase our longevity. But, we have been misled....intentionally.

Since supplements tend to be most perceived for their apparent medicinal qualities, that is where the problems start. They are classified as "food" and not drugs.

The FDA will not remove a supplement from the market until it has been shown to be harmful to people and there is a lack of a program to report adverse effects of these agents and according to Michael McCann, the FDA fails to learn of over 99 percent of adverse consumer reactions. Thus, people serve as guinea pigs until it becomes obvious that these supplements are harmful. I believe that time is now.

Actually, the fact is that the FDA has all the legal authority it needs to remove supplements that contain illegal drugs or have been shown to be harmful from the market. The FDA has failed to do its job, and there are companies selling dietary supplements that contain prescription drugs and I have found hundreds of studies showing the ineffectiveness and harmful potential of the antioxidant vitamins.

The "supplement loophole" in the FDA's regulatory authority needs to corrected and the FDA should serve to protect ever gullible citizens from the potential risk and old-fashioned fraud by the hucksters of unproven and dangerous products. Deliberately fraudulent health claims are everywhere. We now have the most sophisticated snake oil salesmen of all times.

The following was taken from: Office of Dietary Supplements, National Institutes of Health. http://ods.od.nih.gov/pubs/DS_WhatYouNeed-ToKnow.pdf. Accessed 12-14-10.

"Many supplements contain active ingredients that can have strong effects in the body. Supplements are most likely to cause side effects or harm when people take them instead of prescribed medicines or when people take many supplements in combination. Some can increase the risk of bleeding or they can affect a person's reaction to anesthesia or interact with certain prescription drugs in harmful ways. Antioxidant supplements, like vitamins C and E, might reduce the effectiveness of some types of cancer chemotherapy. Keep in mind that some ingredients found in dietary supplements are added to a growing number of foods, including breakfast cereals and beverages. As a result, you may be getting more of these ingredients than you think, and more might not be better. Taking more than you need is always more expensive and can also raise your risk of experiencing side effects. For example, getting too much vitamin A can cause headaches and liver damage, reduce bone strength, and cause birth defects. Excess iron may cause nausea and vomiting and may damage the liver and other organs. You can report adverse supplement effects to the FDA by calling 800-FDA-1088 or completing a form at http://www. fda.gov/Safety/MedWatch/HowToReport."

Laughingly, this NIH site also makes this statement, "The federal government can take legal action against companies and Web sites that sell supplements when the companies make false or deceptive statements about their products, if they promote them as treatments or cures for diseases, or if their products are unsafe."

It is readily apparent that false and deceptive statements are everywhere, especially when they claim medicinal qualities.

The 21st century is becoming the golden age of dietary supplement quackery.

As it relates to the antioxidant supplements, they have been erroneously anchored on the swamp-mud foundation of Harman's free radical theory. The beauty of the Free Radi-Crap Theory of oxidative stress and aging (as I like to call it) is that it is testable and it has miserably failed the test hundreds of times. Yet, sycophant zealots cling tenaciously to its flawed precepts.

There are those scientists who believe that to prevent aging would also prevent the occurrence of all diseases. However, this completely fails to explain the development of childhood diseases or the presentation of diseases at birth.

If the free radical theory was correct, antioxidants should and would prevent/reverse/cure all of the 100-200 diseases attributed to oxidative stress and stop/reverse aging. But, antioxidants have repeatedly failed to do so. They have been a huge disappointing flop.

Your voice needs to be heard to counter the predatory financial influence pharmaceutical and supplement companies wield over Congress. I am counting on you to work with me to bring the truth about the antioxidant vitamins to all of the people, such that they can safely and reasonably decide it they want to use them or not.

What is one to do?

What's a conscientious person to do? Pop more vitamin pills and go on your way?

Not so fast, says Howard Sesso, ScD, MPH, an associate professor of medicine at Harvard Medical School and project director of the Physicians' Health Study II, which followed nearly 15,000 male doctors over the course of 10 years to evaluate the potential health benefits of four of the most popular vitamins: C, E, beta carotene, and multivitamins.

Sesso told WebMD, "Studies over the last few years have suggested that individual supplements don't have benefits."

In one large study, Sesso and his fellow researchers found that neither vitamin E or C lowered the risk of cardiovascular disease. That study was published in The Journal of the American Medical Association (JAMA) in November 2008. In a study published in JAMA in January 2009, the same team reported that taking supplements of vitamins E and C did not lower a man's risk of developing prostate or total cancers.

"You have to look at the totality of evidence in order to come up with recommendations," says Andrew Shao, PhD, senior vice president of scientific and regulatory affairs at the Council for Responsible Nutrition, a trade organization that represents the nearly $27 billion-a-year supplement industry (figures vary and go all the way $23 to $27 billion). They also say that, "There is no magic bullet."

"The promise of supplements is to reduce the risk of disease and maintain health and wellness," Shao says. But he says a good diet "should take a food-first approach."

I agree.

Shao also said, "If people are taking a multivitamin and they're expecting to see some specific result in a short period of time, they are probably going to be disappointed," Dr. Shao said. "It's not a drug and it's not intended to be a drug."

I have looked at the "totality of the evidence" and it is contained in this book. In short, the use of the antioxidant vitamins is likely a waste of money and they are likely endangering your overall health. We seem to be getting "too much of a supposedly good thing."

People need to re-think their expectations about what antioxidants and multivitamins can actually do. They are merely and only supplements to your diet and not magical drugs. You need to be careful of how much you cumulatively take in because supplements make excessive amounts easier to consume. Some vitamins, such as vitamin A, are exceeding their upper safe limits and others are in danger of doing the same. Thus, stay away from mega-dose or high-potency vitamins.

Defenders quickly respond

Vitamin pushers are quick to defend against studies showing harm from the antioxidant vitamins. Researchers from the University of California reported on March 2, 2000, that people who took 500 mgs of ascorbic acid had a 2.5 times faster progression of thickening of the carotid artery (hardening of the arteries) than people who took no supplement.

The director of the study astutely observed that "when you extract one component of food and give it at very high levels, you just don't know what you are doing to the system, and it may be adverse." Other researchers were quick to add that the research shows the uncertainties of picking out a single vitamin among the plethora of nutrients in a healthy diet. They added that it is a challenge to pick out nutrients that may make people live longer because if we are wrong, *we can do harm*.

Obviously, this flies in the face of all the false claims by all the synthetic vitamin manufacturers who state that vitamins can't hurt you, will never cause harm, are always beneficial, and will cure everything from a cold to cancer. The fact is that isolated, synthetic, or fractionated high-dose "vitamins" are unnatural and ineffective and can cause harm. In the case of ascorbic acid, it is feasible that high doses may cause problems.

Norman Krinsky, Ph.D., chair of the Institute Of Medicine's Panel on Dietary Antioxidants and Related Compounds, has concluded, "There has been much confusion about the value of taking antioxidant supplements. **Many people are likely to continue to believe that these compounds have many health benefits, including the prevention of chronic disease, but "we were not able to find definitive proof of that hypothesis."** Dr. Krinsky is a professor of biochemistry at Tufts University Boston.

CHAPTER ONE

TO SUPPLEMENT OR NOT TO SUPPLEMENT

Dr. Denham Harman is famous as the "founder" of a form of hooey known as the free radical theory.

The half century occurrence of the free radical theory will merely represent a moment of confusion in the overall history of redox thought, aerobiosis and oxygen appreciation.

R. M. Howes M.D., Ph.D.
1/19/09

I ask, "How many times must this non-science/non-sense be repeated, before investigators admit that the Free Radi-Crap theory is wrong?"

Why most supplemental antioxidants and antioxidant vitamins are a waste of money:

1) They do not work and

2) They can be quite harmful.

When I wrote my book, *Death in small doses?*, I had hoped that the expression of my views on the subject would promote discussion and debate and I am glad to see that this has occurred.

The free radical theory (FRT) has been invalidated. Why then do scientists from around the world continue to cite the FRT as the basis for antioxidant investigations decades later? This is precisely why I felt compelled to write the book.

As I stated in my book, I do not think studying antioxidant vitamins has been a total waste of time, rather it has improved our understanding of how oxidation serves to protect us from pathogens and cancer. I agree that I was not able to evaluate all of the pertinent literature within the confines of one book. But it is also true that over the past several years, an increasing number of authors are casting doubt on the FRT.

Antioxidants may cause cancer. Bardia et al, showed that regular intake of supplements containing beta-carotene may increase cancer incidence and cancer deaths among smokers, according to a large systematic review and meta-analysis published in 2008. The same report also showed that selenium supplementation may have cancer-fighting effects in men, while vitamin E supplementation had no effect on cancer incidence and mortality (Bardia et al, 2008).

Antioxidants can be bad for the heart. In a report published in 2008, researchers cautioned that cancer patients should avoid use of antioxidant supplements during radiation and chemotherapy. According to the report's authors, antioxidant supplements may reduce the anticancer effects of therapy (Lawenda et al, 2008).

Further, researchers from the University of Washington reported that patients taking antioxidant vitamins in addition to statin and niacin therapy failed to increase their HDL cholesterol (the "good" cholesterol) as much as patients not taking antioxidants. These results, reported in the August 9, 2001 issue of *Arteriosclerosis, Thorombosis, and Vascular Biology*, are but just a few in a long series of disappointing (failures) results in trials examining the ability of antioxidants to prevent heart disease.

A study from the University of Washington brings up the possibility that antioxidant therapy may do more than merely fail to halt the progression of coronary artery disease. This new study suggests the possibility of harm. The study results showed that the increase in HDL levels seen in patients receiving statin-niacin therapy was eliminated when they also received the antioxidants. That is, in these patients the antioxidants were potentially harmful. The primary endpoints of the study also suggested that antioxidants blunted the benefits seen with statin-niacin therapy. While patients receiving statin-niacin had a 4% reduction in coronary artery blockage, those who received antioxidants in addition to statin-niacin had a 7% increase in blockage.

Antioxidants can even increase your risk of dying. Taking antioxidant supplements containing beta-carotene, vitamin E, and vitamin A may be linked to an increased risk of death, according to a 2007 review and meta-analysis of 68 trials including a total of 232,606 participants. Although no increased mortality risk was associated with vitamin C supplementation, researchers didn't find any evidence that vitamin C supplements increased longevity either (Bjlakovic pp. 842-57 et al, 2007).

Does anyone still have to ask if they should take antioxidants?

Does anyone still have to ask if antioxidant vitamins are worth the money?

Admittedly, within the constraints of a single book, I was not able to expound upon my overall theories regarding prooxidant protection and electronically modified oxygen derivative (EMOD) insufficiency, nor can I give it proper justice here. My work must be viewed in the context of my magnum opus of collective books, available at www.iwillfindthecure.org.

In order for us to construct a comprehensive model that clarifies and drives the field forward, the building blocks that go into the complex biochemical architecture of such an innovative model must be generated with care.

In summary, the purpose of my book was to expose false claims with over whelming scientific data and express an opinion. Had I been composing a scientific review of the role of antioxidants, I would have included a comprehensive analysis of the literature and not an acknowledged "selective review."

My previous books have examined in detail the dangers of the antioxidant vitamins and the dangers associated with EMOD insufficiency. Thus, logically, there should be safe ways to correct this situation. They are the basis of this book and I will share them with you.

All of my discussions are merely suggestions and not recommendations. Legal liabilities are so common that one must begin medical discussions with disclaimers.

I do not believe that antioxidants are inherently harmful. In fact, I believe that they frequently serve as pre-oxidants or co-oxidants. We must maintain sufficient electron-donating antioxidants in order to form adequate protective levels of electron-accepting prooxidants.

The harm occurs when there is sufficiently large quantities of antioxidants, which result in an EMOD insufficiency state. The resultant EMOD insufficiency allows for the manifestation of disease states and blocks our ability to protect ourselves against pathogens, neoplasia and coexisting diseases.

It appears that **antioxidants and prooxidants participate in two part harmony**. Problems develop when the antioxidants drown out the oxidants, with resultant cacophony (disease).

Oxidants and antioxidants sing in the choir
of life. It is a two part harmony.
When their voices blend, it is a blissful thing:
a beautiful state of well being.

R. M. Howes, M.D., Ph.D.
12/11/10

It is well established that EMODs are utilized by the body to fight infections and to kill cancer cells via EMOD induced apoptosis and that antioxidants can block this process.

Oxygen in a sealed container remains stable. Curiously, oxygen requires the donation of electrons from antioxidants to produce the full EMOD species family. Thus, without these electron donors (oxidizable substrates or components, i.e., antioxidants), we could not form the ROS or EMODs and oxygen would remain in its bi-radical state. Contrary to the teachings of the FRT, antioxidants do not "mop up" or capture EMODs, but instead, they provide the electrons necessary for the progressive reduction of ground state oxygen and the further reduction of EMODs. Thus, terminology such as "free radical captors or neutralization systems" is technically incorrect and it would be more correct to refer to them as pre-oxidants or co-oxidants.

It is said that, "A paradox in metabolism is that, while the vast majority of complex life on Earth requires oxygen for existence, oxygen is a highly reactive molecule that damages living organisms by producing reactive oxygen species." **This is not true because oxygen is not highly reactive and although addition of electrons to it is thermodynamically favored, it is prevented by the laws of quantum mechanics.**

Please allow me to get technical for just a moment. Molecular oxygen has two unpaired electrons which have parallel spin states. The parallel spins prevent oxidation by 2 electron transfers. Organic molecules that serve as substrates for oxidation do not usually contain unpaired electrons. Their bonds are in the stable form of two electrons with anti-parallel spins.

For O_2 to accept a pair of electrons from an organic substrate, one of the electrons of oxygen or one of the electrons from the donating substrate has to invert its spin. There is a large thermodynamic barrier to such spin inversions. As a result, two electron oxidations by molecular oxygen have to occur stepwise by two single electron transfers. The large barrier to spin inversions keeps us from spontaneously combusting in our O_2 atmosphere.

Now, let's get back to more mundane considerations.

TEN KEY LIES DOMINATE THE MAINSTREAM MEDIA

Lie #1 - Antioxidant vitamins are completely safe and free from harm

Lie #2 - There have never been any deaths attributable to any of the antioxidant vitamins

Lie #3 - The antioxidant vitamins can cure, reverse or prevent cancer

Lie #4 - The antioxidant vitamins can cure, reverse or prevent heart disease

Lie #5 - The antioxidant vitamins can cure, reverse or prevent strokes

Lie #6 - The antioxidant vitamins will increase your life span and prevent aging

Lie #7 - The antioxidant vitamins can cure, reverse or prevent eye diseases, such as cataract formation or macular degeneration

Lie #8 - Oxygen free radicals are toxic and lethal

Lie #9 - Oxidation is destroying cells by blowing holes in them

Lie #10 - (and THE BIGGEST WHOPPER OF ALL):

Oxygen is killing all of us and will bring death to all humans!

Always get the facts and think for yourself.

Even though the antioxidant vitamins are not capable of diagnosing, treating, curing or preventing any disease, customers are lining up, like lemmings at a cliff, to buy them on a daily basis, absent any proof of safety or efficacy whatsoever. Health food stores and pharmacies are filled with "troughs of supplements" to feed the massive herds of human guinea pigs.

The injudicious use of the antioxidant vitamins could be the beginning of a modern medical disaster, because the federal authorities do not require safety data or large scale testing for efficacy of these products.

Studies demonstrating the harmful side of the antioxidant vitamins are always referred to as being "disappointing, surprising or shocking." But, they should call it exactly what it is, "ANTIOXIDANT TOXICITY and POTENTIAL ANTIOXIDANT LETHALITY."

They should refer to these results as being "deeply concerning, dangerous and potentially fatal." But they do not and the profits keep rolling in, the "sheeple" keep acting like guinea pigs, and Big Pharma runs the operation like a corrupt, cigar-smoking Mafiosi mob boss.

TEN THINGS YOU ARE NOT SUPPOSED TO KNOW ABOUT ANTIOXIDANT VITAMINS

#1 - They are not tested by federal agencies for safety or efficacy

#2 - Many deaths are attributable to antioxidant vitamins

#3 - They can not prevent or cure cancer

#4 - They can not prevent or cure heart disease

#5 - They can not prevent or cure strokes

#6 - They can not prevent or cure eye diseases

#7 - They do not increase the life span or prevent aging and they may increase overall mortality

#8 - Over eighty seven scientific studies have shown their wide ranging harmful effects

#9 - Oxygen free radicals are of low toxicity and essential for normal metabolism

#10 - Oxygen is our most essential ally in sustaining a healthful condition, in fighting pathogens and in killing cancer cells

Basically, the antioxidant vitamins are today's snake oils. They have unknown benefits with known harmful effects. Patient safety, and not profits, should always be the priority but drug and supplement manufacturers only look at financial return to their stockholders.

Ultimately, the harm or safety of antioxidants will be determined by the scientifically based evidence and I believe that current scientific evidence presents a convincing argument that the antioxidant vitamins are ineffective, unpredictable and harmful.

Their use should be restricted until their safety is confirmed. If they are not proven to be safe, then they should be removed from the diet of humans. If they have the effects of drugs (as claimed by supplement manufacturers and peddlers), then they should be regulated as drugs.

Because of the fortification of such a wide variety of foods with antioxidants, we have no way to know how much we cumulatively take in and this makes the avoidance of hypervitaminosis more difficult than ever, if not impossible.

Common sense observations

Proponents for the daily use of the antioxidant vitamins espouse their wondrous effects upon normal cells (everything from preventing or reversing all manner of diseases, increasing immunity to prolonging the life span). Logically, one must assume that these same beneficial effects help the survival of cancerous cells. The data has shown that to be the case.

One, then, questions if electronically modified oxygen derivatives (EMODs) also benefit cancer cells and the answer is likely "NO." Studies have proven that high EMOD levels cause EMOD-induced apoptosis and the death of cancer cells. In fact, antioxidants, such as vitamin E and NAC, have been proven to block the EMOD-induced killing of cancer cells.

Jack Chellam was told by Dr. Denham Harman that taking too many antioxidant vitamins would result in fatigue, due to the fact that these agents can block the electron transport chain and the production of ATP, our main energy source. That is a no-brainer because the electron transport chain, which generates superoxide anions, is our main and predominant energy source for ATP.

Radicophobes can ignore the truth or they can reject the truth but they can not change the magnificent truths regarding the crucial role of EMODs in the life process of all aerobes or the inherent splendor of oxygen.

R. M. Howes M.D., Ph.D.
1/26/09

Five common antioxidant killers: uric acid, cholesterol, bilirubin, estrogen, testosterone

Both uric acid and cholesterol are the two most common antioxidants in the body and elevated levels of both are associated with a high risk of cardiovascular diseases and increased mortality. The other two common antioxidants are estrogen and bilirubin, both of which can be quite harmful, if not lethal. Quite literally, these predominant, common antioxidants, when in excess, are killers.

Actually, it appears that these antioxidants in excess amounts could be responsible for a systemic EMOD insufficiency and are therefore, responsible for the manifestation of common diseases, such as cancer, atherosclerosis, diabetes, arthritis, gout, etc.

These simple observations are an alarming indictment of the potential harm associated with prolonged and injudicious and excessive ingestion of antioxidants.

The ATBC study (#29,133 participants), the CARET study (#14,254 heavy smokers plus 4,060 asbestos workers participated) and the SE-LECT studies (#35,533 participants) **were all shut down nearly two years early, due to the obvious fact that the antioxidant agents being tested were causing shocking and unexpected harmful adverse effects, to the point that the supervisory physicians terminated the studies.** Enough said!

Furthermore, antioxidants can cause prolonged adverse effects after discontinuation of their use. **The results of CARET and ATBC emphasize that chemoprevention trials require careful monitoring of all disease endpoints ... even after the study intervention is discontinued."** (Goodman et al, 2004).

In the 1980s, an injectable for of vitamin E, known as E-Ferol, was responsible for the deaths of 38 babies. This was verified by court hearings. Please remember that research has tragically shown that surviving infants who received E-Ferol injections were at an increased lifetime risk for reproductive problems, cervical and vaginal cancer, and other health problems.

Ergo, maintaining sufficient EMOD levels is protective in maintaining a state of good health and high antioxidant levels connote potential problems and harm. Low EMOD levels (i.e., chronic granulomatous disease, chronic steroid use, AIDS, etc.) are tied to over all poor health and an increased risk of mortality. Basically, it may be that simple.

Paradoxically, **many well-established components of the heart-healthy lifestyle are prooxidant, including polyunsaturated fat, exercise and moderate alcohol consumption.** (Williams, K.J. and Fisher, E.A., 2005.

FIVE Common Beneficial Factors with Prooxidant Activity: 1) ground state di-radical oxygen, 2) exercise,

3) alcohol in moderation, 4) polyunsaturated fat, 5) vitamin D3.

TEN Common Harmful Antioxidants: 1) cholesterol, 2) bilirubin, 3) uric acid, 4) estrogen, 5) testosterone, 6) vitamin E, 7) vitamin A (its precursor is beta carotene), 8) multivitamins, 9) selenium, 10) NAC, N-acetylcysteine.

Bjelakovic's analysis found that beta carotene, vitamin A and vitamin E, taken singly or combined with other antioxidant supplements, were associated with increased all-cause mortality. The supplements increase the likelihood of dying by about 5 percent, as a conservative estimate.

Vitamin A increased death risk by 16 per cent, beta carotene by 7 per cent and Vitamin E by 4 per cent. (Bjelakovic et al, 2007).

Further, **meta-analyses of randomized clinical trials have not shown that antioxidant supplements reduce cancer incidence** (Bjelakovic et al, Cochrane Database Syst Rev. 2004) (Bjelakovic et al, Lancet. 2004) (Caraballoso et al., 2003) (Bjelakovic et al., 2006).

Inhibition of apoptosis by antioxidants may explain why, in heavy smokers, **vitamin E and beta-carotene enhanced carcinogenesis in the lung** (De Luca, L. M. & Ross, S. A., 1996).

EMODs regulate the signaling for apoptosis and are capable of activating apoptotic pathways upstream. Many of the drugs and treatments that we use to kill cancer cells (chemotherapy, PDT and radiation) work by generating EMODs (ROS) to activate apoptotic pathways and kill cells. EMODs are involved in final common pathways for cellular suicide.

Various cancer chemopreventive agents can encourage apoptosis in premalignant and malignant cells in vivo and/or in vitro, which is an anticancer mechanism. Evidently many of these apoptogenic agents function as prooxidants in vitro. Reactive oxygen species and cellular redox tone appear to be exploitable targets in cancer chemoprevention via the stimulation of cytoprotection in normal cells and/or the induction of apoptosis in transformed cells.

There is an inherent danger in blocking EMODs which are responsible for initiating apoptosis and tumoricidal activity. I believe that these antioxidants are dangerous in patients with neoplasia or precancerous conditions.

I believe that this is the same tumoricidal pattern that I have seen over and over again with EMOD producing compounds. In short, EMODs kill cancer and antioxidants tend to block this activity, unless they also have prooxidant potential.

David Schardt, a nutrition expert with the consumer advocacy group, the Center for Science in the Public Interest, has said, "Antioxidants are not the magic bullets that the supplement industry would like consumers to believe."

Some authors argue that the hypothesis that antioxidants could prevent chronic diseases has now been disproved and that the idea was misguided from the beginning. (Hail N, Cortes M, Drake EN, Spallholz JE, 2008).

In actuality, free radicals perform a crucial role in normal, healthy physiological processes like our immune system and promote beneficial oxidation. It is important to realize that many vitamins and supplements classified as antioxidants (or so-called antioxidants) are actually *redox agents*, meaning they act as antioxidants in some instances and pro-oxidants in others. This markedly increases the difficulty of intrepreting redox data and is seldom addressed in the literature.

Further reasons to avoid excessive antioxidants

EMODs can induce cellular apoptosis and can therefore function as anti-tumorigenic species (Valko et al, 2007).

Experimental data and clinical studies support this hypothesis, with **some clinical data also suggesting that cancer patients who use antioxidant supplements during radiation or chemotherapy have worse survival than those who do not.** (Lesperance et al, 2002) (Bairati et al, 2006) (Ferreira et al, 2004) (Bairati et al, 2005 Aug 20).

Many experts logically conclude that **the use of supplemental antioxidants during chemotherapy and radiation therapy should be discouraged.** (Howes, Philica. Feb 7, 2009).

Yet, dietary supplement use is higher among individuals with health concerns, especially those diagnosed with cancer. Supplement use is widespread among cancer patients and longer-term survivors. (Velicer and Ulrich, 2008).

The crucial reasons to avoid excess antioxidants

The postulated mechanism of action for many forms of chemotherapy, radiation therapy, photodynamic therapy, ozone therapy, hyperbaric oxygen therapy, intravenous mega-dose of vitamin C, the Howes singlet oxygen cancer therapy system and hydrogen peroxide therapy is the generation of electronically modified oxygen derivatives (EMODs). (Howes R : Cancer Therapy, 2010) (Howes R : Hydrogen Peroxide: 2010).

The presence of certain antioxidants repeatedly blocks therapies based on EMOD generation. The take-home message is that cancer patients should use extra caution to avoid ingestion of excessive amounts of antioxidants.

The production of EMODs leads to the stimulation of various signaling pathways, and in particular, stress-responsive signal transduction pathways are strictly regulated by the intracellular redox state. (Matsuzawa and Ichijo, 2005) (Han et al, 2001).

Also, please remember the insidious effect of an antioxidant overload. Both cancer and heart disease have prolonged latency periods and the effect of an antioxidant overload and EMOD insufficiency may not be appreciated or realized or manifested for many years. An overwhelming antioxidant could have an acute damaging effect, but the gradual effect may be of even more concern to the overall populous.

At least 90% of a human is his animal half.

R. M. Howes, M.D., Ph.D.
9/27/10

CHAPTER TWO

THE KEY WORD IS "CAUTION"

Medical history is rife with examples of failed theories or seemingly rational notions that have delayed medical progress for decades or even for centuries. The most egregious of these was the "doctrine of laudable pus" by Galen, surgeon of the gladiators. It held medicine at a standstill for 1,400 years; whereas, the current free radical theory has blocked progress for merely half a century. (Howes RM: "The Free Radical Fantasy," 2006).

No aerobic life form on Earth can live without di-radical oxygen, especially the obligate aerobe, man. We swim in a sea of oxygen di-radicals and are continuously internally bathed in a biochemical broth of oxygen radicals, generated by normal metabolonics. This automatically tells you, in and of itself, oxygen is not an evil entity. In fact, it is our greatest ally. Stop oxygen intake and the life process stops summarily. (Howes R : Hydrogen Peroxide: 2010).

My Opening Salvo

The print and broadcast media have failed their primary mission of truthfully informing the general public about the potential dangers of the antioxidant vitamins and have betrayed the very audience they claim to serve. Big Pharma now owns a large portion of the supplement business and the media is afraid to upset their corporate string pullers, which might threaten their own financial survival.

The truth about the antioxidant vitamins has been systematically hidden from the public and distortions of the so-called "wonders of the antioxidant vitamins" have been proclaimed everywhere. This represents one of the greatest media frauds ever perpetuated upon an unknowing public.

False glowing claims regarding the antioxidant vitamins are no longer about science, they are about marketing, – pure and simple. Media coverage is about advertising dollars rather than legitimately informing hordes of unsuspecting victims of clever marketing campaigns. The public must know the truth and then they can decide if they are going to waste their money on ineffective or harmful products.

We must ask ourselves, "Why does the truth rarely make it into print or is seldom broadcast to the public?" Why isn't the public constantly informed about the serious and well documented side effects of the antioxidant vitamins? Mainstream media must do the right thing and not simply serve as a corporate mouthpiece, whoring itself out to the highest bidder.

I believe that Big Pharma rules and controls the media outlets with a "gold-plated iron fist."

Perhaps the biggest offender of truth is the supplement industry itself. Study after scientific study points out the ineffectiveness and dangers of a wide variety of dietary supplements, including the antioxidant vitamins. Yet, those selling these potentially dangerous products forge full steam ahead and spew forth more lies than a six year old caught stealing a Tootsie Roll.

Many of their sales people know the truth but they ignore it. The truth would hurt sales. They are aware of the facts but they deny them. Bald faced lies are everywhere.

Death: a day at a time

A vitamin craze has swept America and large populations of the developed world. People are interested in the relationship that supplements, vitamins, and nutrients have to specific diseases and cancer. Thus, research on these areas gets plenty of attention.

However, no one study provides the final word on any subject, and individual news reports may overemphasize conflicting results. Reporters seldom put new research findings in their proper context. The best advice about diet and physical activity is that it is rarely, if ever, advisable to change diet or activity levels based on a single study or a sensationalized news report.

As regards antioxidant vitamin supplementation, if one does not have a deficiency state and you consume a balanced diet, there are few, if any, indications to take these supplements. Otherwise, you may be encouraging "a slow death, a day at a time."

In February 2007, the Journal of the American Medical Association published a large, well-researched study which showed that antioxidant vitamins A and E do not prevent cancer, strokes or heart disease and that they actually increase the incidence of these same diseases. In fact, they increase overall mortality (increased death rates) by a conservative estimate of five percent.

Patients with heart disease and cancer may be wise to avoid these agents. I placed an extensive article on the internet at the www.medi. philica.com website, which suggested legal culpability of vitamin manufacturers and distributors. The promises of the antioxidant vitamins have proven to be hollow. I discuss the science behind their failure at my website www.thepundit.com. I believe that knowledge of the truth beats out blissful ignorance every time.

For many decades, people have taken vitamins, even if unintentionally because they have been routinely added to fortify foods such as bread, cereals, canned goods, and other food products. Add to this the vitamins taken as supplements and people are reaching hypervitaminosis levels. That can be the "compounded source" of today's problem.

Antioxidants are advertised with reckless abandon. But, a 2010 study in JAMA showed that people are ingesting such high dosages of these antioxidants that they're beginning to actually harm their over all health. The study of over 200,000 showed that the addition of large amounts of vitamins and other antioxidants to food not only lacked a beneficial effect, but it increased the rate of mortality as compared to a placebo. In short, treatment with beta carotene, vitamin A, and vitamin E appears to increase mortality. (Bjelakovic et al, 2007).

It does not matter if it is a drug or an antioxidant vitamin, if scientific evidence shows that it produces increased risk of common serious diseases, this product is a public health menace and threat.

If study after scientific study shows that the same product repeatedly causes harm, this is evidence par excellence that there is cause and effect relationship and that this product poses unnecessary dangers, especially if it has been shown to have negligible or no benefits. A placebo effect would tend to show a good effect; whereas, a harmful product repeatedly shows damaging effects.

Such is the established case with the antioxidant vitamins.

There is continually accumulating evidence for antioxidant harm. In 2010, I published my ground breaking pair of books, *Death In Small Doses? and Antioxidant Vitamins Are Making A Killing*, in which I had compiled 181 studies, involving over 8,000,000 human participants and which showed either negligible, null or harmful effects of the common antioxidant vitamins A, C and E. (Howes RM. Death in Small Doses: Book One, 2010) (Howes RM. Death in Small Doses: Book Two, 2010)

Antioxidants: known harm for unknown benefit.

R. M. Howes M.D., Ph.D.
2/11/09

Death in Small Doses?: observations and conclusions as of 6-24-10

Some authors speak of synergism of the antioxidants and use this point to discount antioxidant studies showing no effect or harmful effects. In reviewing the studies, it is apparent from the study results that the antioxidant vitamins alone have somewhat limited numbers of adverse effect such as follows:

- Vitamin A has 7 effects: **vitamin A could increase risk of lung cancer, heart disease, increased total mortality, osteoporosis and fractures, polyp recurrence and transfer of HIV.**

- Vitamin E has 8 effects: **vitamin E could increase the risk of mortality, increase hospitalizations and heart failure, decrease platelet function, increase blood vessel blockages, increase tuberculosis and pneumonia in smokers and falls in Alzheimer's patients.**

- Vitamin C has 3 effects: **vitamin C could increase the risk of cardiovascular disease in female diabetics, block the good effects of exercise and increase cataracts in women.**

- But the studies utilizing **combinations of A, C and E** have huge numbers (over 40) of harmful side effects. Thus, it appears that "antioxidant synergism" or "antioxidant networking" is seen in the production of a wide range of adverse effects. Unfortunately, the synergism has not proven to reduce adverse effects, but conversely, the combined antioxidant vitamin interactions have been seen to increase the number of adverse effects dramatically.

Additionally, this indicates that combinations of antioxidant vitamins such as C and E may aid in their recycling and further add to an EMOD insufficiency. Likewise, it indicates a dramatic "cumulative adverse effect" produced by adding more than one antioxidant. **This is, indeed, the height of "unintended consequences."**

Some other conclusions from *"Death In Small Doses?"*:

- Antioxidant vitamins cause harm...widespread harm
- They increase the risk of common cancers, such as breast, prostate and lung
- They increase total mortality
- They increase stroke mortality
- They increase risk of various forms of heart disease, i.e., heart failure, ischemia, non- fatal myocardial infarction
- They accelerate atherosclerosis and plaque formation
- They increase risk of bone fractures
- They increase disease risks for smokers, diabetics and those exposed to asbestos

- They increased the risk of falling
- They increased the risk of low-birth-weight babies
- They increased the risk of gestational hypertension
- They damage sperm DNA
- They do not perform as advertised in keeping disease at bay
- They do not prevent aging
- They shorten life span, due to increased mortality and disease incidence
- They are not recommended by the vast majority of major medical and scientific organizations

(Howes RM. Death in Small Doses: Book One, 2010) (Howes RM. Death in Small Doses: Book Two, 2010).

Friends do not let friends
injudiciously ingest antioxidants.

R. M. Howes M.D., Ph.D.
2/11/09

More Cautions Indicated for Fortified Foods (Franken-foods?)

In order to sell more product, manufacturers are dressing up so-called junk food with vitamins and supplements. These products are called "functional foods" or "nutraceuticals." I call them Franken-foods.

Functional foods have sales of over $27 billion annually. Coca Cola Inc. and Tropicana Pure premium juices are big in the dosed-up vitamin drinks.

Additives include vitamins A, C, E, B6, caffeine, chromium and ginkgo. They fortify ice cream with calcium and bacteria called probiotics and load candy bars with caffeine and B vitamins. Many such products are packed with fats and calories.

Everything from sports drinks to margarines to sugary cereals are being pumped full of supplements and additives to make them sound healthier. People will pay premium prices for products seen as preventing illness or health problems.

More and more studies are showing that the common vitamins, A, C and E do not prevent or reverse cancer, heart disease or strokes. In fact, they have been shown to increase the risk of these very same diseases and increase overall mortality (your risk of dying). This news seems shocking because we have been so brainwashed into thinking that anything called a "vitamin" is naturally good for us and that anything called a "therapy" must be great.

However, our best scientific studies are showing that we have been misled and that we must recognize the potential for harm for some of these products. The latest vitamin to cause great concern is the B vitamin, folic acid . A Tuft's nutrition expert recently said, "Folic acid is 'uncharted territory' because so many foods now are fortified with it. We don't actually know how high you can go and be safe."

Investigators in Norway found that patients were more likely to die from cancer it they took folic acid and B-12 supplements. It appears that folic acid given over a period of more than three years stimulates the growth of cancers and this raises serious concerns about the benefits of fortifying food with folic acid.

Since 1998, the U.S. has added folic acid to flour and other grain products because it was found to be crucial for women before pregnancy to prevent birth defects such as spina bifida and neural tube defects. Surprisingly, lung cancer rates were 25 percent higher among those taking the B6 and B-12 supplements.

Norway does not fortify their foods with folic acid. So many Americans are taking daily multivitamins and supplements and are getting unknown quantities from fortified foods that they may be exceeding upper tolerable limits, especially in children. Recently, ConsumerLab. com tested a vitamin water and discovered that it contained 15 times the stated amount of folic acid and drinking one bottle would exceed the tolerable limit for an adult.

We must try to educate ourselves about vitamin and supplement safety and to their potential harm. These vitamins do not prevent cancer or heart disease. So, save your money and you may save your life.

With the antioxidant vitamins and EMODs, the only battle is a war between science-based evidence and ignorance.

R. M. Howes, M.D., Ph.D.
10/17/10

Frequently, resistance to these established theories has been registered by a lone voice, dissenting before the recognized medical establishment. **Overall, medicine is reluctant to open its mind to new or creative ideas and, in fact, it tries to squelch or trample loners.** (Howes RM. Reactive Oxygen Species vs. Antioxidants: 2010).

For instance, in 2005, Barry Marshall and Robin Warren were awarded the Nobel Prize in Physiology or Medicine for their discovery that peptic ulcer disease (PUD) was primarily caused by *Helicobacter pylori*, a bacterium with affinity for acidic environments, such as the stomach. As a result, PUD that is associated with *H. pylori* is currently treated with antibiotics used to eradicate the infection. For 30 years prior to their discovery it was widely believed that PUD was caused by excess stomach acid. During this time, acid control was the major method of treatment for PUD, to only partial success. For many years, many scoffed at the idea that a bacterium was the causative agent....but they were wrong.

Dr. Robert Atkins, inventor of the Atkins Nutritional Approach, is another example of a lone voice that was marginalized for years. The **Atkins diet** is a low-carbohydrate diet created by Robert Atkins from a research paper he read in the *Journal of the American Medical Association* published by Gordon Azar and Walter Lyons Bloom. Atkins stated that he used the study to resolve his own overweight condition.

He later popularized it in a series of books, starting with *Dr. Atkins' Diet Revolution* in 1972. A review study published in the Lancet concluded that there was no metabolic advantage and dieters were simply eating fewer calories because of boredom. Professor Astrup stated, "The monotony and simplicity of the diet could inhibit appetite and food intake."

In his second book, *Dr. Atkins' New Diet Revolution*, he modified or changed parts of the diet but did not alter the original concepts. However, even at the time of his death, his approach was hotly debated by organized medicine, but subsequent studies have proven that he was on the right track. Many now believe that the Atkins' diet has essentially eliminated the need for drugs in many with uncomplicated diabetes and has been a boon to weight loss programs.

Organized medical and scientific groups reward conformity and punish innovation. But, it is far better to be the lone voice of truth than to join in with the choir of ignorance. A wasted mind is a tragic thing; whereas, an open mind is a thing of wonderment.

It is far, far nobler to be the heckled and jeered lone voice of truth, than to join the voices singing in the cacophonic choir of ignorance.

R. M. Howes, M.D., Ph.D.
11/25/10

A wasted mind is a tragic and common thing; whereas, an open mind is a rarity of brilliance and wonderment.

R. M. Howes, M.D., Ph.D.
11/25/10

Although I am seriously out-gunned by the powerful $27 billion supplement industry, I know that I am right to fight to let people know that they are frequently wasting their money and endangering their health and the health of their loved ones with the injudicious intake of the antioxidants in general but especially so with the antioxidant vitamins. **I will not be scared off.**

Fruit and Vegetables May Not Dramatically Reduce Disease

Here we go again. New studies may be exposing another "medical myth."

Investigators, writing in the Journal of the National Cancer Institute, are now telling us that fruits and vegetables do not dramatically lower the risk of common diseases, including cancer.

Since the early 1980s, the dietary guidelines for Americans, published jointly by the USDA and the DHHS, have reflected the accumulated scientific research concerning diet and health. Early 1980 guidelines pertaining to nutrition and cancer were to "eat a variety of foods" and "eat foods with adequate starch and fiber."

In 1990, "eat a variety of foods" remained a guideline but "choose a diet with plenty of vegetables, fruits, and grain products" replaced the starch and fiber reference. This mirrored the growing data suggesting a lowered risk of cancer with increased vegetable and fruit consumption.

But, in 1995, grain products were placed ahead of vegetables and fruit in the guidelines to better reflect the structure of the USDA food pyramid.

Other recommendations included the 1989 National Research Council *Diet and Health* report supporting consumption of 5 fruit and vegetable servings per day and the 1991 National Cancer Institute– DHHS sponsorship of the 5-A-Day Program. Public health guidelines for food oriented toward high vegetable and fruit consumption continues up to the present.

This scenario led to the rising popularity of vitamin supplements from the 1980s until today, but there have been huge problems with these trends.

First, the vitamin supplements were shown to lack the effect of vitamins acquired through the diet and second, vitamins A (beta carotene) and E (alpha tocopherol) were shown to have particularly harmful potential. For in depth discussions, see *www.iwillfindthecure.org*.

Yet, recommendations promoting vegetable and fruit consumption remained a center piece, until now. A study of 500,000 Europeans joins a growing body of evidence undermining the high hopes that pushing "five-a-day" might slash Western cancer rates and **it estimated that only around 2.5% of cancers could be averted by increasing fruit and vegetable intake**.

In short, research has failed to substantiate the suggestion that as many as 50% of cancers could be prevented by boosting the public's consumption of fruit and vegetables.

Randomized intervention trials enlisting millions of participants have demonstrated the ineffectiveness and potential harm of supplemental vitamins A and E. This entire body of evidence has to be reinterpreted and we must open our minds to the results and not be misled by aggressive marketing and advertising.

It appears that the kind of people who ate more fruit and vegetables lived healthier lives in many other respects too, which was the basis for any lowered rates of chronic diseases. Still, I believe that fresh fruits and vegetables are overall darned good for us.

So, does eating fruit and veg really work? **"Despite decades of research, it is currently impossible to state what, if any, contribution is made to the health-promoting effects of fruits and vegetables by the antioxidants present,"** says anitoxidant expert, Barry Halliwell.

Even multivitamins are under fire

Indeed, it is disconcerting to learn that dietary supplements, that we were led to believe were good for us, may be either harmful or of no benefit for disease prevention or health maintenance. Unfortunately, such may be the case for multivitamins.

This is an important public health issue because multivitamins are taken by the majority of our citizens, especially those who have been diagnosed with cancer.

A 2008 study linked heavy multivitamin use to fatal prostate cancer, and other research has shown beta-carotene pills can heighten smokers' risk of lung cancer. Confusion is everywhere, which is frequently the case for conflicting articles appearing on the same publishing dates (i.e., one article will say that vitamins are good for you and another will say that they are harmful). Who is one to believe?

Your best bet is to try to follow the suggestions of the best and most reliable scientific studies, as opposed to testimonials or paid advertisements.

No doubt, a vitamin deficiency can cause serious problems but if you are not in a deficient state, you may be wasting your money or putting yourself in harm's way. The largest study to date was <u>published in the February 2009 issue</u> of The Archives of Internal Medicine, where researchers analyzed data from 68,132 women who were enrolled in a clinical trial and 93,676 in an observational study. (Neuhouser et al, 2009).

They were followed for about eight years to track the health effects of multivitamins. The researchers found that the supplements had no effect on the risk for <u>breast cancer</u>, <u>colorectal cancer</u>, <u>endometrial cancer</u>, lung cancer, <u>ovarian cancer</u>, <u>heart attack</u>, stroke, blood clots or mortality. In short, they were surprised to find that the multivitamins did nothing to prevent or protect against heart disease or cancer. In conclusion, nutrition expert, Marian L. Neuhouser, said, **"Consumers spend money on dietary supplements with the thought that they are going to improve their health, but there's no evidence for this."**

We are becoming more aware of the fact that marketing can be misleading or blatantly false. Heavy marketing has made the notion, that multivitamins may be of no benefit or harmful, a difficult concept for the uninformed to grasp or accept.

We should endeavor to get our vitamins by eating a well balanced diet containing fresh fruits and vegetables and not from commercial chemical concoctions. All that one needs to maintain good health is a well balanced nutritious diet. The public has been repeatedly victimized by reprehensible persuasive advertising. So, buyers beware (Caveat emptor).

CHAPTER THREE

FALSE CLAIMS ARE EVERYWHERE

Regarding antioxidant vitamins, you do not have to follow
the science. All you have to do is .... follow the money.

R. M. Howes, M.D., Ph.D.
10/22/10

Herbal Supplement, Ginkgo, Fails to Prevent Alzheimer's Disease

Dietary supplements extol their wondrous claims everywhere. The
Food and Drug Administration (FDA) estimates that there are 29,000
supplements on the market, with 1,000 new ones introduced annually.

In 2005, it was estimated that U.S. dietary supplement sales were at
$20.9 billion. Now, it is estimated to be $27 billion.

There is no mandate for the FDA to screen or test the never-ending
stream of supplements entering or on the market for either safety or
effectiveness.

However, investigators at University of Virginia School of Medicine
and Wake Forest University Baptist Medical Center helped conduct
the "Ginkgo biloba for the Evaluation of Memory (GEM)" study. They
evaluated the effects of ginkgo, an antioxidant, on the occurrence or
prevention of dementia.

Ginkgo is one of the world's most widely advertised herbal supplements claiming to improve memory and cognition. The GEM study

showed that 240 mg of **ginkgo daily had no effect on the onset of dementia or development of Alzheimer's**.

Ginkgo supplements are among the best-selling herbal medications in the U.S. and Europe and it ranks as a top medicine prescribed in France and Germany. Chief study investigators said, "The results were disappointing and surprising."

Unfortunately, ginkgo's widespread use, based on the belief that it helps memory function, does not hold up to scientific scrutiny.

According to the National Institute on Aging, Alzheimer's affects nearly 4.5 million Americans and it will claim one in 10 baby boomers. Nearly a half-million new Alzheimer's cases will be diagnosed annually.

Even worse, with the three main drugs Aricept (donepezil), Exelon (rivastigmine) and Reminyl, Razadyne (galantamine), which are approved for use in mild-to-moderate Alzheimer's disease, not one of six clinical trials conducted by Italian researchers found that these drugs significantly reduced the rate of progression from mild cognitive impairment (MCI) to dementia.

In short, advertising works but neither ginkgo nor the current medications have proven to be effective.

Alzheimer's remains an incurable disease with a slowly progressive mild memory loss, which ends horribly with severe brain damage and death. Experts increasingly advise reliance on keeping mentally and physically active and not being taken in by false hopes of unproven supplements or drugs.

With no cure available or in sight, we must push for more government sponsored research on all forms of dementia. Do it, before we forget to do it.

Vitamin E confusion

A new study is claiming that vitamin E is beneficial in treating non-alcoholic fatty liver disease in obese patients. This may be the first study in which a vitamin supplement has been shown to help treat a major ailment not caused by a vitamin deficiency, but this was a small study and I am very skeptical of the results.

After all, the study was conducted with the help of a vitamin-producing drug company and the lead investigator receives consulting fees from Takeda and other drug companies.

My research of past scientific studies has found that vitamin E does not reduce risk of developing breast cancer, prostate cancer or colon cancer; has no benefit in reducing risk of stroke, cardiovascular diseases, ischemic heart disease, non-fatal myocardial infarction, cancer or total mortality; does not delay progression from mild cognitive impairment to Alzheimer's disease; does not prevent the development or progression of early or later stages of age related macular degeneration (eye disease); does not reduce the incidence of or progression of cataracts; and provides no significant benefit for type 2 diabetes in initially healthy women.

Not only is vitamin E ineffective in preventing diseases, it can cause serious side effects.

Unfortunately, vitamin E has been shown in scientific studies to increase the overall mortality rate by 4%; increase the incidence of heart failure and hospitalization for heart failure; increase the rate of vessel blockages; increase the rate of falling in Alzheimer's patients; increase the risk of tuberculosis and pneumonia; and supplementing the general public with vitamin E results in loss of quality-adjusted life years (loss of about four months).

Studies of combinations of antioxidant vitamins C and E found that they do not ward off cancer or heart disease and the vitamin E appeared to raise the risk of bleeding strokes. A 2008 study showed that the use of 400 mg of vitamin E daily resulted in an increased risk of developing lung cancer, particularly in smokers. For details, please visit *www.iwillfindthecure.org*.

Instead of taking vitamin supplements that have known potentially harmful consequences, we should try to improve our diets, lose some weight (if needed) and increase our exercise levels.

In February 2007, the Journal of the American Medical Association published a study showing that antioxidant vitamins A and E do not prevent cancer, strokes or heart disease and experts were shocked to find that A and E actually increased the incidence of these same diseases and increased overall mortality (increased death rates) by over five percent. Do not believe the unsupported hype on antioxidant vitamins and please remember that they can be harmful. Try to rely on natural nutrients and exercise and not on popping pills.

B-Vitamins Fail to Live Up to Claims

Two overly used sales buzz words are "antioxidants" and "vitamins." They have been touted as being "cure-alls" and incredible disease prevention agents. Unfortunately, unless one has a vitamin deficiency, none of these overstated claims have held up to scientific evaluation.

Nonetheless, TV and printed media pump out lies or misleading ads faster than Congress can tell us another whopper. What is one to believe?

Your best bet is to rely on randomized controlled trials (RCTs), which are the gold standard for medical studies, even though they can also arrive at incorrect conclusions. Increasingly, investigational reports are showing that vitamins and antioxidant dietary supplements are failing to curtail or decrease the incidence of many of the diseases they have claimed to help prevent or to cure.

Most alarming of all, some of the largest studies indicate that these vitamins and dietary supplements actually increase the incidence of cancer, heart disease, strokes and overall mortality in certain groups of patients, especially smokers or those exposed to asbestos. Antioxidant vitamins, such as vitamins A, C and E, have repeatedly failed to prevent cancer, heart disease and strokes.

Advertisers profiting from these sales never let scientific facts get in their way and they have created the deceptive notion that these products are really good for you.

The latest to fall from grace are the B-vitamins, specifically B12, B9 (folic acid) and B6 as prevention agents. A *Cochrane Systematic Review* of eight trials involving a total of 24,210 people found that "none of the eight trials individually supported the idea that giving B-vitamin supplements could prevent cardiovascular disease. Together the data show that B-vitamin supplements, whether compared with placebos or standard care, have no effect on the incidence of heart attack, stroke or death associated with heart disease."

Another current scientific article, published in a recent *FASEB Journal,* states that, "Using too many products enriched with vitamin A could lead to negative, even fatal, consequences."

We must avoid taking potentially harmful, costly, unnecessary supplements or vitamins, unless we have a documented vitamin deficiency. This is particularly important as combinations of foods, health drinks, cereals, and nutritional supplements containing added vitamins and antioxidants make an overdose more possible than ever before and genetic engineers are altering foods to contain many times their normal content of antioxidants.

These products are not medicines (although they make false medical claims) but are more like quack suggestions to get your money. Get moderate daily physical exercise and obtain your vitamins from a well rounded diet containing fresh fruits and vegetables, not from synthesized, chemically concocted "supplements."

Dangers of Antioxidant Vitamins A & E

Vitamin E today ranks as the second highest single vitamin consumed in the world after vitamin C, following highly promoted marketing campaigns extolling its anti-oxidative properties. Anti-oxidation is today a key phony marketing buzzword for the growing market segment of anti-aging dietary supplements.

According to Wellcome Trust there is no evidence in humans that anti-oxidative vitamins (A, C and E) slows aging. An editorial from the American Journal of Clinical Nutrition in 2006 concluded that intervention studies did not support a beneficial effect of antioxidant supplements, and there was a growing body of evidence that with anti-oxidant vitamins, "just enough" was more than adequate (Traber, 2006).

Prof Randolph M. Howes MD, PhD

The question therefore remains: **is it at all justifiable to use "killer" doses of a supplement that has no demonstrable benefits at all above its physiological limits?** http://brainblogger. com/2008/04/28/killer-anti-oxidant-vitamins-when-excess-could-be-dangerous/

Being made aware of facts which contradict a lifetime of erroneous teaching is at the least disturbing, if not "stunning." It requires an open mind to consider the strength of the current scientific data on commonly consumed vitamins, such as A and E.

Fifteen years ago, I was also taking these so called "wonder drugs," with the assumption that they were both beneficial to my overall health and that they may be a preventative of common diseases, such as cancer, heart disease and stroke.

Years of intense study on oxygen metabolism exposed me to data which questioned the accuracy of a preponderance of non-scientific publications praising dietary supplements, especially the antioxidant vitamins. Thus, I researched scientific studies which demonstrated antioxidant vitamin failures.

Frankly, I was surprised at the high number of double blind, randomized clinical trials (RCTs, which are the scientific gold standard) which showed the lack of beneficial effects and the potential harm of the antioxidant vitamins. These are the best studies that exist today.

Yet, proponents of vitamins A and E, especially those peddling these products for profit, attacked these studies with a wide variety of trumped up excuses as to the reasons that the vitamins repeatedly failed to repeatedly demonstrate widespread beneficial health effects (i.e., synthetic vs natural, wrong species tested, wrong statistical analysis, wrong concentrations, etc.). In short, the "vitamaniacs" did not let the facts get in their way.

In fact, the data against antioxidants vitamins was so strong that two of the largest studies had to be terminated 21 months early due to their readily apparent harmful consequences (*The beta-Carotene and Retinol Efficacy Trial - CARET*) (Omenn et al., 1996) *and the alpha-Tocopherol, beta-Carotene Cancer Prevention Study - ATBC)* (Heinonen et al, 1994).

76

Since then, the *Selenium and vitamin E chemoprevention trial (SELECT)* study was also shut down early because it was proving to be harmful to the participants (Lippman et al, 2009).

RCTs have repeatedly failed to confirm the glowing predictions touting the alleged benefits of vitamins A and E.

Following huge marketing campaigns, many patients have taken antioxidant vitamins to assure good health and have nonchalantly assumed that these antioxidant vitamins would not cause them any harm, even if it did not prevent disease. That was a bad assumption.

Many health-related committees and major health organizations, such as the American College of Cardiology, the American Heart Association (AHA), the AHA Nutrition Committee, the US Preventive Services Task Force, the Institute of Medicine, and the American Heart Association Science Advisory statement, and the American Diabetes Association do not recommend that individuals take these vitamin and antioxidant supplements, in the absence of a vitamin deficiency.

Foods contain tens of thousands of chemical compounds and to ascribe their healthful contributions to a select few vitamins is nonsense/nonscience.

Additionally, our immune system protects us from pathogens and cancer development primarily via oxidative mechanisms involving electronically modified oxygen derivatives (EMODs). Antioxidant vitamins can and do block this crucial prooxidant protective system.

Many, if not most, oncologists recommend not taking antioxidants during chemotherapy and irradiation treatments, since both of these processes require the generation of oxygen free radicals to effectively kill cancer cells. Antioxidant vitamins block the killing of these mutagenic cells.

I have study after study to document these facts at www.thepundit. com, www.iwillfindthecure.org and at www.medi.philica.com. True recklessness is to give unsupported health advice and to perpetuate medical misinformation. **There should be legal culpability for giving medical advice which does not have patient safety as its number one priority**.

In 2005, Johns Hopkins expert, Simeon Margolis, M.D., Ph.D., stated "I urge you not to be taken in by unproven claims that a dietary supplement can treat diabetes – or any other disorder, for that matter." Similar sentiments have been echoed at the Mayo Clinic website and the Heart and Vascular Institute of the Cleveland Clinic.

We must get our health information from the most reliable scientific sources available and realize that as our database changes, so may our conclusions. What was recommended five years ago may seem foolhardy or even absurd today. This is the case with the antioxidant vitamins A and E.

Amused and annoyed in equal measure, I peruse the antioxidant vitamin ads. Quotes are inspired by the marketing and business milieu, which distort the facts to score a selling point…. so much for science. Let's hear it for sales.

R. M. Howes M.D., Ph.D.
2/11/09

Vitamin C may blunt cancer therapy

In 2008, it was shown that vitamin C supplements may substantially reduce the benefit from a wide range of anti-cancer drugs. Thirty to 70% less cancer cells in a lab were killed by a range of drugs, after pretreatment with vitamin C. **Follow-up chemotherapy tests found tumors grew more rapidly in mice given cancer pretreated with vitamin C.** http://news.bbc.co.uk/2/hi/health/7643533.stm.

Scientists recently discovered that **cancer cells contain large amounts of vitamin C, which appears to protect them—just as it protects healthy cells—from oxygen damage to the genes. Cancer cells readily take up vitamin C** *in vitro* (Baader et al, 1994) (Spielholz et al. 1997).

Studies have demonstrated high vitamin C concentrations in neoplasms compared with the adjacent normal tissue (Langemann et al, 1989).

As reported on 2-04-09 in the journal Nature, Stanford researcher, Robert Cho, found that breast cancer stem cells make much higher levels of protective antioxidants than other cancer cells. Use of a drug to block the antioxidant, glutathione, caused the cancer stem cells to become far more vulnerable to radiation. Using cells from mice and human breast cancer, the antioxidant glutathione protected the cancer cells from being killed by radiation EMOD-induced apoptosis.

I believe that this is why cancer cells accumulate vitamin C, just as with glutathione and lactate, it is protective for the cancer cell from EMOD induced apoptosis.

It may also be that since atheromatous plaques contain high levels of antioxidants, they are protected from oxidation and excretion.

Prior to these studies, **another mouse study suggested that tumor cells need high amounts of vitamin C to thrive.** Moreover, years ago, **two human studies found that smokers with high levels of beta-carotene in their blood had a higher risk of lung cancer (ATBC and CARET studies),** compared with smokers with low levels of the antioxidant. I believe that this supports my contention that antioxidants lower apoptosis-inducing EMOD levels and can protect cancer cells.

In short, data has shown that antioxidants block the kill of the following cancers:

- **human metastatic melanoma**
- **murine retinoblastoma**
- **human breast cancer**
- **human lymphoma**
- **human melanoma**
- **human leukemia**

- **human prostate cancer**
- **human hepatocellular liver carcinoma**
- **human colon adenocarcinoma**
- **human multiple myeloma**
- **Burkitt's lymphoma**
- **human chronic lymphocytic leukemia**
- **human acute myeloid leukemia**
- **human non-small cell lung cancer**
- **human hepatoma**
- **murine pheochromocytoma**
- **human pancreatic cancer**
- **human colon cancer**
- **human endometrial cancer**
- **human colorectal carcinoma**

(Howes, Philica. Feb 7, 2009).

However, we must remember that mega-doses of intravenous vitamin C kill cancer, but it does so because it generates hydrogen peroxide. Ergo, vitamin C actually kills cancer cells in mega-doses "prooxidatively" (Howes R : Cancer Therapy, 2010) (Howes R : Hydrogen Peroxide: 2010).

Vitamin C mega-doses and H_2O_2

Also, mega-doses given intravenously can generate anti-cancer hydrogen peroxide. Vitamin C (ascorbate, ascorbic acid) has had a controversial history in the prevention of cancer. Much of this work was based on the pioneering work of Dr. Hugh Riordan and there have been some significant recent developments.

One clinical case report by Drisko et al showed that vitamin C together with other oxidants, when added adjunctively to first-line chemotherapy, prevented recurrence in two ovarian cancer patients. (Drisko et al, 2003).

This high dose, intravenous vitamin C therapy was shown to operate through the generation of hydrogen peroxide. Ascorbate-mediated cell death was due to protein-dependent extracellular H_2O_2 generation (i.e., prooxidant EMOD generation).   Ascorbate, an electron-donor in such reactions, ironically initiates prooxidant chemistry and H_2O_2 formation. It was concluded that **ascorbate at pharmacologic concentrations in blood is a pro-drug for H_2O_2 delivery to tissues**. (Buettner and Jurkiewicz, 1996) (Halliwell, 1990).

Prooxidant vitamins add more confusion

Vitamins that are reducing agents can be pro-oxidants. Vitamin C has antioxidant activity when it reduces oxidizing substances such as hydrogen peroxide, (Duarte and Lunec. 2005) **however, it can also reduce metal ions which leads to the generation of free radicals through the fenton reaction.** (Carr and Frei. 1999) (Stohs and Bagchi. 1995).

These enzymes produce EMODs and ascorbate acts as a cosubstrate for them and thus, acts as a prooxidant. (Chen et al. 2005).

Chen et al showed that at pharmacologic concentrations, ascorbate acts as a prooxidant, hydrogen peroxide generating agent, which exhibits selective cytotoxicity towards a wide variety of cancer cells *in vitro* and *in vivo*. (Chen et al. 2007) (Chen et al. 2008).

Even though there is much to be discovered in the ascorbate and hydrogen peroxide system, this appears to be an area of great potential. (Levine et al. 2008) (Howes R : Hydrogen Peroxide: 2010).

The relative importance of the antioxidant and pro-oxidant activities of antioxidant vitamins are an area of current research, but vitamin C, for example, appears to have a mostly antioxidant action in the body (Carr and Frei. 1999).

Could there be advantages in not synthesizing vitamin C?

We must ask, what are the advantages of not synthesizing vitamin C? Does ascorbate have a role in the modulation of both pro- and

anti-carcinogenic mechanisms? In other words, is there an evolution-
ary advantage to not synthesizing vitamin C? If there is no advantage
to not making ascorbate, then why did we stop? In short, if it had
been advantageous, by Darwinian law, we would still be making vitamin C.

We do not make the other two most important small molecular
weight antioxidants, beta carotene or vitamin E, either, "Why not?" If
they are so important, why do we not synthesize them; after all, lowly
plants do. After all, many humans inhabit arid lands where vitamin rich
plants are scarce.

We must also ask, "If EMODs are harmful or toxic, why do we normally make EMODs in such large quantities all of the time?"

Also, keeping antioxidant uric acid levels and cholesterol levels low
may help keep the oxidative capacity at an optimal level. The higher
levels of uric acid and cholesterol, the lower the EMOD levels and
the greater risk of disease occurrence. Also, the salutary effects of
lowered cholesterol could well be attributed to the fact that overall
antioxidant levels have been lowered, thus allowing a slightly higher
oxidative capacity, which would re-establish an EMOD sufficiency.

CHAPTER FOUR

AMERICANS WILL SWALLOW ANYTHING

13 Ineffective antioxidants

At this point, my studies have shown the following 13 anti-oxidants can be ineffective, many of which have shown considerable harmful potential in those without known vitamin deficiencies:

- Vitamin A, beta carotene
- Vitamin E, alpha tocopherol
- Vitamin C, ascorbic acid
- Selenium
- Ferulic acid
- Quercetin, a flavonol
- Lycopene, a carotenoid
- N-acetylcysteine, NAC
- Pine bark extract, antioxidant oligomeric proanthocy-anidin complexes
- Grape seed extract or EGCG, polyphenols decrease iron absorption
- Pomegranate juice
- Multivitamins (contain multiple antioxidants)
- Prenatal vitamins

8 potentially harmful endogenous antioxidants

Also, high levels of the following 8 endogenous antioxidants can be associated with harm:

- **Cholesterol (atherosclerosis and heart disease)**
- **Uric acid (gout and heart disease)**
- **Bilirubin (brain damage)**
- **Estrogen (breast cancer, oral cancer)**
- **Testosterone (prostate cancer)**
- **Glutathione (heart failure)**
- **Catalase (CAT)**
- **Glutathione peroxidase 1 (GPx1)**

The public must be made aware of the drawbacks of antioxidants.

Comprehensive Rejuvenating Antioxidant
Program: C.R.A.P.
Yes, this is their antiaging plan.
There are CRAP creams, CRAP pills, CRAP
supplements, CRAP shampoos, etc.
In short, it's all a lot of CRAP.

R. M. Howes M.D., Ph.D.
2/22/09

Supplements and Pills: What Will Americans Swallow?

When it comes to advertisements and supplement pills, Americans will pay premium prices to swallow darned near anything.

Estimates vary but, by some estimates, we spend up to a whopping $27 billion annually on supplements that have not been tested for safety, effectiveness or quality. With over 40,000 products on the market, who can possibly keep an eye on this gargantuan market?

The Food and Drug Administration (FDA) can not regulate our medicines properly, let alone the additional load of the supplement industry. Dietary supplements, antioxidants, vitamins and neutraceuticals are gobbled up faster than a sizzling T-bone by a starved dog.

We buy fish oil that doesn't even come from fish, lead-laden ginkgo pills, vitamin laced water, dressed up junk food and arsenic tainted herbals at premium prices.

We do this because we have been misled to believe that these products really are "ancient Chinese discoveries," "anti-aging pills," "instant weight loss medicines" or "miracle cures" that orthodox medicine wants to hide from us.

Actually, most of the scientific studies that have been done on many of the antioxidants and vitamins have shown that they totally lack effectiveness and that they are potentially harmful. The only place that they actually do some good is in folks with known vitamin deficiencies.

Additionally, with today's foods being "fortified" with antioxidants and vitamins, and with consumers taking literally tons of these supplements, experts are warning about the possibility of over dosing on many of these products.

According to a 2002 report in the New England Journal of Medicine, "Tens of thousands of supplement-related health problems are handled by U.S. poison control centers each year." Not until 2008 were supplement makers required to report problems to the FDA, and then it was only for serious problems.

The FDA estimates that there are over 50,000 safety problems yearly related to supplement use.

Fungal toxins have been found in red yeast and a water parasite was in herbal supplement oils to relieve colic and teething pain. Popular Indian herbal medicines, ayurvedics, often contain hazardous metals. In fact, in 2004, experts tested 70 ayurvedic remedies in Boston, Houston, Chicago, San Francisco and New York City and found that one in five had potentially harmful levels of lead, mercury or arsenic. Yes, we will swallow just about anything.

We must insist on better quality control of the entire vitamin and supplement industry. Perhaps, we should worry more about the supplements that we humans scarf down, than we do about the anti-freeze in our Chinese-made dog food.

Supplements Losing Support

Progressively, dietary supplements are being shown to be ineffective and pharmaceutical drugs are appearing more and more dangerous. What is one to do?

The best answer is to take only what is necessary or if you are proven to be in a deficiency state.

Usually, Mother Nature seems to know best and our bodies usually can select from a nutritious, balanced diet those compounds which it needs and excrete or remove the others that are harmful or surplus.

Some recent headlines illustrate the "current state of confusion" as it relates to supplements: Popular joint supplements do not work (Glucosamine and chondroitin sulfate); B-Vitamins fail another test; Beware these dietary supplements; Calcium supplements increase the risk of heart disease in the elderly; B-vitamin pills have no effect on heart disease prevention.

A 2010 British Medical Journal article reported, "In a review of trials involving 3,803 patients with knee or hip osteoarthritis, researchers found that there was 'no clinically relevant effect' of chondroitin, glu-cosamine, or the two in combination on perceived joint pain. Global sales of glucosamine supplements reached almost $2 billion in 2008.

In 2010, in The Lancet Neurology, researchers reported that "partici-pants who took the B-vitamins had lower homocysteine levels. But those taking the B-vitamins were not significantly less likely to suffer a stroke, heart attack or to die from any cause during the 3.4-year study."

Also in 2010, a Consumer Reports investigation revealed what the magazine called the 'dirty dozen' of dietary supplements - ones that may harm your health, and that you should consider avoiding." They were the following: aconite, bitter orange, chaparral, coloidal silver, coltsfoot, comfrey country mallow, germanium, greater celandine, kava, lobelia and yohimbine.

More than half of the adult U.S. population has taken dietary supplements hoping to increase their life span, improve their sex lives, make them healthier or to lose weight.

However, people rarely realize that supplement manufacturers routinely, and legally, sell their products without first having to demonstrate that they are safe and/or effective. All they have to do is to follow the guidelines of the industry-friendly 1994 Dietary Supplement Health and Education Act (DSHEA). The DSHEA prohibits them from any claims that the supplements can "diagnose, prevent, cure or treat" any disease condition. Yet, they can claim to "support, bolster, improve or strengthen" almost anything or any condition.

Confusion rules and consumers are wasting billions of dollars annually on ineffective, if not dangerous, products. Scams are everywhere. Please do your homework and research the products you take or talk to your doctor. It is for your own good and protection. Do not continue to be misled. Stop supplement fraud, now.

Supplements Fail....Again....and Again....and

In 2008, a huge review of 67 studies, with over 230,000 participants, results showed that antioxidant vitamin supplements taken by millions do not increase life expectancy and may raise the risk of a premature death. In fact, vitamin A was linked to a 16% increased risk of dying, beta-carotene to a 7% increased risk and vitamin E to a 4% increased risk.

So, forget about taking these vitamins as "anti-aging" miracles.

The evidence with vitamin C suggested that it was no better than a dummy pill. We must base our conclusions on scientific evidence and not on testimonials or statements of those selling these products.

The Cochrane data suggested that antioxidant supplements are either useless or harmful. That should be the end of the story, but world citizens continue to gulp down these scam pills faster than a bass can suck-up minnows.

The supplement industry and marketers of health foods would have you believe that *antioxidants* are the panacea of modern times but vitamin C, if injected intravenously, has a *"prooxidant"* alter ego that can benefit arteries or fight cancer, because it reacts with oxygen to generate hydrogen peroxide. In contrast, vitamin C taken orally has been found to be primarily ineffective at preventing cardiovascular disease, because it is quickly filtered out by the kidneys.

It may come as a surprise to learn that vitamin C, a well-known antioxidant, has a "pro-oxidant" alter ego that can benefit arteries by *increasing* the production of nitric oxide and hydrogen peroxide, an EMOD. That's the conclusion of new research from the University of Cardiff, recently published in the journal Cardiovascular Research. Hydrogen peroxide can also act to increase the strength of electrical signals from the blood vessel's lining telling the surrounding muscle to relax and dilate them.

As of December 2010, the FDA is expanding its reach to crack down on supplements used for weight loss, body building and sexual enhancement. They believe that manufacturers are deceptively labeling products and hiding harmful ingredient contents.

FDA Commissioner Margaret Hamburg said, "The manufacturers selling these tainted products are operating outside the law. These tainted products can cause serious adverse effects, including strokes, organ failure and death."

Dietary supplements have gotten away with these shenanigans for decades because, unlike drugs, they do not have to be approved by the FDA before they are marketed. In other words, manufacturers are responsible for the safety of their products and can keep selling them until they have been proven to be harmful.

So, line up the guinea pigs, folks.

Since 2007, because of links to strokes, kidney failure, liver injury and death, the FDA has "pressured" companies to recall nearly 200 "inappropriately-formulated" products, including 80 body building supplements. Actually, the FDA does not have the power to "force" recalls and instead it issues warning letters to draw attention of illegal products.

We are aware that dozens of weight loss products containing sibutramine have been withdrawn from the market for causing increased risk of heart attack and strokes. Even body builders and athletes frequently do not research the potentially dangerous products they take everyday.

Folks, do you homework and do not be a victim.

Even Supplements and Vitamins Need Testing

Because of the increasingly large number of prescription medications, the Food and Drug Administration (FDA) has a daunting task in testing the safety of current drugs prior to their sale. However, our pill popping nation is also taking daily handfuls of dietary supplements and vitamins.

Unlike drugs, the manufacturers that make supplements are not required to prove to the FDA that their supplements are safe or effective, as long as they do not claim that the supplements can "prevent, treat, or cure any specific disease."

In fact, some such products may not contain the amount of the herb or substance that is written on the label, and some include other substances, contaminants or toxic agents. Actual amounts per dose vary between brands or even between different batches of the same brand.

Consumer Lab.com recently tested multivitamins and found that more than 30 percent contained significantly more or less of an ingredient than claimed, or were contaminated with lead. Importantly, the privately held Consumer Lab.com states that it is neither owned by nor has a financial interest in any companies that make, distribute or sell consumer products.

Additionally, they found that several multivitamin products tested, including three for children, exceeded tolerable upper limits established by the Institute of Medicine for ingredients such as vitamin A, folic acid, and niacin. Some men's multivitamin products contained too much folic acid, which may increase the risk of prostate cancer, while another was contaminated with lead.

Among four women's multivitamins tested, one provided only 66 percent of its claimed vitamin A and one of five seniors' multivitamins tested contained only 44 percent of its vitamin A. Tests revealed a wide range of inaccuracies of stated dosage levels.

Please keep in mind that most such supplements have not been tested to find out if they interact with medicines, foods, or other herbs and supplements. Even though some reports of interactions and harmful effects may be published, full scientific studies of interactions and adverse effects are rarely available. These products clearly state that they do not "prevent, treat, or cure any specific disease" and *that* you can believe.

We must be cautious of taking unnecessary or unneeded chemical substances (supplements and vitamins) into our bodies, even if they are cleverly marketed as containing only "natural ingredients" and as being "perfectly safe."

Actually, the truly safe thing is not to take them at all unless you have a proven vitamin deficiency. Instead, eat a well balanced diet with lots of fresh fruits and vegetables.

Monitoring Drug Safety is a Daunting Task

Because of the large number of currently marketed drugs, keeping up with their harmful or lethal side effects is a daunting task. Everyday, news reports implicating the dangers of medicines hit the airways and the internet.

Complicating the matter is the unreliability of the data released by drug manufacturers and their reluctance to publish negative studies. Just recently, there were reports of dialysis patients in Germany, who had gotten sick using the blood thinner, heparin. This was a different brand from the heparin that was linked to 19 American deaths.

Hundreds of allergic-type reactions have been linked to Baxter International's U.S.-sold heparin injections, which are derived from pig intestines and are produced in China. Large doses of heparin are commonly used for dialysis, heart surgery and to prevent clot formation in patients with thrombosis or atrial fibrillation.

Another report showed that Eli Lilly and Co. failed to adequately warn doctors and patients of dangerous side effects associated with its widely used drug Zyprexa, prescribed to treat schizophrenia and bipolar disorder. Lawyer Scott Allen said that, "If they put a warning on this product, their sales would fall. They would lose money. People would choose another drug, and they decided not to disclose what they knew."

Zyprexa has been given to over 23 million patients and brought in $4.8 billion in sales last year. Nine states are suing Lilly over Zyprexa including Alaska, Utah, Pennsylvania, West Virginia, Montana, Louisiana, New Mexico, Mississippi and South Carolina. Drug companies may have misled patients by inadequate warnings about the risk of developing diabetes, elevated blood sugar and severe obesity.

If your medications cause any unusual or untoward symptoms, you must consult your physician immediately. Do not end up being a fatality statistic as a footnote to a drug warning report.

CHAPTER FIVE

FALSE CLAIMS EXPOSED

Many faux theorist on aging subscribe to the free radical theory, which is like the theory of Bigfoot, only with less credibility or substance.

R. M. Howes M.D., Ph.D.
3/28/09

Vitamin E does not prevent prostate cancer

Antioxidants are constantly touted as being able to fight a wide variety of diseases, including cancer and heart disease. Yet, study after study fail to show their benefits and many studies indicate a significant increase in the risk of cancer, heart disease, stroke and overall mortality with the use of common antioxidants, such as vitamins A, C and E.

The beneficial predictions of antioxidants on combating disease are based on the flawed free radical theory.

Antioxidant popularity is driven by multi-billion dollar annual sales of these ineffective and potentially dangerous products, as evidenced by the latest study released by the National Cancer Institute. Investigators studied more than 35,000 men over age 50 in the SELECT trial. Each participant was randomly assigned to take a supplement, either selenium, vitamin E, a combination, or a placebo to determine whether vitamin E or selenium could prevent prostate cancer (Lippman et al, 2009).

After an average of five years, **the study found no lower risk of prostate cancer in men taking the supplements, either alone or together.** In fact, **men who were taking only vitamin E actually had a slightly higher risk of developing prostate cancer and men taking only selenium seemed to have a slightly higher risk of developing diabetes.** This is the same trend found in other reliable scientific studies.

Likewise, some of these large randomized controlled trials have had to be shut down early due to the increased risk of diseases in the group taking the antioxidants.

I have researched oxygen metabolism, free radicals and antioxidants extensively and have concluded that oxygen free radicals are essential in protecting us from recurrent infections and the development of cancer. My books can be found at www.thepundit.com and www.iwillfindthecure.org and some of my scientific papers at www.medi.philica.com.

In my opinion, antioxidants should be controlled just like other drugs and there should be legal liability associated with their use, due to their significant potential to be harmful. Nonetheless, today antioxidants are casually fortified in many food products, cereals, bread, soft drinks, so-called health drinks, chewing gum, hair products, skin products and even dog food.

Any need for antioxidants is covered by eating a well balanced diet containing fresh fruits and vegetables. Studies repeatedly show that synthetic supplements do not work and are only recommended in cases of known vitamin deficiencies.

Do not be bamboozled by cleverly crafted ads. Guard against being tricked or deceived by those interested only in profit. Any food additive should be proven to be beneficial and free of harm. I firmly believe that taking antioxidant supplements is a "radical mistake." Do not be misled.

Selenium Is Losing Its Magic

Dietary supplements, including multivitamins and the antioxidant selenium, are taken daily by tens of millions of Americans in hopes of bolstering their health and warding off diseases such as cancer and heart disease. Annual supplement sales are over $25-27 billion and there are over 40,000 products on the current market, with thousands of new products entering the market each year.

According to a 2002 by De Smet and Peter, reported in the New England Journal of Medicine, tens of thousands of supplement-related health problems (especially herbal supplements) are handled by U.S. poison control centers each year.

The FDA estimates that more than 50,000 safety problems a year are related to supplement use and until last year, supplement makers were not required to report problems to the FDA, and even now they must report only serious ones. There are no requirements to report lack of benefit or ineffectiveness of these supplements.

Last year, nearly 200 people were sickened by supplements containing up to 200 times the amount of selenium stated on the label. Symptoms included loss of hair, discolored and painful fingernails, joint and muscle pains and diarrhea and fatigue.

In October 2008, a study of 35,000 men showed vitamin E and selenium did not work together or alone to prevent prostate cancer. **Both supplements are antioxidants** and there were slightly more cases of prostate cancer in men taking only vitamin E and slightly more cases of diabetes in men taking only selenium, according to the National Cancer Institute (Lippman et al, 2009).

Now, a consumer group is threatening to sue Bayer-Healthcare, the manufacturer of One-A-Day vitamins (which contain selenium), who claims selenium reduces the risk of prostate cancer. David Schardt, the group's senior nutritionist, said, "The largest prostate cancer prevention trial has found that **selenium is no more effective than a placebo**. Bayer is ripping people off when it suggests otherwise in these dishonest ads." (Lippman et al, 2009).

Pharmaceutical drugs must show evidence of effectiveness before they go on sale but supplements do not. Even so-called "safe" supplements can be harmful. According the National Cancer Institute, users of the antioxidant, beta carotene, still had increased rates of lung cancer, six years after the study was stopped. Supplement suppliers must say that their products "are not intended to diagnose, treat, cure, or prevent any disease." Yet, their ads can readily mislead consumers.

We must educate ourselves as to the true effectiveness of all supplements and vitamins. Advertising is out of control and the supplement industry has grown exponentially. Supplements are not a "cure-all" and people have been misled to believe that they are magical.

Ideally, 70 micrograms of selenium can be taken per day. Selenium overdose as a result of a large dose or because of taking too much on a daily basis can cause some dangerous effects.

Such toxicity effects include brittle nails and hair, bad breath, exhaustion, loss in weight, hair loss, heart attack, cardiac arrest, hypothyroidism (inefficient production of thyroid gland), infertility in males, skin cancer, allergies which can be of food, dyes or preservatives and death

Tea and The Truth

A big marketing ploy is to push "tea" as being a near cure-all, because of its antioxidant content, especially polyphenols. So, let's evaluate the scientific data.

I have previously pointed out the 2009 report in Proceedings of the National Academy of Sciences which showed that the antioxidant vitamins C and E can "undo" the benefits of exercise, weaken the body's own exercise-induced free radical defense system and increase the risk of diabetes by decreasing insulin sensitivity. Another surprising antioxidant study found that vitamin C supplementation decreased training efficiency because it prevented some cellular adaptations to exercise and it significantly hampered endurance capacity.

Recently, the Advertising Standards Authority asked tea-maker, Tetley, to withdraw their advertisement for green tea because it implied that the tea had some general health benefits, like exercise, beyond hydration, due to its antioxidants.

Although some studies have suggested green tea protects against breast cancer, a number of studies have found no such link and a new Japanese study of 54,000 women, in the journal Breast Cancer

Research, suggests that green tea intake, within a usual drinking habit, is unlikely to reduce the risk of breast cancer. They found, "**There was no difference in the number of cancer cases among the women, regardless of their level of tea consumption** - even between the women who drank more than 10 cups a day and those who drank half a cup or less a week."

Yet, other studies have linked the tea to a decreased risk of other types of cancers, including bladder, ovarian, stomach and colorectal cancers, according to the University of Maryland Medical Center.

In a warning letter on Aug. 30, 2010, the Food and Drug Administration issued warnings to the makers of Canada Dry ginger ale and Lipton tea for making unsubstantiated nutritional claims about their green tea-flavored beverages. Confusion still reigns!

We must be cautious about the continual portrayal of antioxidants as a comprehensive health panacea, in the absence of meaningful scientific data. Every second, our cells are actively conducting tens of thousands of different types of life-saving oxidation reactions. Far from being "harmful", oxidation and oxygen free radicals are fundamental to sustaining life and health.

Please check out my book, *Death In Small Doses? Antioxidant Vitamins A, C and E in the 21st Century: A Health Impact Statement*, available at Amazon.com to make sense of the whole antioxidant question (Howes RM. Death in Small Doses: Book One, 2010) (Howes RM. Death in Small Doses: Book Two, 2010).

Cancer patients must be especially cautious with ingestion of large amounts of antioxidants because of the possibility of interfering with treatment. Yet, the conflicting scientific evidence does not mean that people should stop drinking tea. Simply, do not expect it to be a miraculous cure-all, because it is not.

Resveratrol

According to Aaron Saenz, new data by <u>Pfizer</u> and <u>Amgen</u> cast doubt on the manner in which health supplement resveratrol is said to work.

Resveratrol is a substance found in moderate quantities in red wine, and is believed to help prevent the negative side effects of aging.

Prominent researchers, like David Sinclair, believed that it worked by activating a certain gene, SIRT1. This activation is thought to produce the benefits of a caloric restriction diet even among those with high fat and high caloric intake. In the October 2009 volume of Chemical Biology and Drug Design, Amgen offered experimental results that indicate resveratrol does not, in fact, activate SIRT1. Pfizer, in the January 2010 volume of the Journal of Biological Chemistry, offers similar results, showing that resveratrol (and related substances such as SRT1720) do not active SIRT1 and did not reduce blood sugar in mice fed a high fat diet.

This last result is in direct contradiction to previous resveratrol research published by David Sinclair of Harvard University in Nature. To simplify: Pfizer and Amgen are saying that resveratrol doesn't work in the way people thought, and may, in fact, not work at all.

http://singularityhub.com/2010/01/19/two-new-studies-cast-doubt-on-resveratrol/ (accessed 12-25-10).

Considering the complexity of this research, it's going to take many more years of research, and analysis of conflicting results, before anyone is likely to conclusively know if and how resveratrol works on mice...let alone humans. Those proponents of the substance should take heart in the fact that SIRT1 activation is just one possible mechanism by which resveratrol could induce the benefits of a caloric restriction (CR) diet.

Opponents should point out that Pfizer's mice didn't show any benefits of CR, so that no matter what mechanism resveratrol is supposed to be using, it didn't seem to work. Pfizer also points out that resveratrol (and especially related substance SRT1720) did not improve mitochondrial capacity, and had many other effects on cells, some of which could complicate its use in humans.

Critical scientists, like myself, are happy to call attention to a potential conflict of interest. Pfizer and Amgen are competitors with GSK, one of the companies spending millions of dollars in clinical trials to see how resveratrol works. One would think that Pfizer and Amgen had something to gain by proving that GSK's potential products wouldn't work. That being said, they would have even more to gain if they found that resveratrol does work and if they could determine a way to market a SIRT1 activator themselves.

There should be a "wait and see" policy to resveratrol and the other antioxidants. There are very few health supplements, including the antioxidants, with undeniable scientific support.

Even Vitamin D and Fish Oil are having to be re-evaluated at the moment. In the meantime, I still recommend the proven benefits from regular exercise as tolerated, eating a nutritious diet and living as stress free as possible.

Resveratrol (3,5,4'-trihydroxy-trans-stilbene), one of the major antioxidative constituents found in the skin of grapes, has been considered to be responsible in part for the protective effects of red wine consumption against coronary heart disease ('French Paradox'). Rat pheochromocytoma (PC12) cells. PC12 cells treated with hydrogen peroxide (H_2O_2) underwent apoptotic death. **Resveratrol pretreatment attenuated hydrogen peroxide-induced cytotoxicity, DNA fragmentation, and intracellular accumulation of EMODs** (Jang JH, Surh YJ. 2001).

Again, this illustrates the fact that antioxidants can block the protective apoptotic effect of H_2O_2 and that antioxidants could allow for rapid neoplastic growth. H_2O_2 is well suited to act as cellular messenger since it does not randomly react with all molecules, as most other EMODs do, but instead primarily targets cysteine residues.

I believe the simple fact that tumors are rare in the brain, heart, thyroid and the retina, even though they have the highest oxygen consumption levels in the body, with high EMOD generation (and low antioxidant levels) argues powerfully against the free radical theory. Ergo, tumorigenesis is hardly related to EMOD levels.

This issue is discussed in detail and is available in "The Howes Selective World Library of Oxygen Metabolism." (Available at www.iwillfindthecure.org)

If oxygen is the cause of aging, then infinitely dividing cells, such as neoplasia, should also age and die, even though most cancer cells are relatively hypoxic. This alone discounts the free radical theory of aging. Even though these cancer cells use oxygen, they are immortal. In fact, they have a higher EMOD level than do normal cells and yet, they have immortality! Additionally, hypoxia is usually associated with increased ROS production, which should rapidly end the life of cancerous cells, but it does not. It must reach an "apoptotic trigger point."

Grape seed extract or EGCG decreases iron absorption

A study on grape seed extract and EGCG in the August 2010 *Journal of Nutrition*, showed that **eating polyphenols decreased iron absorption.** Okhee Han, assistant professor of nutritional sciences, studied the effects of eating **grape seed extract and epigallo-catechin-3-gallate (EGCG) found in green tea.** They used cells from the intestine – where iron absorption takes place – to assess the polyphenols' effect and found that **polyphenols bind to iron in the intestinal cells, forming a non-transportable complex.** This iron-polyphenol complex cannot enter the blood stream. Instead, it is excreted in the feces when cells are sloughed off and replaced. (Ma et al. 2010).

People already at risk for iron deficiency (such as pregnant women and young children) increase that risk if they consume high amounts of grape seed extract or EGCG. **Iron deficiency is the most prevalent nutrient deficiency in the world.**

According to my theories, iron deficiency anemia, and it associated decreased oxygen transport to the tissues, should be a condition of EMOD insufficiency and conducive to development of cancer or "allowance" of disease manifestation. This prediction is upheld by the following data:

Severe Iron Deficiency Anemia (ADI) Warns of Cancer

A 2002 study showed that severe anemia defined by a ferritin level of 20 ng/mL or less, or a hemoglobin level of 12.5 or less, is a **sign of cancer risk**. Charts were reviewed for **308 patients** who had colonoscopy. They defined severe iron deficiency anemia (IDA) as ferritin values 20 ng/mL or less, or ferritin between 21 and 50 ng/mL and hemoglobin 12.5 or less.

Results showed that **severe anemia incurred a cancer risk of 7.7 percent. Milder anemia had a 1 percent risk of cancer associated with it. Severe iron deficiency anemia had a positive predictive value for cancer of 9 percent, a negative predictive value of 99 percent, sensitivity of 94 percent, and specificity of 34 percent.**

Mild anemia carries no added risk for cancer. **All of the upper gastrointestinal (GI) cancers were in the group with severe iron deficiency anemia.** These results were presented on May 20 at the 103rd annual meeting of the American Gastroenterological Association and Digestive Disease Week (DDW).

According to the Office of Dietary Supplements, **iron deficiency anemia symptoms include lethargy, slow cognitive ability, glossitis** (inflamed tongue), spoon nails (thin and concave fingernails) and decreased immune function. (Office of Dietary Supplements, NIH. Dietary supplement fact sheet. (Available online: http://dietary-supplements.info.nih.gov/factsheets/iron.asp).

ADI is also associated with preterm deliveries and I have seen increased risk of preterm deliveries associated with antioxidant vitamin use. (Scholl et al, 1992).

CHAPTER SIX

ANTIOXIDANTS PROVE INEFFECTIVE

Glutathione (an antioxidant) and heart failure

A study published in the August 10th 2007 issue of Cell says that **too much of a certain antioxidant, glutathione** (one of the body's most powerful antioxidants**), may cause heart disease**. An overload of natural antioxidants could actually lead to heart failure. In some people, a mutated gene can disrupt the fine balance, causing the cells to produce too much glutathione.

In the study of laboratory mice with failing hearts caused by mutant alpha B-Crystallin, researchers found increased activity of the biochemical pathway leading to high levels of reduced glutathione in the animals. To establish the connection between reduced glutathione and heart failure, Dr. Ivor Benjamin mated mutant alpha B-Crystallin mice that carried too much G6PD with mice that had far lower levels.

The resulting offspring had normal levels of reduced glutathione and did not get heart failure and dramatically changed the survival of these mice. The myopathic hearts show an increased recycling of oxidized glutathione (GSSG) to reduced glutathione (GSH), which is due to the augmented expression and enzymatic activities of glucose-6-phosphate dehydrogenase (G6PD), glutathione reductase, and glutathione peroxidase.

The researchers also added that **although many people take antioxidants to prevent heart and other protein-aggregate diseases, there actually is scant evidence to prove they work.**

Prof Randolph M. Howes MD, PhD

"This field of medicine has not appreciated reductive stress and its influence on disease," investigator Ivor Benjamin said. (Radasekaran et al, 2007).

Taking antioxidant supplements irresponsibly is dangerous and going into GNC and aimlessly picking bottle after bottle that are popularly marketed antioxidants is nonsense/nonscience. The old and uninformed belief that supplements can't hurt you because they are natural is *bovine excreta*. Rattle snake venom and mercury are natural but I beg you not to take them. Some of the most dangerous substances in the world are natural antioxidants.

Lycopene (an antioxidant) is under scrutiny

Epidemiological trials have suggested that higher intake of the lycopene-containing foods (carotenoids from primarily tomato products) or blood lycopene concentrations are associated with decreased cardiovascular disease and prostate cancer risk. Of the carotenoids tested, **lycopene has been demonstrated to be the most potent in vitro antioxidant.** But, **there is limited support for the in vivo antioxidant function for lycopene.** Moreover, **tissue levels of lycopene appear to be too low to play a meaningful antioxidant role.** Investigators concluded that **there is an overall shortage of supportive evidence for the "antioxidant hypothesis" as lycopene's major in vivo mechanism of action.** (Erdman et al, 2009).

Other antioxidants are also failing to act as predicted by the free radical theory. A selenium study in humans was shut down early after it was found increase the risk of developing a second primary tumor and decreasing the life span.

Ferulic acid and quercetin (plant-based antioxidants), under scrutiny

In rat studies with ferulic acid, quercetin (a flavonol), it appeared that they developed more advanced forms of kidney cancer in diabetic rats. The study appeared in the September 2010 American Cancer Society's bi-weekly *Journal of Agricultural and Food Chemistry*. In an article entitled, "Quercetin and Ferulic Acid Aggravate Renal Carcinoma in Long-Term Diabetic Victims," researchers suggested that quercetin could contribute to the development of cancer. They found that diabetic laboratory rats fed either quercetin or ferulic acid developed more advanced forms of kidney cancer, **and concluded the two antioxidants appear to aggravate or possibly cause kidney cancer. Quercetin aggravated, at least, if not directly caused, kidney cancer in rats.**

They concluded that the U. S. Food and Drug Administration should reevaluate the safety of all plant-based antioxidants.

Chocolate anitoxidant flavonoids poorly absorbed

Millions of chocoholics, including myself, are rejoicing at a July 4, 2007 article in the Journal of the American Medical Association (JAMA), which claimed that "...inclusion of small amounts of polyphenol-rich dark chocolate as part of a usual diet efficiently reduced blood pressure." Some believe that chemicals contained in cocoa, called polyphenols or flavonoids (antioxidants), are responsible for its purported cardiovascular benefits.

However, a statement in 2005 from the Pennington Nutrition Series stated that at that time, **"there are no trials demonstrating a protective effect of cocoa polyphenols on cardiovascular disease."**

JAMA reported that only thirty calories of dark chocolate – roughly one Hershey kiss – could help lower high blood pressure. Not white chocolate, but dark chocolate appeared to lower systolic (top number) blood pressure by about three points and diastolic (bottom) pressure nearly two points.

However, according to WebMD.com, **the study doesn't say high blood pressure will be reduced by dark chocolate alone, but should be used in combination with a healthy diet, exercise, reduced salt intake and losing excess weight.** Actually, this very small study was not "blinded" and the small changes in blood pressure make the results questionable.

Cocoa must be chemically processed to make it palatable, which destroys most of its flavonoids. Further, according to the Linus Pauling Institute, **flavonoids are poorly absorbed (usually less than 5%)** and the small amounts that do get into the circulation are rapidly broken down and excreted. Nonetheless, my fellow chocoholics, let's enjoy these tasty treats but watch out for the added calories from their sugar and fat content. So-called scientific conclusions are always subject to change as new data is collected.

I rest my case!

Pomegranate Claims Violate The Law

Recently, I read an advertisement in *Discover* magazine for pills made from pomegranate juice, which called their "pompills or POMx" the "Antioxidant Superpill." It went on to say that they have spent $34 million in medical research, documented POMx's unique and superior antioxidant power and "revealed promising results for prostate and cardiovascular health."

WOW! However, in very small print at the bottom of the page, they state, "These statements have not been evaluated by the FDA. This product is not intended to diagnose, treat, cure or prevent any disease." Yet, their logo replaces the "O" in POM with a symbol of the heart and their article is written as though pomegranate juice or POM pills can prevent prostate cancer and protect against heart disease.

Neither of these insinuations are true.

In fact, the FDA says, "Pomegranates may be full of antioxidants, but **there is no evidence that POM Wonderful's pomegranate products prevent heart disease, prostate cancer or erectile dysfunction.**"

In February of 2010, the FDA issued a warning about the health claims the POM company made online about its products, which stated that its 100% pomegranate juice was shown to reduce blood pressure and reduce the risk of prostate cancer in scientific studies, using language that is only permissible for FDA-approved drugs and therefore in violation of the Federal Food, Drug and Cosmetic Act.

In September of 2010, the Federal Trade Commission (FTC) filed a complaint against POM Wonderful for its printed health ads claiming its product produces a "30% decrease in arterial plaque and promotes healthy blood vessels." The FTC says these overstated claims are both false and unsubstantiated.

According to the Chicago *Tribune*: "The labor-intensive and messy pomegranate was stuck on the sidelines of the American fruit market until 2002 when Beverly Hills billionaires Stewart and Lynda Resnick planted enough of the fruit to quadruple the market, simultaneously introducing POM Wonderful juice to consumers." In short, they jumped on the "antioxidant band wagon."

The Director of the FTC's Bureau of Consumer Protection said, **"Any consumer who sees POM Wonderful products as a silver bullet against disease has been misled."** As expected, the POM company disagrees with these charges.

Echinacea

Some authors have claimed that the antioxidant properties of echinacea make it a valuable medicinal agent.

Echinacea roots and derivatives are a good source of natural antioxidants and could be used to prevent free-radical-induced deleterious effects (Pellati et al, 2004) (Hu and Kitts, 2000).

According to the Mayo Clinic website, people with allergies to plants should use caution and multiple cases of anaphylactic shock and allergic rash have been reported with echinacea taken by mouth. Allergic reactions including itching, rash, wheezing, facial swelling, and anaphylaxis may occur with more commonly in people with asthma or other allergies and are not recommended in children. Echinacea injections have caused severe reactions and are not recommended.

Some discourage the use of echinacea by people with conditions affecting the immune system, such as HIV/AIDS, some types of cancer, multiple sclerosis, tuberculosis and rheumatologic diseases. Long-term use of this herb may cause low white blood cell counts. Liver transplant patients who consume large amounts of echinacea may have increased liver enzyme activity, indicating liver damage.

In vivo studies have indicated that all Echinacea species significantly decreased inflammatory mediators (Zhai Z et al, 2007). **I believe that this clearly shows the unfavorable effects of the antioxidant echinacea, in that it blocks bacterial killing and blocks apoptosis by blocking the inflammatory mediators.**

If you want to know the truth about antioxidants, read my new book, *Death In Small Doses? Antioxidant Vitamins A, C & E in the 21st Century: A Health Impact Statement.* (Howes RM. Death in Small Doses: Book One, 2010). It is available at Amazon.com, Barnes and Nobles and Borders bookstores and online. Let the truth protect you and do not be a chump for clever marketing and false claims. Many will lie to you for profit but I will tell you the scientific truth and let you decide for yourself.

Are vitamin supplements beneficial in patients with breast cancer?

A new cohort study by Nechuta et al is fresh off the press and it is likely to stimulate considerable discussion. Thus, I have included it, along with my analysis of it.

Vitamin supplement use during breast cancer treatment and survival: a prospective cohort study.

Antioxidants may protect normal cells from the oxidative damage that occurs during radiotherapy and certain chemotherapy regimens, however, the same mechanism could protect tumor cells and potentially reduce effectiveness of cancer treatments. Investigators evaluated the association of vitamin supplement use in the first six-months after breast cancer diagnosis and during cancer treatment with total mortality and recurrence. **METHODS:** They conducted a population-based **prospective cohort study of 4,877 women** aged 20-75 years diagnosed with invasive breast cancer in Shanghai, China between March 2002 and April 2006. Women were interviewed approximately six-months after diagnosis and followed-up by in-person interviews and record linkage with the vital statistics registry. **RESULTS:** During a mean follow-up of 4.1 years, 444 deaths and 532 recurrences occurred. Vitamin use shortly after breast cancer diagnosis was associated with reduced mortality and recurrence risk, adjusted for multiple lifestyle factors, sociodemographics, and known clinical prognostic factors. Women who used antioxidants (vitamin E, vitamin C, multivitamins) had 18% reduced mortality risk and 22% reduced recurrence risk. **The inverse association was found regardless of whether vitamin use was concurrent or non-concurrent with chemotherapy,** but was only present among patients who did not receive radiotherapy. **CONCLUSIONS:** Vitamin supplement use in the first six months after breast cancer diagnosis may be associated with reduced risk of mortality and recurrence. Impact: Our results do not support the current recommendation that breast cancer patients should avoid use of vitamin supplements (Nechuta et al, 2010).

My analysis:

- patients who used antioxidants (vitamin E, vitamin C, multivitamins) had an 18% reduction in their mortality risk
- the risk for recurrence was decreased by 22%. This association was observed whether vitamin use was concurrent or non-concurrent with chemotherapy
- this benefit was only seen in patients who did not receive radiotherapy
- complete information was not available for dosages taken
- 2 studies that examined the use of multivitamins and breast cancer risk came to very different conclusions: One study found that their use decreased the risk for

breast cancer, and the other study showed that vitamin supplementation actually increased the risk for breast cancer
- this study is not a randomized trial
- this study was conducted in a population of women in Shanghai, China, so there may be issues such as diet, culture, genetics, and so forth that could affect outcome
- the risks have always been theoretical
- this study does not settle the question of complete safety
- results from this single observational study are not adequate to change the guidelines of vitamin use during cancer treatment
- women who did undergo radiotherapy showed slightly worse outcomes, but the results were not statistically significant
- patients treated with radiotherapy and who used antioxidant vitamins also had non-significant increased risk for mortality and recurrence

The use of antioxidant vitamins in cancer patients is so controversial that I am writing a book on just this subject alone. Since a major means of killing cancer cells is EMOD induced apoptosis, there is a solid theoretical basis that cancer patients should use caution in taking any antioxidants, which would likely produce an EMOD insufficiency and negate the treatment.

There is scant evidence that antioxidants are doing anything to directly combat the cancer itself (unless they are going through a prooxidant stage), even though they may help alleviate some of the adverse effects of chemotherapy and radiotherapy.

So, if you are a cancer patient or have a premalignant condition, proceed with the use of antioxidants with extreme caution.

CHAPTER SEVEN

A HISTORY OF MISTAKES

Certain self evident truths need not require additional evidence or proof, such as the low toxicity of EMODs, as evidenced by their omnipresent ubiquity.

R. M. Howes M.D., Ph.D.
7/15/09

Medicine's historical mistakes

History recalls numerous flawed theories, which confused bacterial or viral etiologies, infectious versus chemical causation and hypotheses which were completely off the mark. Diseases of old, such as scurvy, pellagra, puerperal or childbed fever and newer diseases, such as sub-acute myelo-optic neuropathy, HIV/AIDS and mad-cow syndrome fall into the more current examples.

Frequently, **the one to put mankind on the proper track, dies with rejection and without recognition and it is decades or longer before the truth of his/her genius is recognized. Such may be the case with the flawed free radical theory.** (Howes RM: "The Free Radical Fantasy," 2006).

The erroneous concept that "antioxidants are good and prooxidants are bad" is so engrained into the world orthodoxy that change is ever so slow and is resisted at every turn. The flaws flow freely and are openly supported in so-called scientific forums, even though I have amassed irrefutable data (science-based evidence) against the nullified free radical theory.

> Any old consensus of acceptance of the free
> radical theory has been fractured.
> My book, Death In Small Doses?, splintered it and my fol-
> low up book should lay it to rest, with
> the decaying corpses of other fallen theories.
>
> R. M. Howes, M.D., Ph.D.
> 12/11/10

This nonsense/nonscience must stop. The public must be protected and the antioxidant vitamins must be regulated. To that end, I will continue my crusade.

The confusion and data inconsistencies of the results of the antioxidant studies is due to the fact that they are based on the disproved free radical theory of Harman. The free radical theory repeatedly fails the scientific method due to its lack of predictability. Prooxidants are essential for pathogen and neoplasia protection and are of low toxicity, since they are present in all aerobic cells in steady state levels.

Please see details at www.iwillfindthecure.org, http://www.thepundit.com or http://www.medi.philica.com.

Antioxidants may serve as co-oxidants and are useful in that regard but randomized, controlled, blinded studies have shown the ineffectiveness of antioxidant supplementation and their potential to do harm by causing a prooxidant deficiency state.

Singular antioxidants extracted from fruits and vegetables (supplements) fail to have the same biochemical effects as when they are incorporated in the entire fruit and vegetable biochemical matrix. My book, Death In Small Doses? Antioxidant Vitamins A, C and E in the 21st Century: A Health Impact Statement, presented 181 of the world's best randomized, controlled scientific trials which show that the antioxidant vitamins have marginal or no effects different from placebo or dummy pills. Sixty of these studies showed the harmful potential of these antioxidant vitamins. They can increase the risk of cancer, heart disease, stroke and over all mortality. Denial of the facts is unacceptable and ignorance is no excuse. (Howes RM. Death in Small Doses: Book One, 2010) (Howes RM. Death in Small Doses: Book Two, 2010).

My new book, Antioxidant Overkill, adds 69 more studies showing that antioxidant vitamins are no more effective than a placebo pill for a total of 250 studies. I also add more studies showing the harmful effects of these antioxidants for a total of 80 studies. A study of this magnitude has never been done before. It is unique and it is a first. Be informed and be safe.

If you are taking an antioxidant or an antioxidant vitamin, or are thinking of going on antioxidants, consider the information in my fully referenced book before you do. **The undeniable legacy of antioxidant vitamin use at today's high doses is an assemblage of confusing and conflicting studies and reports of bad side effects in hordes of unsuspecting victims.** (Howes RM. A, C & E: Equivocal Scientific Studies. 2006) (Howes RM. Hydrogen Peroxide Monograph. 2006).

Only by knowing this information, reviewed in consultation with a knowledgeable healthcare professional, can you make an informed decision about your well being. If you are a user of antioxidant vitamins A, C or E, or multivitamins, this book contains vital information for you.

Most of the antioxidant side effects discussed are likely unknown to your busy doctor. In fact, a higher percentage of the members of the healthcare team take more antioxidant vitamins than those taken by the general population. Although they are knowledgeable about routine medical problems, few have heard of increased risks for cancer, heart disease, and strokes caused by use of these vitamins; fewer still associate increased mortality with antioxidants.

As a surgeon, medical research scientist, biochemist and practicing doctor, I have been appalled by the lack of information in the medical community on the full range of side effects of the antioxidant vitamins. Antioxidant Vitamins A, C, and E in the Twenty-first Century offers a selective reference source and summary demonstrating the ineffectiveness and adverse side effects of the antioxidant vitamins A, C, and E. Howes RM. Death in Small Doses: Book One, 2010).

Prof Randolph M. Howes MD, PhD

This, my latest book, *Your Protection Against Antioxidant Harm: A Health Impact Update*, offers readily available, safe, effective and inexpensive ways to prevent antioxidant harm.

My work leads the global field in medical research on the complexities of oxygen metabolonics and redox signatures in disease allowance, coexistence and prevention.

R. M. Howes, M.D., Ph.D.
11/9/10

Antioxidants have failed to block, reverse or prevent diseases, such as cancer, strokes and cardiovascular disease, in randomized clinical trials with over eight million participants and clearly show that the free radical theory lacks predictability and had been invalidated because it fails to meet the requirements of the scientific method. I have researched this extensively. (Howes RM. Death in Small Doses: Book One, 2010) (Howes RM. Death in Small Doses: Book Two, 2010).

Basically, **oxygen free radicals are of low toxicity and are crucial metabolic agents for pathogen and neoplasia protection. The antioxidant study failures were due to the fact that they were based on a flawed and out dated theory.** (Howes RM. 2007).

This needs frequent repeating.

Be Cautious of What You Take

More than 30 years ago, former Merck CEO, Henry Gadsden, established the aim of the entire pharmaceutical industry and dietary supplement companies when he said, "I want to sell drugs to everyone. I want to sell drugs to healthy people. I want drugs to sell like chewing gum."

114

In this time of aggressive, misleading drug and dietary supplement marketing, a courageous patient advocate like myself, may be more important than ever!

R. M. Howes, M.D., Ph.D.
11/7/10

Killer drugs and medical SNAFUs

We should turn an ear of caution to the nearly unrestrained marketing from pharmaceutical and dietary supplement companies, which produce the drugs that are responsible for the 106,000 annual deaths from adverse reactions to medications. Yet, hospitals appeared to be a bastion of safety and security from the harms of the world and illness, but that may not be the case.

According to a new federal government study, hospital care-related problems contribute to the deaths of about 15,000 Medicare patients each month or 180,000 annually. They claim that, "One in seven patients suffers harm from hospital care, including infections, insulin-mismanagement, over-sedation, excessive bleeding from blood-thinning drugs, and bed sores."

In another one in seven patients, temporary harm occurred but was detected in time and corrected. Peter Pronovost of Johns Hopkins University, co-author of the book, *Safe Patients, Smart Hospitals,* said, "Medical mistakes are an enormous public health problem."

100,000 Americans die each year from adverse reactions to prescription drugs – the USA's fourth-leading cause of death – and that is just among hospital patients (Jason et al, 1998).

Estimates suggest that pharmaceuticals are responsible for 199,000 additional deaths among out patients (Weingart et al, 2000).

Barbara Starfield's JAMA article, " Is US Health Really the Best in the World?" gives very large estimates of death due to medical treatment. A total of 225,000 deaths are attributed to various iatrogenic causes.

This figure puts them at the 3rd highest cause of death, only after heart disease and cancer. Thus, **there are 106,000 deaths due to "non-error adverse events of medications".** (Starfield B. 2000).

The medical burden of fatal adverse drug reactions (FADRs) is significant. Hemorrhages were seen in a majority of the FADRs; antithrombotic agents or NSAIDs were implicated in most of these events. These results suggest that **preventive measures should be taken to reduce the number of deaths caused by drugs.** (Wester K. et al, 2008).

The drugs most frequently associated with ADRs were diuretics, opioid analgesics, and anticoagulants. In conclusion, **approximately one in seven hospital in-patients experience an ADR,** which is a significant cause of morbidity, increasing the length of stay of patients by an average of 0.25 days/patient admission episode. The overall burden of ADRs on hospitals is high, and effective intervention strategies are urgently needed to reduce this burden (Davies et al, 2009).

This astonishingly totals about 486,000 annual deaths from medicines and hospital mistakes. Folks, be careful. Be very careful! Bear in mind that about 2.5 million deaths occur annually in the USA. These estimates put iatrogenic causes at almost 20% of deaths and most of these deaths are preventable. So, why aren't we doing more about it?

CHAPTER EIGHT

MY PERSONAL QUEST

My Goals

For over four decades, I have studied the arcane science of oxygen metabolism. I have published (free on line at *www.iwillfindthecure.org*) a magnum opus of about 6,000 pages, with tens of thousands of scientific references, which corrects the myth that electronically modified oxygen derivatives (EMODs) are inherently destructive. In fact, they are normally of low toxicity and are absolutely essential for subcellular signaling and energy production. (Howes, 2004) (Howes, 2005).

It is unprecedented to accuse an essential normal product of normal metabolism, in normal levels, to be toxic or lethal.

I believe that an EMOD insufficiency is the basis of disease allowance with diseases such as cancer, atherosclerosis, diabetes, arthritis, HIV/AIDS, Alzheimer's disease and malaria. (Howes, 2008) (Howes, Cardiovascular Disease. 2006) (Howes, Diabetes. 2006).

An adequate EMOD level is also essential for controlling neoplastic or cancerous growths by the induction of cellular apoptosis (cellular suicide). This feature offers a unique site for selectively killing cancerous cells and not injuring normal cells. (Howes, Cancer, Apoptosis. 2007).

Please also remember that **anaerobes thrive in a reducing environment**, whereas an oxidizing environ will kill them. We use oxidation ponds to cleanse and sanitize the effluent from municipalities, not reduction ponds!

My father died from cancer and my mother had Alzheimer's disease and as a physician, I felt helpless to significantly change their fatal course. I went on a personal mission to develop innovative new theories to combat such diseases and I found a commonality of causes, which was related to a reduction in their overall oxidative capacity and EMOD levels.

My goal is to get my methods and techniques to the patient's bedside in my lifetime. Thus, I have got to hurry. Oxygen and its free radicals have been erroneously demonized for over five decades and the time has come to correct misconceptions and half truths regarding their beneficent character.

Antioxidants have been praised as guarding against wanton radical destruction and harmful prooxidants and responsible for preventing and curing diseases such as cancer, heart disease and strokes. Yet, the scientific data reveals that the common antioxidant vitamins, such as A, C and E, can actually increase the risk of developing cancer, heart disease and stroke and overall mortality (your risk of dying). (Howes, Philica. Feb 7, 2009) (Howes, Death. 2007).

Shockingly, **interference from antioxidant vitamins and N-acetylcysteine have been shown to block prooxidant killing of cancer cells with chemotherapy, radiation therapy and photodynamic therapy. The antioxidants can protect malignant cells against the prooxidant killing of neoplastic cells.** (Howes, Philica. Feb 7, 2009) (Howes, Cancer, Apoptosis. 2007).

The role of antioxidant vitamins demands further evaluation and cautions, such that they are regulated the same as drugs. Antioxidants have unproven benefits and known harmful potential. I believe that their injudicious use is an insidious killer, in that they reduce EMODs and allow deadly diseases to manifest themselves. (Howes, Harm. 2007).

Antioxidant vitamins should also be used with caution (or not used at all) in patients with pre-malignant conditions or with known cancer. EMODs hold a central and prominent role in cancer therapy. (Howes R : Cancer Therapy, 2010).

There is considerable evidentiary proof of a link between common diseases and the antioxidant vitamins, especially vitamins A (beta carotene) and E (alpha tocopherol).

The public health sector is just whistling past the graveyard, which is also the approach of most doctors with the antioxidant vitamins. They have not researched this subject and accept erroneous dogma and have been swayed by clever advertising. Actually, many intentionally overlook the scientific data. The difference between myself and most doctors? I actually checked the data, with over 4 decades of extensive research.

Generalities

A healthy lifestyle consists of abstinence from smoking, keeping a low body mass index, moderate alcohol consumption, regular exercise, and a healthy, nutritious, well balanced diet, which has been consistently associated with substantially reduced risk of common diseases. **Intake of antioxidant vitamin supplements may not further add to disease risk reduction and carries significant potential for harm.**

We must inform patients that there is little or no clinical evidence that taking a multivitamin or the antioxidant vitamins every day will help protect the average healthy adult from disease and infection or increase their lifespan. While there is no clinical proof of their benefits, taking excessive daily vitamins has repeatedly been shown to be harmful.

However, antioxidant vitamins and multivitamins may offer some clinical benefit to certain subgroups of populations, including people with known vitamin deficiencies, malabsorption syndromes, women who are pregnant, the elderly, and people with chronic conditions.

Prof Randolph M. Howes MD, PhD

Surprisingly, as recently as 2002, no less an authority than the Journal of the American Medical Association recommended that "all adults take one multivitamin daily." In glaring contrast, **many experts no longer recommend multivitamins to their patients nor do they take them themselves.** As of November of 2010, Dr. Isadore Rosenfeldt no longer recommends vitamin E to any of his patients.

Being a physician, surgeon and a scientist, I am driven to introduce improved alternatives for the prevention and treatment of cancer and heart disease. I can not sit idly on the side. I must be "proactive for prooxidants." Oxygen derivatives, EMODs, offer new therapeutic modalities which are readily available, safe, effective and inexpensive. However, to get prooxidants through clinical trials will require re-education of medical scientists and the general public. **Injudicious antioxidant use is so common, especially amongst medical personnel, that it is a serious global healthcare issue.**

Unrestrained antioxidant vitamin advertising has convinced the public to continue to spend their money for these products, even though they have a significant downside.

Our species has evolved over the past 2.4 million years as omnivores, consuming a wide variety of flora and fauna. Yet, industrialized food processing and fortification has received the blessing of the FDA and antioxidants have been legally introduced (forcefully crammed) into all of our diets, whether you want them there or not. This has been done because of the erroneous belief that these highly refined and processed foods containing these antioxidants are benefiting our health. However, accumulating data is showing that may not be the case.

Vitamin and Food Supplements Overstated

It is bad and it gets worse everyday. Unrestricted, aggressive advertising extolling the hyped benefits of food and beverage additives drowns out the facts and numbs common sense evaluation of the exuberant claims by supplement marketers.

Herbal remedies and vitamin-laced water products are commanding significant consumer dollars as people seek quick fixes in a high-tech society. Consumer watchdogs say people are wasting their money and are buying "untested" products that could harm them. There is no proof of safety with vitamin, fiber, herbal and mineral food additives or fortifications.

Today, these products are everywhere and they do not need proof of safety or effectiveness. Studies have found that about 44 cents out of every dollar spent on alternative medicine was spent for products like fish oil, glucosamine and echinacea.

Much of the so-called fish oil does not come from fish but actually comes from plants. Consumers spent nearly $15 billion, or about a third of what Americans spend out-of-pocket for prescription drugs.

Unfortunately, the major reliable scientific studies show that most of these products are ineffective and some show that they may be harmful. A new report from research firm Pricewaterhouse Coopers states that, "….some that are little more than dressed-up junk food."

Advertising is so strong that people will pay premium prices for products that they have been led to believe are good for their health. Amazingly, a recent study found that people would continue to take vitamins and supplements, even if studies show them to be harmful. Such is the incredible power of advertising.

When antioxidant studies fail to show benefits or even show harm, investigators state that the results are "disappointing." However, for the people who had a 28% increased risk of developing lung cancer as a result of taking the antioxidant, beta carotene, I believe that such a result is tragic and crosses over to being criminal.

These so-called "nutraceuticals or functional foods" account for more than $27 billion in sales a year and sales are growing faster than America's waist line. A spokesperson at the Center for Science in the Public Interest said, "People are going to be deceived into thinking a lot of these products are especially healthy for them when there's little evidence they are."

We must not be duped by false advertising for vitamins, antioxidants, nutraceuticals, vitamin-enhanced waters and sports drinks, etc.

Unless you are vitamin deficient, health benefits come from eating whole, nutritious foods and not from chemically concocted extracts. These products are not medicines but are, in actuality, quack suggestions to get the money from your pocket into their pocket. Please, keep an open mind.

Tax credit for vitamins: What?

The contribution you make to your Health Savings Account (HSA) is 100% tax deductible up to a limit of $6,150 for a family, and $3,050 for an individual. Your HSA-qualified health insurance must be in place by December 1st in order to qualify for a 2010 tax deduction. Since they first became available in the beginning of 2004, Health Savings Accounts have rapidly gained popularity, particularly among individuals and small businesses. Charges incurred as part of a preventive health program could include vaccines, blood tests, metabolism tests, and other lab tests, and even fees paid to a health institute or **vitamins if prescribed by a doctor**.

CHAPTER NINE

SUPPLEMENTS AND ENZYMES SHORT-COMINGS

Synthetic antioxidants not recommended

Exceeding the daily recommended doses of supplemented, or synthetic, Vitamins A and E, and beta carotene can be extremely detrimental to your health. Major medical organizations say the following about synthetic antioxidants:

The Mayo Clinic website:"… There's no proof that antioxidants in pill form can improve your general health or extend your life. In fact, they can have the opposite effect."

The American Diabetes Association (ADA) does not advise antioxidant supplements due to long term safety concerns and insufficient evidence to prove their effectiveness.

The American Heart Association (AHA) recommends obtaining antioxidants from food sources, and not from synthetic supplements.

Failures of the Big Three Antioxidant Enzymes: Catalase, Superoxide Dismutase & Glutathione Peroxidase

Without oxygen, we die. Further, without electronically modified oxygen derivatives (EMODs), we die.

The big three antioxidant enzymes (i.e., catalase, CAT, superoxide dismutase, SOD and glutathione peroxidase, GPx) fail to support the invalidated free radical theory and may have negligible effects or harmful potential. These endogenous (internally generated) antioxidant enzymes are more potent in preventing free radical damage than are dietary antioxidant vitamins, such as vitamins A, C and E.

Any agent which interferes with fundamental bodily biochemical processes must be taken seriously and substances, such as dietary antioxidants and antioxidant enzymes, which indiscriminately attack essential cellular signaling agents (i.e., electronically modified oxygen derivatives, EMODs) must be viewed with considerable caution. Such is the case for protecting essential EMODs and preventing their annihilation by antioxidant vitamins, low molecular weight antioxidants and antioxidant enzymes. The antioxidant enzymes, which also attack EMODs, have more specificity but they also more vigorously attack these same vital EMOD signaling molecules.

Various isoforms of CAT, SOD and GPx are dispensable (expendable, nonessential, unessential, unneeded, unnecessary, superfluous) and not needed for normal growth and survival.

CAT, with **hydrogen peroxide is its only substrate,** is believed to be one of the fastest and most perfect catalysts and is believed to be the predominant H_2O_2-removing enzyme in human erythrocytes. Yet, we can live normally without it. GPx is the powerful scavenger of oxygen free radicals. CAT is the unsurpassed, highly efficient scavenger of hydrogen peroxide and SOD is the scavenger of superoxide anion. **Humans with genetic deficiency of catalase ("acatalasemia") or mice genetically engineered to lack catalase completely, suffer few ill effects.**

My conclusions on the big three, CAT, SOD and GPx are that CAT and GPx are both dispensable (expendable, superfluous, unessential, unnecessary, replaceable, surplus to requirements, etc.), since **both can be eliminated and the animal can live a normal life**; whereas, SOD is not an antioxidant enzyme at all, since it generates hydrogen peroxide from superoxide.

Even ecSOD is somewhat expendable since mice without the extracellular SOD have minimal defects (only being sensitive to hyperoxia).

This is in contrast to species which lack **NOX, NADPH** oxidase, which generate superoxide. They are prone to repeated infections, granulomas and die an early death.

There are at least four different glutathione peroxidase isozymes in animals. **Glutathione peroxidase 1 is the most abundant and is a very efficient scavenger of hydrogen peroxide, while glutathione peroxidase 4 is most active with lipid hydroperoxides. Surprisingly, glutathione peroxidase 1 is dispensable, as mice lacking this enzyme have normal lifespans**, but they are hypersensitive to induced oxidative stress.

CHAPTER TEN

ALWAYS ASK QUESTIONS

Multivitamins

In 2002, the Journal of the American Medical Association recommended that "all adults take one multivitamin daily." However, in light of accumulating scientific evidence, that view is rapidly changing and being abandoned.

In the National Health and Nutrition Examination Survey (NHANES) 1999-2000, 52% of adults reported taking a dietary supplement in the past month, and 35% reported regular use of a multivitamin-multimineral (MVMM) product. Women (versus men), older age groups, non-Hispanic whites (versus non-Hispanic blacks or Mexican Americans), and those with a higher education level, lower body mass index, higher physical activity level, and more frequent consumption of wine had a greater likelihood of reporting use of MVMM supplements in NHANES 1999-2000.

Of great concern to me, among adults with a history of breast or prostate cancer, usage rates for dietary supplements in general and MVMMs are considerably higher (e.g., 56-57% for MVMMs). (Rock, 2007).

In October 2007, an online survey was administered to 900 physicians and 277 nurses by Ipsos Public Affairs for the Council for Responsible Nutrition (CRN), a trade association representing the dietary supplement industry. The "Life...supplemented" Healthcare Professionals Impact Study (HCP Impact Study) found that **72% of**

physicians and 89% of nurses in this sample used dietary supplements regularly, occasionally, or seasonally. Regular use of dietary supplements was reported by 51% of physicians and 59% of nurses. The most common reason given for using dietary supplements was for overall health and wellness (40% of physicians and 48% of nurses), but more than two-thirds cited more than one reason for using the products. **When asked whether they "ever recommend dietary supplements" to their patients, 79% of physicians and 82% of nurses said they did.** (Dickinson et al, 2009).

In 2010, Perlman et al. found that the in-school daily consumption of an MVM supplement by third- through sixth-grade inner-city children did not lead to improved school performance based upon standardized testing, grade point average, and absenteeism. Multivitamin/Mineral supplementation does not affect standardized assessment of academic performance in elementary school children. (Perlman et al. 2010).

A 2010 study of Swedish women found that those who took multivitamins were 19% more likely to be diagnosed with breast cancer over a 10-year period than those who didn't.

In 2007, de Souza et al. found that multivitamins do not improve radiation-related fatigue in patients with breast cancer and that no significant changes were elicited with the use of multivitamins. (de Souza et al. 2007).

A 2007 paper in the Journal of the National Cancer Institute found that men who took multivitamins along with other supplements were at increased risk of prostate cancer.

A study in the Aug. 6, 2005 issue of the *British Medical Journal* found multivitamins failed to protect elderly patients from infection. The randomized, double-blind, placebo-controlled trial of 910 men and women, ages 65 and older found no significant differences between the two groups and the number of times they visited a physician for infection.

Four months earlier in another issue of *BMJ*, British researchers led by Alia El-Kadiki, a researcher at Royal Hallamshire Hospital, conducted a meta-analysis of the literature and concluded there was not enough evidence to recommend that the elderly take multivitamins to ward off infection.

Another study found that the multivitamins didn't improve fatigue among breast cancer patients undergoing radiation therapy.

And inner-city schoolchildren who took a multivitamin did not perform any better on tests or have fewer sick days than students who didn't take one.

A review of 63 randomized, controlled trials (the gold standard research method) on multivitamins, published by the Agency for Healthcare Research and Quality found that multivitamins did nothing to prevent cancer or heart disease in most populations (the exception being developing countries where nutritional deficiencies are widespread).

Marian Neuhouser, PhD., a scientist at the Fred Hutchinson Cancer Research Center, published a paper in 2009, which followed 160,000 postmenopausal women for about 10 years. The researchers' conclusion: "Multivitamins failed to prevent cancer, heart disease, and all causes of death for all women. Whether the women were healthy eaters or ate very few fruits and vegetables, the results were the same."

Let me repeat the words of Miriam Nelson, PhD, director of the John Hancock Research Center on Physical Activity, Nutrition, and Obesity at Tufts University, who said, "The multivitamin as insurance policy is an old wives' tale, and we need to debunk it."

A 2005 report showed that routine multivitamin and multimineral supplementation of older people living at home does not affect self reported infection related morbidity. (Avenell et al. 2005).

And other research has linked excessive folic acid intake to higher colon cancer risk in people who are predisposed.

As Dr. David Katz said, the obvious question is,"Why expose yourself to any product with an increased risk of disease, if you are not benefiting from it (i.e., vitamin supplements)?"

Just remember that a pill is no substitute for a healthy diet and that much of the data on vitamins is only observational.

No proof exists as to their benefits except in cases of known vitamin deficiencies or malabsorption syndromes or pregnant females.

The American Academy of Family Physicians backs up the U.S. Preventive Services Task Force's sentiment that there's a lack of proof multivitamins provide any clinical benefits to average healthy adults.

Thomas Barringer, M.D., medical director of the center for cardio-vascular health at Carolinas Medical Center in Charlotte, N.C. said, "I don't know why doctors recommend them (MVMMs). But it's very time-consuming trying to talk someone out of doing something that's pretty innocuous." "There's no evidence, no hard evidence that in the nutritionally replete, the person who consumes some fruits and vegetables every day, benefits."

Yet, even today, whether a daily multivitamin provides any clinical benefit to the average healthy American depends on whom you ask. Most people are uninformed and go along with a false impression placed in their minds by aggressive marketing. They have been misled. They have been brainwashed by years of advertising.

People erroneously believe that multivitamins support their overall health and well being. They have been duped….again!

General recommendations of the USDA and the FDA are as follows: take fiber, omega-3s, and vitamin D3. At this point, unless the data changes, this sounds reasonable.

Vitamin D3

There is Good News and bad news for Vitamin D3

In 2007, Canadian researchers reported that children, later diagnosed with multiple sclerosis, had far lower levels of vitamin D than other youngsters and this was the first study to show links between the "sunshine" vitamin and a childhood disease, other than rickets.

Multiple sclerosis is a nervous system disease caused by damage to the myelin sheath that protects nerve cells and it affects 2.5 million people globally. Vitamin D is necessary for the effective absorption of dietary calcium, which becomes deposited in bones and teeth.

Your individual requirements depend on your age, the amount of sunlight exposure you get, liver and kidney function and medical conditions. Generally, the recommended amount has been 400 IU a day for people ages 51 to 70, but that amount is increasing. For those over age 70, the recommendation was 600 IU a day but, in addition to modest sun exposure, adults can take up to 2,000 IU of vitamin D per day, which is the "tolerable upper intake level" set by U.S. health officials.

More than 2,000 IU a day can cause toxicity problems including excessive urination, high blood pressure, nausea, weight loss, fatigue, calcium deposits in soft tissues (kidney stones) and kidney damage. Vitamin D3 is found in fatty fish like salmon and is added to milk and other foods. Data suggests it helps lower blood pressure, reduces inflammation and boosts the immune system.

High doses of vitamin D3 have been linked to lower risks of cancer, arthritis, tuberculosis and diabetes. Lower rates of breast, colon, ovarian, prostate, pancreatic and lymphomatous cancers are seen in patients with higher vitamin D3 levels and vitamin D3 helps prevent cancer cells from growing and spreading.

We must rely on safe means of protecting ourselves from disease and the judicious intake of vitamin D3 seems to be on target. The D3 form appears to be most effective and it is readily available and inexpensive. However, do not assume that "more is always better." Use good common sense, exercise, eat fresh fruits and vegetables and avoid unnecessary pharmaceuticals whenever possible.

Vitamin D: Up to 800-1,000 IU daily (less if you live in a year-round warm climate and get 15 minutes of unblocked sun every day). Get it from a separate pill or with calcium. Vitamin D and calcium go hand in hand.

It is hard to consume 600 IUs of vitamin D from food alone. A cup of D-fortified milk or orange juice has about 100 IUs. The best sources may be fatty fish — some servings of salmon can provide about a day's supply. Other good sources are D-fortified cereals.

However, a study on 11-30-10 by the Institute of Medicine recommends: "Most people in the U.S. and Canada — from age 1 to age 70 — need to consume no more than 600 international units of vitamin D a day to maintain health, the report found. People in their 70s and older need as much as 800 IUs. The report set those levels as the "recommended dietary allowance" for vitamin D."

A National Cancer Institute study last summer was the latest to report no cancer protection from vitamin D and the possibility of an increased risk of pancreatic cancer in people with the very highest D levels.

Super-high doses, above 10,000 IUs a day, are known to cause kidney damage.

Dr. Joann Manson of Harvard Medical School, who co-authored the Institute of Medicine's report, pointed to history's cautionary tales: "**A list of other supplements — vitamins C and E and beta carotene — plus menopause hormone pills that once were believed to prevent cancer or heart disease didn't pan out, and sometimes caused harm, when put to rigorous testing."**

As for calcium, the report recommended already accepted levels to go along with your daily D — about 1,000 milligrams of calcium a day for most adults, 700 to 1,000 mg for young children, and 1,300 mg for teenagers and menopausal women. Too much can cause kidney stones; the report said that risk increases once people pass 2,000 mg a day.

Calcium: Up to 1,000 mg total from food and supplements. If you don't eat 3 servings of milk/dairy, take the equivalent in a supplement that contains vitamin D3.

More Vitamin D Recommended for Kids

In 2009, the American Academy of Pediatrics doubled the recommended daily dose of vitamin D for children and teens up to 400 units per day, which is equivalent to drinking four cups of milk.

Vitamin D has been receiving great press and has been **fortified in milk since 1933 for the prevention of rickets.** Estimates are that 60,000 cases of colon cancer and 85,000 cases of breast cancer could be prevented every year in the U.S. for those who maintain a vitamin D level of at least 55 ng/mL.

Vitamin D improves muscle strength and is necessary for the effective absorption of dietary calcium, which becomes deposited in bones and teeth. Individual vitamin D requirements depend on your age and your amount of sunlight exposure.

New research indicates that teens with the lowest vitamin D levels are more than twice as likely to have high blood pressure and high blood sugar, which sets them up for hypertension and diabetes. Teens in the study were also four times more likely to have a dangerous condition called "metabolic syndrome."

However, the Johns Hopkins Bloomberg School of Public Health reminds us that these are "strong associations" and not proof of causality. Experts say that getting about 15 minutes of sunlight exposure a few times a week is generally enough and point out that vitamin D is found in fatty fish like salmon and is added to milk. Other studies suggest that it helps lower blood pressure, reduces inflammation and boosts the immune system.

My research indicates that vitamin D3 has such wide ranging beneficial effects because of its strong prooxidant activity (www.iwillfindthecure.org).

We welcome medical news which offers preventative measures for major health problems such as hypertension, cancer and diabetes. Currently, increasing vitamin D levels seems to be one such measure. More importantly, it has minimal downside and adverse effects, although over dosage can carry health hazards. As always, check with your physician regarding questions. Please remember, "Treat your body like it belongs to you."

Vitamin D deficiency doubles the risk of fatal stroke in whites but not in blacks

A November, 2010 report in the Los Angeles Times said vitamin D deficiency doubles the risk of fatal strokes in whites, but has no effect on the risk in blacks, even though blacks are more likely to have vitamin D deficiencies and are 65% more likely to die from strokes, researchers said Sunday. The results were puzzling, said Dr. Erin Michos of the Johns Hopkins School of Medicine in Baltimore. "We thought maybe the lower vitamin D levels might actually explain why blacks have higher risks for strokes," she said.

Stroke is the third leading cause of death in the United States, killing more than 140,000 Americans annually and permanently disabling more than half a million.

Vitamin D, a fat-soluble vitamin involved in bone health, helps prevent rickets in children, protects against severe bone loss in adults, and may lower the risk of heart disease, cancer, multiple sclerosis, diabetes and other medical conditions. Natural sources include exposure to ultraviolet B rays in sunlight and eating fatty fish, egg yolk, and fortified foods such as milk and breakfast cereals.

Michos and her colleagues analyzed health records of 7,981 black and white adults who participated in the Third National Health and Nutrition Examination Survey of Americans, conducted between 1988 and 1994, following the participants for a median of 14 years. They reported at a Chicago meeting of the American Heart Assn. that, among the participants, 6.6% of whites and 32.3% of blacks had severely low levels of vitamin D in their blood, classified as levels below 15 nanograms per milliliter. During the period of the study, 116 whites and 60 blacks died of stroke. Accounting for age and other risk factors, blacks were 65% more likely to suffer a stroke. Higher levels of diabetes and hypertension probably account for some of the increased risk, but not this much, Michos said. "Something else is surely behind this problem. However, don't blame vitamin D deficits."

The lack of sensitivity to low levels of vitamin D may be an adaptation to historic low levels associated with the sun-blocking effects of skin pigments, she added. The blacks in the study also had fewer incidents of bone fracture and greater overall bone density than whites. "In blacks, we may not need to raise vitamin D levels to the same level as in whites to minimize their risk of stroke," she concluded

Now, for the bad news.

On December 1, 2010 the following study was released: **Vitamin D studies "inconsistent."**

After reviewing about 1,000 studies on the supposed links between low vitamin D levels and higher risk of serious diseases, a panel of US and Canadian doctors concluded that they showed inconsistent results, sometimes due to shoddy research methods. **The only sure benefit of the combination of calcium and vitamin D is bone health.**

The experts also issued **new guidelines**, the first since 1997, for North Americans, saying **people should take between 700 and 1,300 milligrams of calcium and anywhere from 600 to 800 international units of vitamin D each day**. The panel's establishment of new guidelines offer a more solid recommended daily dose than the 1997 approach of suggesting adequate intake (AI) amounts.

Glenville Jones, a Canadian doctor who was on the 14-member committee for the US-based Institute of Medicine, said, **"Vitamin D deficiency is quite rare in North Americans at this point in time."**

Humans need calcium to help clot blood and for proper functioning of muscles and nerves, and vitamin D is necessary for the body to absorb calcium. Inadequate calcium has been shown to lead to bone fractures and osteoporosis. And some populations are likely to need more Vitamin D than other groups, including breastfed babies, people with dark skin and those living in northern latitudes where daylight exposure is limited.

"Our dilemma is that there are mixed reports that are not all consistent," said Jones, who is a professor of biochemistry at Queens University in Kingston, Ontario. "Some of the studies are not well controlled," he said.

"We don't want to base public health recommendations upon a mixed conclusion where some studies say there is a benefit in cancer and other studies say they don't," he added.

The panel also set upper limits for both calcium (2,000 milligrams per day) and vitamin D (4,000 IUs per day), beyond which point risks such as kidney and tissue damage begin to mount. "Higher levels have not been shown to confer greater benefits, and in fact they have been linked to other health problems, challenging the concept that 'more is better,'" the report said.

CHAPTER ELEVEN

SOMETHING SMELLS FISHY

Omega-3 fish oil

For sometime, I have pondered the activity of the omega-3 fatty acids, since it has a double bond and some claim that it is an antioxidant. Finally, I have found the answer, which is the basis for their salutary effects in fighting disease. Omega-3s generate EMODs. Supplementation (polyunsaturated fatty acids (PUFAs) with **n-3 long-chain-PU-FA (n-3 LCPUFAs) significantly increased oxidative stress** at rest and after a judo-training session (Flaire et al, 2010). In short, omega-3s help maintain sufficient EMOD levels for pathogen and cancer protection because they are prooxidants.

Fish Oil Does Not Prevent Alzheimer's Disease

Omega-3 fish oil supplement producers have claimed curative powers for diseases such as cancer, heart disease, dementia, ADD, ADHD, depression, bipolar disorder, dyslexia, dyspraxia, obsessive compulsive disorder, headaches and migraines.

Also, it was claimed to decrease aggressive behavior, prevent learning disabilities and make kids smarter. Unsupported aggressive advertising has led to "soaring sales for fish oil."

However, disappointing studies are now coming forth and supplements do not have the same benefits as do natural foods containing these same ingredients. Even though claims of being "heart healthy" persist, **a large German study gave fish oil or dummy capsules to more than 3,800 people who had suffered a recent heart attack and found that after a year, there was no difference between fish oil pills or placebo**.

But, there is more bad news for fish oil. Even though data from a trial of over 800 older people initially showed that those who eat plenty of oily fish seem to have better cognitive function, a new study has found that omega-3 pills, promoted as boosting memory, did not slow mental and physical decline in older patients with Alzheimer's disease.

This $10 million project studied nearly 300 men and women, aged 76 on average, with mild to moderate Alzheimer's disease. They were randomly assigned to take either the omega-3 fish oil pill (DHA) or dummy pills daily for 18 months. Results were similar in both groups, in that **DHA provided no benefits in slowing Alzheimer's symptoms** nor did the pills work in a subgroup of participants with the mildest Alzheimer's symptoms.

The researchers concluded, "There is no basis for recommending DHA supplementation for patients with Alzheimer disease." Laurie Ryan, program director of Alzheimer's studies at the Institute on Aging, called the results discouraging. Thus, Alzheimer's disease remains basically untreatable and the "fish oil gold rush" may be slowing.

We realize that generally dietary supplements do not work, except in cases of known deficiencies or malabsorption syndromes. Still, sales of dietary supplements bring in about $27 billion annually.

We know that eating more heart-healthy omega-3 fats provided no additional benefit in a study of heart attack survivors who were already getting good care. There is little harm side effects of fish oil when the ratio of omega-6 to omega-3 is properly balanced.

Please remember the words of expert, Dr. Lichtenstein, "We need to be a little more cautious about the prediction of individual benefit of any nutritional supplements. People are so willing to embrace the simple answer, as if it's possible to crack a capsule over a hot fudge sundae and undo the harm of harmful diets and lack of exercise."

But, give me a chocolate sundae. I'll take my chances.

Fish Oils: Is There A Downside?

Please remember, even though there is a current fish oil craze, you can never be too careful about what you put into your body. As I mentioned, fish oil (especially omega-3) proponents have made wild claims for their curative powers for diseases such as cancer, heart disease, dementia, ADD, ADHD, depression, bipolar disorder, dyslexia, dyspraxia, obsessive compulsive disorder, headaches and migraines.

Such unsupported aggressive advertising has led to "a fish oil gold rush." Unfortunately, most supplements do not hold up under scientific testing and pill-forms of agents such as omega-3, vitamin E, beta carotene and vitamin C do not offer the same benefits as do natural foods containing these same ingredients.

When it comes to improving brain function, data from a trial of over 800 older people initially showed that those who eat plenty of oily fish seem to have better cognitive function. But factors such as education and mood explained most of the difference and a UK study has cast doubt on claims that eating oily fish can protect against dementia in old age.

The American Heart Association (AHA) recommends adults eat fish at least twice a week and for people with heart disease, **they advise 1 gram of omega-3 a day**.

Fish oil capsules are not for children or pregnant women, because the pills pose a bleeding risk and capsules should be stopped a week before any surgery.

We must continue to emphasize the basics of eating a balanced diet, exercising more, avoiding stress, not smoking and not being misled by unscrupulous advertisers. Every time we turn on the TV, we are being oversold on the latest miracle meds or supplements, like they were pitching OxyClean or Sham Wow. So, be on guard and protect your wallet and your health.

Omega-3: Up to 1,000 mg daily if you don't reliably eat fish such as salmon 2 or 3 times a week.

Prof Randolph M. Howes MD, PhD

The Fish Oil Gold Rush

Slowly, Americans are becoming more aware that they are constantly being bombarded with unrestricted dietary supplement advertising and unsupported advertising of legal medical drugs but that does not stop their onslaught.

Currently, we are in the midst of "a fish oil gold rush" and the latest mantra is that fish oil (especially omega-3) can cure all varities of diseases. If only all of this were true, it would be a miracle but it is not all true.

Just as you should not rely on synthetic vitamin pills to replace fresh fruit and vegetables, you should not rely on omega-3 pills to replace the ingestion of fish with a high fat content.

These results do not mean that getting more of the essential nutrient has no value because studies have shown fish oil fats may reduce heart disease. Larger randomized studies are needed to clarify the benefits or lack of benefits with omega-3 supplements.

As with marketing techniques for other supplements (such as anti-oxidants), in recent years, omega-3 has been added to or "fortified" in some foods such as margarine and eggs, or labeled to highlight the omega-3 content of foods like tuna fish in efforts to **capture the current fish fat craze.**

Fish oil capsules are not for children, surgical patients or pregnant women, because of a bleeding risk.

We must concentrate on eating a balanced diet, exercising more, avoiding stress, not smoking and not being misled by unscrupulous advertisers. People seem to ignore this advice even when their life depends on it. Get your medical advice from a physician and not from someone who is "pushing" supplements.

Fish oil does not accelerate weight loss

According to an online December 15, 2010 article, in the American Journal of Clinical Nutrition, fish oil capsules won't help boost weight loss if you're already dieting and exercising.

Among a group of overweight and obese adults enrolled in a diet and exercise program, **those who took omega-3 fatty acids didn't lose any more weight than those given placebo** capsules, Dr. Laura F. DeFina of The Cooper Institute in Dallas and her colleagues found.

There is prior evidence from animal studies that omega-3 fatty acids promote weight loss, DeFina and her team note, while studies in people have had mixed results. Because fish oil has many other potential health benefits, including cutting cholesterol, improving insulin sensitivity, and reducing blood pressure, "weight-loss programs associated with the use of omega-3 polyunsaturated fatty acids seemed appropriate to the investigators."

To investigate whether fish oil enhanced the results of a diet and exercise regime, the researchers randomly assigned 128 sedentary overweight or obese men and women to take five fish oil capsules (providing a total of three grams of omega-3 fatty acids) or five placebo capsules every day for 24 weeks.

Participants were also instructed to do 150 minutes a week of aerobic exercise and 20 to 30 minutes of strength exercises at least twice a week.

The people in the omega-3 group lost 5.2 kilograms, or about 11.5 pounds, on average, compared to 5.8 kilograms (nearly 13 pounds) for the placebo group, not a statistically significant difference. People in both groups lost more than five percent of their body weight, enough to produce health benefits.

At the end of the study, there was no difference between the groups in measures of heart disease risk, such as blood pressure and cholesterol levels. However, researchers found that omega-3 blood levels in the fish oil group increased to a level "previously found to have a positive cardiovascular effect."

Not everyone actually completed the 24-week program; there were only 81 participants at the end. But the results were similar when the researchers looked only at those 81 people.

Investigators said, "Whereas one may not enhance weight loss by taking supplements with this level of omega-3 fatty acids, the protective cardiovascular effect should still be realized because of the sheer increase in blood concentrations of the fatty acids."

One online jokester said, "The BP brand of fish oil is going on sale in November." That is not funny for those of us living in Louisiana.

We must continue to search for scientific based evidence to know the truth.

CHAPTER TWELVE

GROWTH HORMONE AND "ORGANIC"

Is Growth Hormone the Fountain of Youth?

In short, the answer is "No." Even though seventy five million baby boomers are rushing to an age whereby they are frantically seeking out the fictional "fountain of youth," they are being misled by clever marketers of ineffective or dangerous products.

Growth hormone is the same substance used by athletes to improve athletic performance, along with anabolic steroids. No doubt, steroids do improve athletic performance.

However, growth hormone can not turn back the hand of time and neither can any other supplement or vitamin concoction, according to our best scientific analysis. Studies suggest that the risks can be substantial and outweigh the possible benefits.

Growth hormone is made by the pituitary gland and its level starts to decline as we enter our 40s. Synthetic human growth hormone can be legally used to treat children with short stature and some other growth problems caused by childhood diseases but bolstering levels of the hormone through injections will not help stave off the effects of aging.

However, according the American College of Physicians, "It's estimated that some patients spend as much as $1,000 to $2,000 a month on growth hormone for anti-aging purposes." The American Association of Clinical Endocrinologists says there's currently no place for the use of growth hormone as an anti-aging agent.

Analysis of data from randomized, controlled trials on growth hormone use in healthy older adults, published last year in the **Annals of Internal Medicine, found suggestions that users of growth hormone had high rates of soft tissue swelling and joint pain, and increased risk of impaired blood sugar control or diabetes**. As I have pointed out many times, there are no magic pills.

I can state that the claimed miracle results of hormonal therapy and antioxidant vitamins have been exaggerated and **there has not been a single product or agent, which has been scientifically proven to prevent or reverse the aging process**. Caloric restriction without malnutrition may offer some hope but it is too early to tell. Do not be scammed. Instead, rely on exercise, a nutritious diet, avoidance of stress and do not smoke. Always make safe decisions regarding your health.

Is 'Organic' Actually Better?

Repeatedly, shrewd marketing makes fools of us faster than we can turn on the evening news. We are constantly being misled by advertising and apparently, the hyped benefits from "all things organic" are just another example.

First, headlines in July of 2009 read, "Organic food is no healthier." London School of Hygiene & Tropical Medicine investigators stated that, "consumers were paying higher prices for organic food because of its perceived health benefits, creating a global organic market worth an estimated $48 billion in 2007."

Researchers performed a systematic review of 162 scientific papers published in the medical literature over the last 50 years. **Their conclusion was that organic food has no nutritional or health benefits over ordinary food.** They also said that a small number of differences in nutrient content were found to exist between organically and conventionally produced foodstuffs, but these are unlikely to be of any public health relevance.

So, another marketing myth has been shot down by the most reliable means available to us for evaluating the veracity of advertising claims. Their article, published in the American Journal of Clinical Nutrition, indicated that there is currently no evidence to support the selection of organically over conventionally produced foods on the basis of nutritional superiority.

To me, that seems counterintuitive but "the results are what they are." Due to increasingly difficult financial times, sales in organic foods have fallen.

Second, in 2008, a consumer watchdog group, the Organic Consumers Association (OCA), found that leading brands of personal care products such as shampoos, lotions and body washes that are labeled "organic" or 100 per cent natural contain an undisclosed carcinogenic toxin 1,4-Dioxane. The chemistry of processing produces the 1,4-Dioxane and it is a known cancer causing agent.

Reportedly, the California Environmental Protection Agency (EPA) classes 1,4-Dioxane as a leading contaminant of groundwater and believes it to be a kidney, nerve and lung toxicant. The objection here is that it was found in so called "natural" and "organic" products, none of which are certified under the US Department of Agriculture's National Organic Program.

The OCA director said, "When it comes to misbranding organic personal care products in the US, **it's almost complete anarchy and buyer beware** unless the product is certified under the USDA National Organic Program."

We do not mind paying more for "organic" products that live up to their claims. Yet, we do not want to unknowingly rub dangerous "natural or organic" toxins all over our bodies. Do not get ripped off by unscrupulous marketing. There are more snake oil salesmen around than there are truth-challenged politicians.

CHAPTER THIRTEEN

INCREASING YOUR OXIDATIVE CAPACITY

Whenever I tell anyone of the emerging dangers of the antioxidant vitamins, they immediately ask, "How can I block or prevent this?", "How can I counter the antioxidants or how can I increase my EMOD levels and my oxidative capacity?" In short, "What can I do to protect myself?"

For years, I have been studying safe, effective, inexpensive and readily available means of doing just that and will expand upon them in this book forthright.

For decades, tens of millions of people have been misled or even lied to via deceptive and duplicitous advertising, as regards the safety and harmful potential of the common synthetic supplemental antioxidant vitamins A, C and E. Also, they have been ingesting unknown quantities of antioxidants in their food.

Consequently, on a daily basis, they ingest these synthetic substances in hopes of improving their overall health, boosting their immunity, fighting cancer and heart disease, increasing their sexual prowess and extending their life span. None of this has proven to be the case.

To the contrary, in over 250 studies and/or reports, I point out the ineffectiveness and dangers of these synthetic antioxidant vitamins. Yet, there are 80 negative studies contain therein showing harm, which continues to be ignored or denied by the swindling antioxidant vitamin peddlers and they continue to tout false claims as though they are well established scientific facts.

Additionally, data continues to accumulate on the harmful potential of antioxidants, used as preservatives, in our food supply. Where does it stop?

In the absence of a deficiency state or a malabsorption problem, there is no justifiable medical rational for taking these potentially harmful synthetic substances.

On 2-6-08, Steve Novella at the www.sciencebasedmedicine.org website wrote, "In the last two decades our increasing knowledge of oxidative stress and natural antioxidants has led to a great deal of legitimate scientific speculation about the role of ROS in degenerative disorders and even natural aging. Before scientists could even write their research grants, however, there emerged from this 'irrational exuberance' a cottage industry of antioxidant products marketed as if they were the very elixir of life." (http://www.sciencebasedmedicine. org/?p=38. Accessed 8-25-10)

It is also possible that nutritional antioxidants may have some benefits but at the same time disrupt certain essential metabolic balances and an extensive review of the literature reveals exactly that. The antioxidants may serve as "pre-oxidants or co-oxidants" and thus, actually help form the family of EMODs necessary to protect us from pathogens and neoplasia. But, excesses of antioxidants can dangerously lower protective EMOD levels.

Most of the data in this book is on actual people and not on *in vitro* studies or animal models. The lackluster clinical data has countered but not quieted the false and exuberant claims for the antioxidant vitamins. Until now, as regarded antioxidant studies, ambiguity, equivocality, uncertainty, doubt, vagueness, and inconsistency have been the rule.

As I said before, keeping all antioxidant levels including the antioxidants cholesterol, uric acid, bilirubin, estrogen and testosterone levels low may help keep the oxidative capacity at an optimal level.

We must keep in mind that even though cholesterol is an effective antioxidant when incorporated into an estrogen molecule, its activity is changed with the addition of side groups and on whether the media is aqueous or lipid. The order of reactivity in scavenging of radicals in the aqueous phase is dependent on the precise cholesterol or estrogenic structure, with phenolic estrogens being more potent antioxidants than catecholestrogens or diethylstilbestrol (Begona Ruiz-Larrea et al. 2000).

The antioxidant activity of an estrogen depends not only on the hydrophilic or lipophilic nature of the scavenged radical, but also on the phenol and catechol structures of the estrogen compound (Begona Ruiz-Larrea et al. 2000).

Surprisingly, natural **estrogens have much greater radical-scavenging antioxidant activity than has previously been demonstrated, with activities up to 2.5 times those of vitamin C and vitamin E** (Begona Ruiz-Larrea et al. 2000).

A direct link between high estrogen levels and the return of a higher risk of breast cancer has been established by U.S. researchers. It was well known that the initial development of breast cancer is linked to more estrogen in the bloodstream.

Breast cancer is the second most common neoplasm in the world.

But, latest study ascertains the fact that women who have a past history of breast cancer have to take a few more steps to lower their estrogen levels. Regular exercise and weight management are amongst the steps included to keep the estrogen levels in check.

It was found that **women whose cancer reappeared had more than double the concentration of estrogen as compared to women who were not affected by the fatal disease.** A special emphasis has been given on regular exercising and weight management because the component estrogen accumulates in the fat and promotes tumors. Therefore, keeping weight down is equivalent to lowering the risk of the cancer growing back.

The findings appear in the March, 2008 issue of Cancer Epidemiology, Biomarkers and Prevention. In short, breast cancer survivors whose bodies make the least estrogen have the lowest chance of breast cancer recurrence, according to this long-term study.

Please remember that, "Fat tissue is the primary non-ovarian site for estrogen production in the body," said Cheryl Rock, PhD, RD, a professor in the cancer prevention program at the University of

California, San Diego. I have discussed the relationship of obesity to the allowance and coexistence of many diseases in my prior books, which are available at www.iwillfindthecure.org.

In the past it was known that several factors, including the size and type of a tumor, and whether the disease had spread to surrounding lymph nodes determined the intensity of cancer. However, the latest revelation concerning estrogen levels adds to the list.

An article in the January, 2011 issue of Cancer Prevention Research, a journal of the American Association for Cancer Research, quotes researchers at Fox Chase Cancer Center who reported that **estrogen may increase the movement of precancerous cells in the mouth and thus promote the spread of the disease within the oral cavity.**

They found that estrogen induces the expression of an enzyme called cytochrome P450 1B1 (CYP1B1), which is responsible for breaking down toxins and metabolizing estrogen. Interestingly, CYP1B1 induction occurred only in precancerous cells, which are neither totally normal nor cancerous. Surprisingly, estrogen did not induce CYP1B1 in cancer cells.

Estrogen also reduced cell death in the precancerous cells, irrespective of the amount of CYP1B1 present. In short, estrogen appeared to promote spread of cancer cells and it tended to block the killing of precancerous cells. I believe that all of this is based on the redox signature of this system, i.e., pro-oxidants kill cancer and antioxidants block this killing ability and, in a sense, protect cancer cells.

An article in the October 2010 issue of JAMA stated, "**Women who took hormone replacement pills had more advanced breast cancers and were more likely to die from them than women who took a dummy pill.**" The findings included 11 years of follow-up from the Women's Health Initiative study, which in 2002 found women who took estrogen plus progesterone for five years had higher rates of ovarian cancer, breast cancer, strokes and other health problems.

One expert said, "Doctors can only be guessing that taking the pills at a lower dose and for a shorter time would be less harmful."

Hyperuricemia, hypercholesterolemia and hyperbilirubinemia (all are antioxidants)

There are two glaring examples of insidious antioxidant threats when one considers hyperuricemia and hypercholesterolemia. Both of these conditions of elevated antioxidant levels connotes serious threats to normal health. This has been clearly proven by past medical observations. **I am the first to view these conditions in terms of their redox signature**, as I have done with three other common antioxidants, hyperbilirubinemia, high estrogen and high testosterone levels.

Obviously, these agents can have a vast range of biochemical effects but we must be mindful of their antioxidant nature and their ability to produce an EMOD insufficiency, with its associated disease "allowances."

Keeping antioxidant uric acid levels and antioxidant cholesterol levels low (normal) may help keep the oxidative capacity operating at an optimal level. Moreover, the salutary effects of lowered cholesterol and uric acid could well be attributed to the fact that overall antioxidant levels have been lowered, thus allowing a slightly higher or increase in overall oxidative capacity, such that EMODs can operate at optimal rates.

New Rules: 11 Ways to increase oxidative capacity

If you do not use antioxidant supplements, don't start!

If you use antioxidant supplements, stop!

Exercise as much as tolerated

EWOT (exercise with oxygen therapy)

Aspirin (ASA is a good prooxidant)

vitamin D3 (a good prooxidant)

peroxide

artemisinin (epoxides generate prooxidants)

curcumin, sulforaphane, cinnamaldehyde (they have considerable prooxidant activity)

hyperthermia

hyperbaric oxygen

Others - methylene blue,

1. **RULE NUMBER ONE:** If you do not currently use antioxidant supplements, don't start! In the absence of a deficiency or a malabsorption syndrome, do not take synthetic supplemental antioxidant vitamins.

2. **RULE NUMBER TWO:** If you currently take antioxidant vitamin supplements, stop!

3. **RULE NUMBER THREE:** Exercise as much as tolerated.

3) Exercise

Antioxidants are the current craze in the marketing of dietary supplements and it is implied that they promote good health, prevent disease risk and fight so-called harmful oxygen free radicals. According to the free radical theory, exercise should kill us. Yet, upon examination of the scientific literature, we find that many of the predicted beneficial claims for antioxidants have been "disappointing."

In short, antioxidants have failed to live up to their hype and, in fact, they have been found to have considerable potential to do harm. Please visit *www.iwillfindthecure.org* for details.

We also hear a lot about the need and the benefits of exercising, which I highly recommend. Exercise is promoted as being one of the best ways of preventing common diseases ranging from cancer to the formation of gall stones. If one avoids the "pounding injuries to joints" of exercises such as jogging, exercise consistently has proven to be valuable and advantageous.

Surprisingly, it is readily conceivable that a person who exercises a lot, could inhale 100 million gallons of diradical oxygen in a life time, because exercise increases oxygen consumption 10-15 times that of a resting state. Because exercise is known to dramatically increase the body's content of oxygen free radicals, it was thought that athletes would benefit from the use of antioxidants, such as the vitamins E and C. However, recent studies have shown just the opposite.

A 2009 report in Proceedings of the National Academy of Sciences stated, "We find that antioxidant supplements prevent the induction of molecular regulators of insulin sensitivity and endogenous antioxidant defense by physical exercise." In other words, the antioxidant vitamins C and E can "undo" the benefits of exercise, weaken the body's own exercise-induced free radical defense system and increase the risk of diabetes by decreasing insulin sensitivity.

In another surprising antioxidant study, vitamin C supplementation decreased training efficiency because it prevented some cellular adaptations to exercise and it significantly hampered endurance capacity.

We realize that there are free radicals, which can wreak havoc in the chemistry lab. But, the living/breathing human cell compartmentalizes, controls and exquisitely regulates their biochemical activity. Thus, the proposed widespread cellular destruction predicted by the free radical theory does not normally occur.

In fact, there are now many who enter their eighth and ninth decades of life and have been free of cancer, have maintained a sharp mind and breathed oxygen throughout. Oxygen proved to be essential to their survival and not the deadly culprit painted by the free radical theory. In fact, I say, "Give me oxygen or give me death." Don't you?

So folks, keep on exercising and breathing that good old life-giving oxygen and enjoy yourself.

Exercise is Always a Good Thing

If there is one thing that is consistently good for one's health, it is exercise. Of course, that does not mean participating in an Iron Man marathon or jogging across America.

Common sense needs to be applied in most situations and extremes are to be avoided. In my many years of medical research, exercise has been shown to decrease the risk of most major diseases, such as cancer, heart disease, strokes, obesity and diabetes. Arguments continue over the mechanism by which exercise is helpful because, according to the teachings of the free radial theory, increased oxygen consumption during exercise should be uniformly harmful and even shorten one's life span or kill you outright.

To the contrary, results of a study published in the Archives of Internal Medicine "clearly support the continued encouragement of physical activity, even among the oldest age groups. Indeed, it seems that it is never too late to start." People even in their mid to late 80s can extend their life by a few years by getting four hours or more of exercise per week.

Reportedly, "As little as four hours a week was as beneficial as more vigorous or prolonged activity." They also found that exercise had improvements even for previously sedentary 85-year-olds because their three-year survival rate was double that of inactive 85-year-olds.

I believe that the most common denominators for the body's responses to exercise are the increases in oxygen consumption and oxygen utilization. Some say that oxygen consumption increases up to 20 times during exercise, resulting in increased oxygen to most organs and tissues of the body. I believe that we should consider exercise to be a "medicine" and that each episode of exercise is equivalent to a substantial dose of oxygen and its subsequent metabolic products, which protect us from bacteria, fungi, viruses, protozoans and cancer.

Aerobic exercises are based on an oxygen boost to improve the immune system, improve overall health and aid in disease prevention. The importance of oxygen could not be more readily apparent. It is the essential sustaining and driving force for all aerobic cellular metabolism.

Routine exercise is widely recognized as one of the most important adjuncts for disease prevention and maintaining overall good health. Risk reduction for chronic degenerative diseases can even occur with low levels of exercise as was pointed out in consensus statements by the Centers for Disease Control and Prevention and the American College of Sports Medicine.

Combinations of a nutritious diet and regular exercise can be extremely important in maintaining health and in reducing overall risk of illness. So, take heart that at any age, even a little exercise can help maintain your health and extend your life. So, why is it so darned hard to do?

Exercise, Good; Antioxidants, Bad

Exercise is consistently seen as being good for overall health, as has eating a diet of fresh fruits and vegetables. Unfortunately, the diet data has been misinterpreted to suggest that the antioxidants contained in fruits and vegetables are the specific agents responsible for their good effects, but that is not the case.

Being made aware of facts that contradict decades of erroneous teaching is at the least disturbing, if not "stunning."

One must have an open mind to consider the strength of the current scientific data on commonly marketed antioxidants, such as vitamins A, C and E. Years of intense study on oxygen metabolism presented me with reliable data which questioned the accuracy of a preponderance of non-scientific publications praising dietary supplements, especially the antioxidant vitamins.

Please remember that dietary supplements are a $27 billion business and their advertising influence is demonstrably powerful.

German scientists from the University of Jena have found that the antioxidant vitamins C and E can undo some of the most important health benefits of exercise and that taking vitamins C and E after a workout appears to prevent physical exercise improvement of the body's energy regulation. These vitamins appear to block the good effect that exercise has on insulin sensitivity, which could lead to Type 2 diabetes and insulin resistance.

The findings add to the growing evidence that antioxidants, including vitamins A, C and E, have complex effects on the body which can do harm as well as good. Also, the much derided oxygen free radicals have been shown to have crucial beneficial effects, including energy production, immunity and protection from cancer and pathogens.

In fact, these often maligned oxygen free radicals are essential for our well being. I have presented a world literature review (free of charge) to document these facts at www.thepundit.com and www.medi.philica.com or www.iwillfindthecure.org.

Presenting unsupported health care advice and perpetuation of medical misinformation is truly dangerous and irresponsible. There should be legal culpability for giving medical advice which does not have patient safety as its number one priority.

We must put away misleading medical mythology. Face the facts, folks.....the medical facts.

Exercise as much as tolerated

The 2007 recommendations state that adults up until age 65 need at least 30 minutes of moderate-intensity activity, five days a week. While the minutes can be accumulated throughout the day, it must be done for at least 10 minutes to be considered toward meeting the goal. The recommendation can also be met by doing at least 20 minutes of high-intensity activity, three days per week. If desired, moderate- and high-intensity activities can be combined to meet the requirement.

New recommendations are also available for those 65 and older. While similar to the recommendations for younger adults, there are some differences. For example, it is recommended that older individuals exercise at a moderate-intensity level rather than a high-intensity level. Stretching exercises that promote flexibility are also stressed, as are activities that promote balance for those at risk of falls.

Also new in the 2007 recommendations was the inclusion of strength-building (resistance training) as part of one's activity regimen. This addition was based on newer evidence showing that resistance training builds muscular strength and endurance, improves the ability to perform activities of daily living, and improves quality of life while reducing disability. To summarize, this targeted set of recommendations emphasizes reducing sedentary behavior through moderate-intensity aerobic activities, strength-building exercise and an individual approach based on medical risks.

The 2007 recommendations provide information about the minimum amounts and types of physical activity adults need to maintain or improve their health. If an individual's goal for being active extends beyond health benefits to include cardiovascular fitness or weight management, the amount of exercise needed extends beyond the 2007 recommendations.

The following is taken from: http://www.cdc.gov/physicalactivity/everyone/guidelines/adults.html#Musclestrengthening (accessed 9-12-10)

According to the CDC (Center for Disease Control), regular physical activity helps improve your overall health and fitness, and reduces your risk for many chronic diseases. Fitting regular exercise into your daily schedule may seem difficult at first, but the *2008 Physical Activity Guidelines for Americans* are more flexible than ever, giving you the freedom to reach your physical activity goals through different types and amounts of activities each week.

Adults need at least: 2 hours and 30 minutes (150 minutes) of moderate-intensity aerobic activity (i.e., brisk walking) every week **and muscle-strengthening activities** on 2 or more days a week that work all major muscle groups (legs, hips, back, abdomen, chest, shoulders, and arms) OR an equivalent mix of moderate- and vigorous-intensity aerobic activity (running) **and muscle-strengthening activities** on 2 or more days a week that work all major muscle groups (legs, hips, back, abdomen, chest, shoulders, and arms).

150 minutes each week sounds like a lot of time, but you don't have to do it all at once. Not only is it best to **spread your activity out during the week**, but you can **break it up into smaller chunks**

---

of time during the day. As long as you're doing your activity at a moderate or vigorous effort for **at least 10 minutes at a time**. Try going for a 10-minute brisk walk, 3 times a day, 5 days a week. This will give you a total of 150 minutes of moderate-intensity activity.

Aerobic activity – what counts and why?

Aerobic activity or "cardio" gets you breathing harder and your heart beating faster. From pushing a lawn mower, to taking a dance class, to biking to the store – all types of activities count. As long as you're doing them at a moderate or vigorous intensity for **at least 10 minutes at a time**.

Intensity is how hard your body is working during aerobic activity.

How do you know if you're doing light, moderate, or vigorous intensity aerobic activities?

For most people, light daily activities such as shopping, cooking, or doing the laundry doesn't count toward the guidelines. Why? Your body isn't working hard enough to get your heart rate and oxygen consumption up.

Moderate-intensity aerobic activity means you're working hard enough to raise your heart rate and break a sweat. One way to tell is that you'll be able to talk, but not sing the words to your favorite song. Here are some examples of activities that require moderate effort:

- Walking fast
- Doing water aerobics
- Riding a bike on level ground or with few hills
- Playing doubles tennis
- Pushing a lawn mower

Vigorous-intensity aerobic activity means you're breathing hard and fast, and your heart rate has gone up quite a bit. If you're working at this level, you won't be able to say more than a few words without pausing for a breath. Here are some examples of activities that require vigorous effort:

- Jogging or running
- Swimming laps
- Riding a bike fast or on hills
- Playing singles tennis
- Playing basketball

You can do moderate- or vigorous-intensity aerobic activity, or a mix of the two each week. A rule of thumb is that **1 minute of vigorous-intensity activity is about the same as 2 minutes of moderate-intensity activity**.

Some people like to do vigorous types of activity because it gives them about the same health benefits in half the time. If you haven't been very active lately, increase your activity level slowly. You need to feel comfortable doing moderate-intensity activities before you move on to more vigorous ones. The guidelines are about doing physical activity that is right for you.

Besides aerobic activity, you need to do things to strengthen your muscles at least 2 days a week. These activities should work all the major muscle groups of your body (legs, hips, back, chest, abdomen, shoulders, and arms).

To gain health benefits, muscle-strengthening activities need to be done to the point where it's hard for you to do another repetition without help. A **repetition** is one complete movement of an activity, like lifting a weight or doing a sit-up. Try to do 8—12 repetitions per activity that count as 1 **set**. Try to do at least 1 set of muscle-strengthening activities, but to gain even more benefits, do 2 or 3 sets.

You can do activities that strengthen your muscles on the same or different days that you do aerobic activity, whatever works best. Just keep in mind that muscle-strengthening activities don't count toward your aerobic activity total.

There are many ways you can strengthen your muscles, whether it's at home or the gym. You may want to try the following:

- Lifting weights
- Working with resistance bands

- Doing exercises that use your body weight for resistance (i.e., push ups, sit ups)
- Heavy gardening (i.e., digging, shoveling, chopping)
- Yoga

If you are an adult with a disability, regular physical activity can provide you with important health benefits, like a stronger heart, lungs, and muscles, improved mental health, and a better ability to do everyday tasks. It's best to talk with your health care provider before you begin a physical activity routine. Try to get advice from a professional with experience in physical activity and disability. They can tell you more about the amounts and types of physical activity that are appropriate for you and your abilities. If you are looking for additional information, visit The National Center on Physical Activity and Disability.

Children and adolescents should do 60 minutes (I hour) or more of physical activity each day. Encourage your child to participate in activities that are age-appropriate, enjoyable and offer variety! Just make sure your child or adolescent is doing three types of physical activity: aerobic activity, muscle strenghtening activity and bone strengthening. Some physical activity is better-suited for children than adolescents. For example, children do not usually need formal muscle-strengthening programs, such as lifting weights. Younger children usually strengthen their muscles when they do gymnastics, play on a jungle gym or climb trees. As children grow older and become adolescents, they may start structured weight programs. For example, they may do these types of programs along with their football or basketball team practice.

Older adults

As an older adult, regular physical activity is one of the most important things you can do for your health. It can prevent many of the health problems that seem to come with age. It also helps your muscles grow stronger so you can keep doing your day-to-day activities without becoming dependent on others.

Not doing any physical activity can be bad for you, no matter your age or health condition. Keep in mind, some physical activity is better than none at all. Your health benefits will also increase with the more physical activity that you do.

If you're 65 years of age or older, are generally fit, and have no limiting health conditions you can follow these guidelines: 2 hours and 30 minutes (150 minutes) of moderate-intensity aerobic activity (i.e., brisk walking) every week **and muscle strengthening activities** on 2 or more days a week that work all major muscle groups (legs, hips, back, abdomen, chest, shoulders, and arms).

Aerobic physical activity is activity in which the body's large muscles move in a rhythmic manner for a sustained period of time. Aerobic activity, also called endurance activity, improves cardiorespiratory fitness. Examples include walking, running, and swimming, and bicycling.

Bone-strengthening activity is physical activity primarily designed to increase the strength of specific sites in bones that make up the skeletal system. Bone strengthening activities produce an impact or tension force on the bones that promotes bone growth and strength. Running, jumping rope, and lifting weights are examples of bone-strengthening activities.

Exercise can decrease cancer risk

It has been known for a long time that exercise cuts your risk of cancers including the breast, colon, esophagus and kidney. Excess body fat sometimes leads to higher hormone levels, which in turn, may elevate the risk of cancer. In 2010, experts at the United States' National Cancer Institute analyzed 14 previous studies and found physical activity cuts the risk of endometrial cancer by 20 to 40 percent when compared to sedentary women. The study was published in the British Journal of Cancer.

However, experts still aren't sure exactly how much physical activity is needed to lower their risk. One study showed more than 20 percent of womb cancers could have been avoided if women had exercised vigorously for about 20 minutes at least five times a week.

Researchers can't say for sure how exercise lowers cancer risk, but exercise increases oxygen consumption, which increases EMOD production, which protects for both pathogens and neoplasia. It may be that simple.

Another new study suggests that regular physical activity can lower a woman's risk of developing cancer, but only if she sleeps more than seven hours a night. I have written for years that exercise increases EMOD levels and stage 4 sleep increases EMODs. Both will help keep cancer cells in abeyance. On the other hand, an EMOD insufficiency allows for cancer (and a plethora of other diseases) to manifest themselves.

Get moving: Cancer survivors better work up a sweat

Among the nation's nearly 12 million cancer survivors, there are hints, although not yet proof, that people who are more active may lower risk of a recurrence. The American College of Sports Medicine convened a panel of cancer and exercise specialists to evaluate the evidence. **Guidelines advise cancer survivors to aim for the same amount of exercise as recommended for the average person: about 2 1/2 hours a week.**

Dr. Lee Jones suspects **that fitness, measured by how well their bodies use oxygen, plays a role. Be as active as you're able.**

Basic recommendations from American College of Sport Medicine and American Heart Association:

Guidelines for healthy adults under age 65

Do moderately intense cardio 30 minutes a day, five days a week

Or

Do vigorously intense cardio 20 minutes a day, 3 days a week

And

Do eight to 10 strength-training exercises, eight to 12 repetitions of each exercise twice a week.

Guidelines for adults over age 65

(or adults 50-64 with chronic conditions, such as arthritis)

Do moderately intense aerobic exercise 30 minutes a day,
five days a week

Or

Do vigorously intense aerobic exercise 20 minutes a day,
3 days a week

And

Do eight to 10 strength-training exercises, 10-15 repetitions of each exercise twice to three times per week

And

If you are at risk of falling, perform balance exercises

And

Have a physical activity plan.

My advise, "Run for your life....er, or at least walk!"

4) Supplemental oxygen

- At sea level, each breath is about 500 ml and contains about 21% O_2.
- Pressure at sea level is 760 mm Hg for air and partial pressure at sea level of O_2 is 160 mm Hg.
- Partial pressure of alveolar air is 100 mm Hg.
- Partial pressure of pulmonary arteries is 40 mm Hg.
- Thus, oxygen diffuses into venous blood to red cells and hemoglobin.
- Hgb leaving the lung is 98% saturated with O_2.
- Hgb O_2 in one liter of blood is about 200 ml, of which 50 ml (25%) is extracted each pass through the capillaries.

- A 60 kg man requires 200-250 ml of pure O_2 per minute.
- Human suffocation occurs at around 7% O_2.
- 100 ml of plasma at 100 mm Hg can hold only 0.3 ml of O_2.
- **Thus, a 60 kg adult has about 20 ml O_2 in their plasma.**
- Our body is at least 80% H_2O which is, which is 8/9 oxygen by molecular weight. Thus, we are composed of over 2/3 oxygen, twice as much as everything else in us combined.

Any condition which decreases one's ability to take in oxygen or to get proper levels to the tissues and organs can be detrimental. This includes the usual decrease in oxygen utilization associated with aging. Smoking, asthma, COPD, emphysema, etc. will decrease one's intake and utilization of oxygen. **Lung capacity decreases roughly 5% with every decade of life.**

These conditions can be helped simply by increasing the concentration or amount of oxygen inhaled. **Even periodic timed deep breathing, yoga and diaphragmatic deep breathing exercises can help.**

Inhalation hyperoxygenation. Use intermittent nasal oxygen; i.e., (3 L/min taken for one hour two to four times a day). The use of intermittent nasal administration of oxygen (2.5 to 3.5 L/min given for periods of one hour two-four times a day) benefits most patients. Oxygen therapy may be under-utilized in the care of patients with primary and spreading malignant tumors.

When used intermittently and in moderate doses, this therapy has been found to be free of adverse effects. If one has access to photodynamic therapy or sonodynamic therapy, use it. If one has access to red light, a red light laser, use them to stimulate endogenous porphyrins to produce singlet oxygen or EMODs insitu.

In the brain, O_2 is the energy source that produces and promotes consciousness. The brain is a "heavy breather" using 20% of the body's total O_2 intake, even though it is only 2% of the body's weight.

5) Aspirin

Aspirin induced oxidative stress

Induction of oxidative stress as a mechanism of action of chemopreventive agents against cancer (aspirin)

Prevention is a promising option for the control of cancer. Cellular redox changes have emerged as a pivotal and proximal event in cancer. In this review, they provide a brief background on redox biochemistry, discuss the important distinction between redox signaling and oxidative stress, and outline the 'multiple biological personalities' of **reactive oxygen and nitrogen species: at low concentrations they protect the cell**; at higher concentrations they can damage many biological molecules, such as DNA, proteins, and lipids; and, as we argue here, **they may also prevent cancer by initiating the death of the transformed cell.**

Nitric oxide-donating aspirin is discussed as an instructive example: it generates a state of oxidative stress through which it affects several redox-sensitive signaling pathways, leading ultimately to the elimination of the neoplastic cell via apoptosis or necrosis. As additional examples, **they discuss the chemopreventive n-3 polyunsaturated fatty acids and conventional nonsteroidal anti-inflammatory drugs, which induce cell death through redox changes.** They conclude that **modulation of redox biochemistry represents a fruitful approach to cancer prevention** (Rigas and Sun, 2008). Division of Cancer Prevention, Department of Medicine, Stony Brook University, Stony Brook, NY. USA.

Low-Dose Aspirin Cuts Colon Cancer Risk

Explain to interested patients that low-dose aspirin use decreased the incidence of colon cancer by about one-quarter and mortality by about a third over a median follow-up of nearly 20 years. Note that further analysis determined that the reduction in colon cancer incidence was limited to the proximal colon.

A report on 10-22-10 showed that the use of long-term low-dose aspirin reduced both the incidence and the mortality associated with colorectal cancer, a 20-year follow-up of randomized trials showed.

Aspirin use for a scheduled mean duration of six years cut the incidence of colon cancer by about one-quarter (HR 0.76, 95% CI 0.60 to 0.96, P=0.02) over a median of 18.3 years of follow-up, according to Peter M. Rothwell, MD, PhD, of the University of Oxford in England, and colleagues.

Moreover, the **risk of death from the disease fell by a third** (HR 0.65, 95% CI 0.48 to 0.88, P=0.005), the researchers reported online in *The Lancet*. **Unlike with colon cancer, aspirin use was not associated with a reduction in incidence of rectal cancer or mortality**.

However, the researchers wrote, **"benefit increased with scheduled duration of treatment. The risk of proximal colon cancer was reduced by about 70% ... and also reduced the risk of rectal cancer."**

Rothwell's group had previously shown that five years of high-dose aspirin use was associated with a 30% reduction in the incidence of colorectal cancer over 20 years.

But high doses can have adverse bleeding consequences when taken for long periods, and the effects of lower doses on colorectal cancer risk had not been established. So the researchers looked at data from **five trials conducted in the U.K. and Sweden that included a total of 16,488 participants.** The trials were designed to assess the effects of aspirin in primary or secondary prevention of vascular events. Two of the trials randomized patients to 75 mg aspirin or placebo daily, a third compared 300 mg or 1,200 mg daily with placebo, and another compared 500 mg daily with no aspirin. The other trial randomized patients to 30 mg or 283 mg of aspirin daily. The researchers confined their data analysis to the four trials that compared aspirin with a control.

Among the **14,033 patients** in those trials, there were 391 cases of colorectal cancer and 240 deaths during a median follow-up of 18.3 years.

Analysis of subsite data determined that **the reduction in colon cancer incidence was limited to the proximal colon:**

- Proximal colon, HR 0.45 (95% CI 0.28 to 0.74, P=0.001)
- Distal colon, HR 1.10 (95% CI 0.73 to 1.64, P=0.66)

Similar risk reductions were seen for mortality:

- Proximal colon, HR 0.34 (95% CI 0.18 to 0.66, P=0.001)
- Distal colon, HR 1.21 (95% CI 0.66 to 2.24, P=0.54)

Case fatality rates also were higher for proximal cases. Differences between proximal and distal colon cancers also have been seen for other treatments, the researchers noted.

"There are many differences in normal physiology between the proximal and distal colon, due partly to their different embryological origins, and in risk factors for cancers in the two sites, in mechanisms of carcinogenesis, and in the molecular and genetic characteristics of the cancers," they explained.

The study had several other important findings, according to the authors. **It showed that 75 mg of aspirin daily was as effective in preventing disease as higher doses, and that the decrease in mortality was "statistically robust and clinically important."** They also pointed out that their seven- to eight-year estimate of the latent period before a mortality effect was seen could have been too long.

The study did have limitations. For instance, the researchers noted that their findings were not generalizable to other regimens, such as alternate-day aspirin use. In addition, patients on aspirin might have had more diagnostic evaluations for problems such as gastrointestinal bleeding that could have led to earlier diagnosis of cancer compared with patients receiving placebo, although in none of the trials was there any evidence of this.

The finding that fewer deaths occurred among the aspirin groups without any evidence of earlier diagnosis suggests that there may be a difference in tumor aggressiveness in patients receiving aspirin compared with nonusers, according to the researchers. "The suggestion of a particular effect of aspirin on more aggressive and rapidly growing tumors might allow less frequent screening, and the prevention of proximal colonic cancers by aspirin, which would not be identified by sigmoidoscopy screening and for which colonoscopy screening is only partly effective, is clearly important," they wrote. In a comment that accompanied the study, Robert Benamouzig, MD, and Bernard Uzzan, MD, of Avicenne Hospital in Bobigny, France, noted that there were other limitations to the study, including the fact that colon cancer was not the primary outcome in the trials and that there was a lack of data on aspirin-associated mortality.

Furthermore, **patients in the trials were primarily men who had cardiovascular risks, so the conclusions can't be extended to women and patients without such risks**. However, the editorialists described the study as "interesting," and said that it "could incite clinicians to primary prevention of colorectal cancer by aspirin, at least in high-risk populations." (Rothwell et al, 2010).

I believe that this supports my theory of having a prooxidant advantage to prevent cancer. **Aspirin (ASA) produces oxygen free radicals.**

6) EWOT (exercise with oxygen therapy)

Multi-step Oxygen Therapy - "The Best Antiaging Gift you can Give Your Body" by Dr. Robert Rowan, MD was the basis for the following EWOT description. I have modified the original article. Dr. Rowen has led the oxidative therapy movement.

Here is how it works. Atmospheric air pressure at sea level is 760 mm of mercury. Since oxygen comprises approximately 20-21 percent of the atmosphere, the pressure component of oxygen, called partial pressure, is 20% of 760, or about **150 mm. The air coming into the lungs, therefore, contains a pressure of O_2 at 150 mm.** However, in the lungs, the oxygen is diluted considerably with carbon dioxide leaving the body. Thus, in the air sacs of the lungs (alveoli), the pressure of oxygen is the 150 mm minus the partial pressure of CO_2 (which is 40) for a net O_2 pressure in the air sacs of about 100-110 mm.

This 100-110 mm is the amount of pressure that helps to drive the oxygen from the lungs into the blood. The blood takes the oxygen by way of the arteries to the extremities and distant parts of the body where it is fed to the capillaries and the tissues. The capillaries release some of the oxygen to support each individual cell along their pathway.

In an ideal situation, the pressure of oxygen in the arteries will almost match the pressure in the alveoli. When we're young, this is the case, with the arterial pressure running around 95 mm. However, as we age, the arterial pressure declines, with the average 70-year-old having an arterial pressure of only about 70 mm. This is due to many factors associated with aging and the overall condition of the lungs.

Unlike carbon dioxide, O_2 is much harder to dissolve in liquids and its solubility is heavily dependent on the pressure driving it. Oxygen is extracted in the capillaries and when the blood comes out the venous end of the capillary, the **average pressure of oxygen in the veins is about 40 mm** early in life and **drops to about 35 mm by age 70**. The difference in the pressure of oxygen between the arterial and venous sides reflects how well the oxygen is delivered and consumed.

In your 30s, the amount of oxygen released to the cells is significantly higher than in your 70s. If you do the math, **a 30-year-old will release 55 mm of pressure (95-40=55), while a 70-year-old will release only 35 mm of pressure (70-35=35).** That's a huge drop (55 vs. 35) in the amount of pressure of oxygen your cells are receiving.

This transfer of oxygen from the blood to the cells is perhaps the most significant underlying factor in whether you live a long and healthy life or not! The more damaged the transfer mechanism becomes, the more likely you will become ill. This is why you are more susceptible to illness as you age! Aging is associated with decreasing ability to get oxygen to the cells and the cells may also have decreasing ability to generate EMODs.

The following is **Dr. Rowen's description of "multi-step therapy." Multi-step therapy is surprisingly simple. All it involves is breathing high levels of oxygen while exercising**. Dr. Rowen has been a leader in oxidative medicine for decades.

Typically, the multi-step therapy consists of an 18-day, 36-hour program. First, a drug-nutrient combination is orally administered 30 minutes before the exercise starts. The combination consists of 30 mg of thiamin (vitamin B1), 75 mg of Dipyridamol (the prescription drug Persantine), and 100 mg of magnesium orotate. These agents help the uptake and utilization of oxygen.

Thirty minutes after taking the combination, you begin exercising while breathing oxygen using a mask and storage balloon at **a flow rate of four to six liters per minute**. This lasts two hours each day for 18 days, giving you a total of 36 hours of therapy time. Every 20 minutes during the two-hour treatment period, the individual pushes the exercise to a comfortable maximum, which enhances cardiac output and oxygen delivery to the needy areas. This procedure is probably best supervised by a doctor, though this is not entirely necessary.

A simpler modification, called **the quick technique, uses the same procedure (including the drug-nutrient combination), but instead of two hours, you do moderate aerobic exercise for only 15 minutes while breathing pure oxygen at 10 liters per minute.**

Oxygen multi-step therapy is definitely something you can do in the privacy of your home and very inexpensively. **To get medical-grade oxygen, you'll need a prescription or** you can use an **oxygen concentrator**, which is available from most medical supply houses. However, you need a minimum of 10 liters per minute with 100% oxygen for the therapy to be of any use, and **the concentrators usually max out at five liters per minute and are typically a little less than 100% oxygen.**

Federal law also prohibits doctors from using commercial-grade oxygen for any medical purpose. Therefore, make sure you read all the safety precautions associated with handling oxygen.

The thiamin and magnesium orotate can be acquired from health food stores. The dipyramidole (Persantine) would have to be obtained through prescription, but Dr. Rowen does not believe that it is an absolute essential.

It is always advisable to consult with a physician familiar with oxygen therapies.

7) Hyperthermia

Many chemical reactions are sped up by increasing the temperature. Such is the case with hyperthermia and it relation to EMOD formation. Hyperthermia can be obtained with the use of electric blankets, saunas, spas, whirlpools, etc. However, overheating can be dangerous, if not fatal and should be done under appropriate supervision.

Hyperthermia is the clinical application of therapeutic heat in the treatment of disease.

Hyperthermia increases EMOD production

Investigators tested the hypothesis that mild intra-operative hypothermia decreases neutrophil phagocytic capacity and generation of reactive oxygen intermediates (a measure of oxidative killing). Mild hypothermia directly impairs numerous immune functions in vitro. Thermal management was randomly assigned in **10 surgical patients**, causing intraoperative core temperatures to range from 33 to 37°C.

Neutrophil oxidative and phagocytic capacities were significantly reduced intra-operatively, compared with preoperative and postoperative values. **Intraoperative**

production of reactive oxygen species was linearly related to core temperature. In contrast, there was no correlation between core temperature and phagocytic activity. **In vitro production of reactive oxygen intermediates increased six fold from 32 to 40°C.** In vitro phagocytic capacity increased fourfold in this temperature range. Production of oxidative intermediates ROS was most closely related to intraoperative core temperature, decreasing nearly fourfold over a 4°C range. This in vivo temperature dependence was matched in vitro. **Impaired neutrophil oxidative killing may contribute to the observed hypothermia-induced reduction in resistance to infection** (Wenisch et al. 1996).

I believe that this argues for the use of hyperthermia as a simple and safe means to increase oxidative capacity. This can be obtained by the use of electric blankets, a sauna, shower or hot tub.

Temperatures which are readily achievable in the clinic (39-41 degrees Celsius) might be optimal for maximizing hyperthermic response. At higher temperatures, these effects are reversed, thereby limiting the therapeutic benefits of more severe hyperthermic exposure (Jackson et al. 2006).

I believe that the increased EMOD release by hyperthermia, alone, can be of great clinical benefit for cancer treatment and it can be added to my techniques for increasing the oxidative capacity.

Cancer clinical experience with hyperthermia

Tumor cells have specific environmental requirements, largely dependent on blood flow. When there is an increase in the temperature around the tumor, there is a corresponding increase in the blood flow to that area, as the hypothalamus attempts to regulate body temperature.

Hyperthermia is recognized as a standard treatment in the management of malignant tumors. It is especially recommended for metastatic tumors where other treatment methods have a poor history of success.

Repeated heating to 107-113 degrees F. can cause the tumor cells to be killed. Tumor response has been found to be from 40 - 80%.

A side benefit of hyperthermia treatment has been substantial pain reduction in a majority of patients.

Hyperthermia is now an FDA-approved cancer therapy for breast cancer.

Experts reviewed the medical records of **421 sessions of hyperthermia treatments in 73 patients treated between 1987 and 1992** at the University Heights Cancer Center and the Indiana University Medical Center in Indianapolis, Indiana.

All patients had previously "failed" conventional radiation therapy, chemotherapy and surgery. Temperatures attained during the course of therapy on each patient were averaged and the results were evaluated for complete, partial or no response.

Responses were defined as:

1. Complete response: Lesions completely disappeared during treatment and response was maintained for a minimum of six months

2. Partial response: Lesions that were reduced in size more than 50%

3. No response: Less than 50% reduction in tumor size during the treatment

Response varied somewhat according to histology and anatomical site of treatment; however,

1. complete response was achieved in 45%;

2. partial response in 48%;

3. and no response in 7% of the patients.

The response achieved varied with temperature attained and a minimum temperature of 40 degrees C for 40 minutes produced the greatest number of responses. Response to hyperthermia was directly related to the temperature achieved and the length of time the temperature was applied.

8) Ingestion of iron (over the counter dosages)

First and foremost, please remember that excess iron may cause nausea and vomiting and may damage the liver and other organs. However, the most common form of anemia is iron deficiency and iron is essential for oxygen uptake and transport. Therefore, maintaining adequate iron levels is essential.

Iron is absorbed in the colon. The colonic lumen is predominantly anaerobic, the mucosal oxygen tension measured by a surface probe was 9 mm Hg compared with 65 mm Hg in serosal tissue (Zabel et al, 1996).

Consumption of 100 mg $FeSO_4$/d was associated with a marked increase in the production of free radicals in feces. Most dietary iron remains unabsorbed and hence may be available to participate in Fenton-driven free radical generation in conjunction with the colonic microflora. This occurred to me to be a great opportunity to safely increase the oxidative capacity of the gastrointestinal tract, which I believe would aid in oxidation of ingested mutagens, pathogenic organisms and reduce incidence of premalignant lesions. Thus, this clearly could increase the oxidative capacity of the GI tract, as I had predicted. This method is safe, inexpensive and readily accessible.

However, others may consider the Fenton reaction generation of the highly reactive hydroxyl radical as being dangerous or even mutagenic, but please remember that two hydroxyl radicals can yield one molecule of hydrogen peroxide of considerably lesser reactivity. Since it is so highly reactive and its diameter of reactivity is so small, it is likely that it may collide with another hydroxyl radical before it encounters other protein or nucleic acid molecules.

Increased copper ingestion may produce the same result (over the counter dosages).

It has been suggested that iron plays an important role in the pathogenesis of atherosclerosis, primarily by acting as a catalyst for the atherogenic modification of LDL. Although some epidemiological data suggest that high stored iron levels are an independent risk factor for coronary artery disease and that iron has been detected in both early and advanced atherosclerotic lesions, the evidence is often **contradictory and inclusive.**

Iron overload (FeO) **but not** iron deficiency (FeD) **decreased plasma cholesterol levels compared with control animals both before (P < .05) and after (P = .055) cholesterol feeding.** Neither FeO nor FeD had a significant effect on the levels of antioxidants and lipid peroxidation products in plasma and aortic tissue or on the susceptibility of LDL to ex-vivo oxidation. **FeO significantly decreased aortic arch lesion formation by 56% compared with controls (P < 0.5), whereas FeD had no significant effect.** These results indicate that in this animal model, **FeO decreased rather than increases atherosclerosis,** likely because iron dextran exerts a hypocholesterolemic effect. The data did not support the hypotheses that elevation of Fe stores increases or that a reduction of Fe stores by phlebotomy decreases the risk of coronary artery disease (Dabbagh et al, 1997).

Further, **I believe that this directly contradicts the Free Radi-Crap theory, which states that increased iron loads should increase EMODs, increase hydroxyl radical production and increase atherosclerosis, but it does not.**

Cancer cells have much higher levels of iron than do normal cells. The surface of cancer cells has 5-15 times more transferrin receptors than healthy cells. Henry Lai, from the University of Washington, **increased the iron-holotransferrin-transferrin levels of breast cancer cells and treated them with artemisinin and found a dramatic effect, especially in breast cancer cells that were resistant to radiation.**

The Free Radi-Crap theory suggests that patients with iron overload should be symptomatic of all of the diseases attributed to high RONS levels, **but out of 410 patients, 27% with iron overload, had no symptoms whatsoever.**

Iron overload has also been implicated in the sequelae of atherosclerosis, although **the data are conflicting and inconsistent, and individuals with iron overload do not suffer from premature atherosclerosis** (Kiechl, S.).

I believe that this is a most important observation, e.g., "individuals with iron overload do not suffer from premature atherosclerosis." In my opinion, this discounts the paranoia of iron, H_2O_2, and the Fenton reaction, even with iron overload. But, why take the risk of over dosing?

I believe that the timing of the increased EMODs is a key factor in understanding the scenario of atherosclerosis and evidence indicates that there is an initial increase in antioxidant enzymes which precedes atherosclerotic changes and "allows" for the formation of lesions. The body then reacts oxidatively to challenge or correct this diseased condition.

The "essential poison" paradox is not limited to oxygen but also includes glucose and iron. I do not believe that any of them are inherently "poisons." Yet, excessive amounts of almost anything can be harmful, if not lethal.

9) Hyperbaric oxygen (HBO$_2$)

While oxygen delivered at high pressure is a promising investigative area, there are a number of problems inherent in such procedures. Some of these problems are: 1) limited duration of patient exposure due to CNS and pulmonary toxicity; 2) compression and decompression hazards; and 3) the expense and space requirements of hyperbaric systems.

In America, HBO$_2$ chambers were first used as a treatment for deep-sea divers who experienced decompression sickness. The Undersea and Hyperbaric Medical Society (UHMS) has evaluated the use and effectiveness of HBO$_2$ for different medical conditions. Currently, the UHMS approves HBO$_2$ for 13 medical conditions as follows:

Air or gas embolism

Carbon monoxide poisoning

Clostridial myositis and myonecrosis (gas gangrene)

Crush injury, compartment syndrome, and acute traumatic ischemia

Decompression sickness

Enhancement of healing in selected problem wounds

Exceptional blood loss (anemia)

Intracranial abscess

Necrotizing soft-tissue infections

Osteomyelitis (refractory)

Radiation injury (delayed)

Skin grafts and flaps (compromised)

Thermal burns

Normally, 97% of the oxygen delivered to body tissues is bound to hemoglobin, while only 3% is dissolved in the plasma. At sea level, barometric pressure is 1 ATA, or 760 mm Hg, and the partial pressure of oxygen in arterial blood (P_aO_2) is approximately 100 mm Hg. At rest, the tissues of the body consume about 5 mL of O_2 per 100 mL of blood.

During HBO$_2$ treatments, **barometric pressures are usually limited to 3 ATA** or lower. **The oxygen content of inspired air in the chamber is typically 95% to 100%.** The combination of increased pressure (3 ATA) and increased oxygen concentration (100%) dissolves enough oxygen in the plasma alone to sustain life in a resting state.

Under hyperbaric conditions, oxygen content in the plasma is increased from 0.3 to 6.6 mL per 100 mL of blood with no change in oxygen transport via hemoglobin. HBO$_2$ at 3.0 ATA increases oxygen delivery to the tissues from 20.0 to 26.7 mL of O$_2$ per 100 mL of blood.

Increased oxygen delivery to the tissues is believed **to facilitate healing** through a number of mechanisms.

American doctors accept **HBO$_2$** for use in **wound healing, bone infection, carbon monoxide intoxication, and air emboli, or air bubbles in the bloodstream due to decompression sickness, open-heart surgery,** and other sources. (Sukoff and Gottlieb. 1989) (Neubauer et al, 1989) (Gottlieb. 1989) (Gottlieb and Neubauer. 1988), including treatment of non-healing wounds, carbon monoxide poisoning, various infections, damage caused by radiation treatments, and all types of diving accidents).

HBOT can also be used for conditions such **as coma resulting from head injuries, bruising of the spinal cord, stroke, and neurological disorders such as multiple sclerosis.** These additional applications have yet to be recognized by the medical establishment in the U.S.

Of interest is the fact that the Baylor group found that intra-arterial administration of H_2O_2 had the same physiological effect on O_2 saturation as did hyperbaric O_2 administration.

Due to the technical and physiological problems inherent with OHP, studies were undertaken in Baylor University Medical Center laboratory to determine the feasibility of administering intravascular oxygen in a regional or systemic system. This approach employees dilute concentrations of hydrogen peroxide given by a variety of routes to provide oxygen. Hydrogen peroxide under the influence of catalase and peroxidases is degraded to oxygen and water. Human blood and tissues contain excess quantities of both enzyme systems. **Hydrogen peroxide provides from 3 to 8 atmosphere equivalents of oxygen which is administered in solution,** thus avoiding the necessity of lung transport (Urschel et al, 1966).

Photodynamic therapy (PDT) is currently approved in the palliation of locally advanced cancers and a few early-stage diseases. **It should now be included for first-line treatment in early malignant and premalignant disease, adjuvant therapy for surgery, and interstitial treatment of deep-seated tumors.** Early observations indicate that **hypoxic or anoxic conditions almost completely reduce the antitumor effectiveness of PDT in vitro** (Henderson and Fingar. 1987).

In other studies it was demonstrated that **hyperbaric oxygen can enhance the effects of PDT.**

Aminoglycosides such as gentamicin, tobramycin, alizarin and netilmicin are oxygen dependent for their antimicrobial activity. The effect of oxygen has been studied in vivo and in vitro using Pseudomonas treated with tobramycin and controls grown aerobically and anaerobically. The aerobic grown Pseudomonas controls had a 51% increase in colonies compared to the tobramycin treated. **Vancomycin is another antibiotic that does not kill microorganisms well under low oxygen tensions. Sulfonamides antimicrobial effect is potentiated in hyperbaric oxygen.**

Similarly, many of the chemotherapeutic drugs are oxygen dependent.

Oxygen is directly lethal to strict anaerobic bacteria because of the organisms inability to detoxify oxygen radicals. Oxygen enhanced environments have been shown to be bactericidal for most clostridia species and inhibit alpha toxin release. Hyperbaric oxygen has been shown to be a beneficial adjunct to therapy in Bacteroides fragilis, Fusobacterium infections and nonclostridial anaerobic infections (Schreiner. 1974).

Hyperbaric oxygen, tissue levels may approach 1200 mmHg, in which increased production of superoxide, peroxide and other oxygen radicals occurs, however, some organisms adapt by producing increased levels of superoxide dismutase. There is no direct antibacterial effect of enhanced oxygen on aerobic organisms. Indirect antibactericidal effects are related to improved PMN function in killing bacteria. **Results with hyperbaric oxygen is similar to that obtained by the Baylor investigators using intra-arterial H_2O_2.**

When subjects are **breathing HBO_2, the cumulative effects of EMODs are well recognized because of their role in CNS O_2 toxicity; yet, adverse reactions to HBO_2 are rare** (Demchenko et al, 2003) (Demchenko et al, 2001) (Tibbles and Edelsberg. 1996) (Torbati et al, 1992) (Torbati et al, 1989).

Accumulating evidence supports the notion that **the CNS responds to a continuum of O_2 tension at both normobaric and hyperbaric pressures**. The direct effects of O_2 on the brain stem need to be considered when hyperoxia is used. Dripps and Comroe (Dripps and Comroe. 1947) first introduced the use of normobaric hyperoxia (100% O_2, 8-min exposure) as a tool for physiological denervation of the carotid body chemoreceptors. They emphasized, however, the following caveat: "It must be remembered that a stimulant effect of oxygen which tends to increase respiration may be acting simultaneously to limit the extent of this immediate depression of minute ventilation."

Hyperbaric oxygen (HBO) treatment of cholesterol-fed rabbits **dramatically reduces the development of arterial lesions**

despite having little or no effect on plasma or individual lipo-protein cholesterol concentrations.

Similarly, in regression studies, **HBO treatment** has no effect on the rate of plasma (or lipoprotein) cholesterol decline but **significantly accelerates aortic lesion regression** compared with no treatment. (Kudchodkar et al, 2000).

In this case, **I believe that the authors made some extremely valuable observations but they came to the wrong conclusion. The plaque regression was not due to increased anti-oxidants but was due to increased EMODs, which are well known products of HBO_2. Further, administration of HBO_2 should, according to the Free Radi-Crap theory, cause increased lipid oxidation and plaque formation. Whereas, just the opposite is the result in experimental animals, whereby HBO_2 causes increased regression of plaque and decreases accumulation of lipid oxidation products. This is one of my most important observations.**

There is some evidence that HBOT can reverse age-related macular degeneration (AMD), the leading cause of severe visual loss in people over the age of fifty. (Bojic, L., Gosovic, S., Kovacecic, H. and Denoble, P. Hyperbaric Oxygenation in the Treatment of Macular Degeneration. Split, Yugoslavia: Split Naval Medical Institute pp 1-4).

Seventy percent of the treated multiple sclerosis (MS) patients either did not deteriorate, had their conditions stabilize, or showed small improvements (Davidson, 1989).

A wound's chances of becoming infected are directly related to how little oxygen there is in the affected tissues (Hunt. 1979).

Under-oxygenation can also reduce the body's ability to heal the wound, especially since healing tissue needs even more oxygen than does healthy tissue (Niinikoski et al, 1972).

HBOT is the best way of increasing the oxygen content of under-oxygenated tissues (Sheffield. 1985) (Strauss et al, 1983) (Strauss et al, 1986) (Skyhar et al, 1986) (Nylander et al, 1985).

The use of **HBOT is a very valuable way of treating difficult wounds** (Hunt and van Winkle. 1976) (Sheffield. 1985).

The earlier and more frequently HBOT is used, the more likely it is that severely injured body parts will be saved (Strauss and Hart. 1984) (Strauss and Hart. 1989).

One of the most respected trauma surgery units in the world is the Department of Microsurgery at the University of Liege Hospital in Belgium. The **Liege doctors were convinced that HBOT helped them heal difficult wounds** and save reattached limbs that would otherwise have not been healed or saved.

HBOT helps to heal bone disorders by stimulating both the osteoclast and the osteoblasts (Hunt et al, 1969) (Strauss. 1987).

Complications

Usual complications of HBO therapy are a result of either barometric pressure changes or oxygen toxicity. The most common complications involve cavity trauma due to change in pressure. Any air-filled cavity that cannot equilibrate with ambient pressure, such as the middle ear when the eustachian tube is blocked, is subject to deformity and barotrauma during pressure changes in HBO therapy.

Pneumothorax is a rare complication of HBO treatment, usually occurring only in patients with severe lung disease.

Air embolism, presumably resulting from a small tear in the pulmonary vasculature, is another rare complication. One hundred percent oxygen under high pressure for long periods is neurotoxic and can lower the seizure threshold and affect central nervous system control of respiration. However, neurotoxicity is rare with the low-pressure, short-duration treatments used clinically in HBO therapy. In one series the incidence was reported as 1.3 seizures per 10 000 treatments.

Pulmonary oxygen toxic reactions can occur with 100% inspired oxygen at less than 1 ATA with prolonged exposure. **Almost all patients will show pulmonary toxicity after 6 continuous hours of inspired oxygen at 2 ATA** (Clark and Lambertson. 1971). No clinical HBO protocol requires this length of continuous exposure to 100% oxygen. However, HBO treatments may contribute to the pulmonary oxygen toxicity seen in critically ill patients who receive high concentrations of inspired oxygen between hyperbaric treatments.

Although a concern in premature newborns, **retrolental fibroplasia has not been noted in infants, children, or adults undergoing HBO therapy** (Nichols and Lambertsen. 1969).

Development of cataracts has been reported in patients receiving more than 150 HBO treatments (Palmquist et al, 1984).

10) Vitamin D3 ($1,25(OH)_2D_3$), a prooxidant (up to 2000/d)

My friend, Dr. Robert Muller says that, "Diagnosis of Vitamin D deficiency is the new garbage bag diagnosis, when they can't determine what truly is the diagnosis. It is replacing fibromyalgia."

My research indicates that vitamin D3 could have wide ranging beneficial effects because of its strong prooxidant activity (www.iwillfindthecure.org).

Please remember that cholesterol is a precursor to vitamin D and inhibiting the synthesis of cholesterol will also inhibit the synthesis of vitamin D. Since sunlight is required to turn cholesterol into vitamin D, avoiding the sun will also undermine your ability to synthesize vitamin D and since vitamin D-rich foods are also rich in cholesterol, low-cholesterol diets are inherently deficient in vitamin D.

Yet, even though cholesterol is an effective antioxidant, vitamin D3 is a capable prooxidant. This is another example of changing chemical reactivity by changing the molecules attached to a central molecule.

Please remember, "Treat your body like it belongs to you."

Now, Vitamin D Confusion

Here we go again. Now, vitamin D is getting the cautionary headlines. For years we have been told of a serious problem with vitamin D deficiencies in America. But, we are getting warnings about taking too much vitamin D.

A report by the Institute of Medicine, could put a halt on the nation's vitamin D craze, warning that super-high levels are risky. New dietary guidelines report, "There's no proof that megadoses (of vitamin D) prevent cancer or other ailments." This reinforces the old adage that, "More is not necessarily better."

The new guidelines state, "Most people in the U.S. and Canada, from age 1 to age 70, need to consume no more than 600 international units of vitamin D a day to maintain health. People in their 70s and older need as much as 800 IUs." Previously, experts had recommended up to 2,000 IUs a day, because studies suggested that low levels of vitamin D were increasing the risk of cancer or heart disease.

Super high doses above 4,000 IUs should always be avoided because of possible kidney damage. Another study showed that those with the highest vitamin D levels had increased risk of pancreatic cancer.

Vitamin D and calcium intake go hand in hand to build strong bones. But, the Institute's two-year study concluded that **research into the possible role of vitamin D in other diseases is conflicting, with some studies showing no effect and others showing harm**.

We know that a vitamin deficiency can cause serious problems but if you are not in a deficient state, you may be wasting your money or putting yourself in harm's way. The take-home message is, "Do not go overboard with any of these vitamins, including antioxidants, multivitamins and vitamin D."

My new book, *Death In Small Doses?*, (Trafford Publishing, available at Amazon.com) presents overwhelming scientific evidence of the potential harm of the antioxidant vitamins A, C and E supplements. In this current book, I have presented 250 scientific studies, with over 8 million participants, showing that the antioxidant vitamins are no more effective than dummy pills.

Eighty of these studies showed harmful effects of these vitamin supplements, including increased risk for cancer, heart disease, strokes and even shortening of the life span. This is shocking news for those of us who have taken these supplements religiously, only to find out that we have been the victims of marketing and clever sales schemes.

Please remember that none of these vitamin supplements are tested for effectiveness or safety by the U.S. Food and Drug Administration. I have been a proponent for vitamin D but my support for it has to change as its data base changes. It is the only honest thing to do.

Low vitamin D levels common in breast cancer

Yet, according to British researchers, more than half of women with breast cancer have low vitamin D levels. The reason for this is unknown but I believe that it at least in part reflects an over all EMOD insufficiency, which allows cancer to grow. Breast cancer cells have vitamin D receptors, and when these receptors are activated by vitamin D, it triggers a series of molecular changes that can slow cell growth and cause cells to die (apoptosis). The results were presented by Sonia Li, MD, of Mount Vernon Cancer Centre in Middlesex, England in December 2010.

11) Artemisinin (20-40 mg each day, which can act as a prooxidant)

Artemisinin (Antimalarial) and Reactive Oxygen Species

Experiments to determine artemisinin's anti-malarial mechanism of action led to tests as an anti-cancer drug. The key turned out to be **a shared characteristic of the malaria parasite and dividing cancer cells: high iron concentrations.** When artemisinin, or any of its derivatives, comes into contact with iron, a chemical reaction ensues, spawning **free radicals,** which attack and bind with cell membranes, breaking them apart and killing the single-cell parasite. **Cancer cells have much higher levels of iron than do normal cells. The surface of cancer cells has 5-15 times more transferrin receptors than healthy cells.** Henry Lai, from the University of Washington, **increased the iron-holotransferrin-transferrin levels of breast cancer cells and treated them with artemisinin and found a dramatic effect, especially in breast cancer cells that were resistant to radiation.**

I have outlined and suggested 11 safe adjuncts, under current laws, which can be used in a combinatorial manner to aid in the treatment of a wide variety of pathophysiologies. Considerations in a wide array of diseases including: primary and metastatic cancer, cardiovascular disease, diabetes, arthritis, viral infection, sepsis, HIV/AIDS, and malaria.

Contrary to the laws of thermodynamics and concepts of entropy and chaos, we operate in the "realm of the miraculous" and, while not invoking religiosity, it could be envisioned as being coordinated by supernatural intervention, performing nigh biochemical miracles, extraordinarily complex electron transfers and marvelous protective antics, doing most of this whilst on auto-pilot and with minimal organismal conscious input.

R. M. Howes, M.D., Ph.D.
8/30/10

CHAPTER FOURTEEN

LEFTOVERS

Controversial possible methods of increasing oxidative capacity:

- Consider H_2O_2 soak/baths (1 pint 3% in bath water, soak 20 minutes)

Possibly study taking H_2O_2 IV (0.03% H_2O_2 given over 1-3 hrs.).

Many clinical and experimental applications of hydrogen peroxide have been demonstrated, especially by the Baylor group (Urschel, Mallams, Finney, Balla) in the 1960s and 70s.

In over 300 patients regional intra-arterial hydrogen peroxide has potentiated the effect of radiation therapy in situations of malignancy involving the head, neck, pelvis and retro-peritoneum (Mallams et al, 1965).

Increased localization of radioactive isotopes in malignant tumors has been achieved by regional and intra-arterial infusion of hydrogen peroxide (Finney et al, 1961) (Finney et al, 1965).

Peripheral bone marrow stimulation has been obtained by carotid artery infusion of hydrogen peroxide experimentally and clinically. (Finney et al, 1965; 16: 62).

Wound healing has been markedly accelerated by the intra-arterial administration of hydrogen peroxide (Balla et al, 1964).

Significant reduction in the morbidity and mortality of experimental and clinical Clostridium welchii infections has been achieved by intra-arterial hydrogen peroxide (Bradley et al, 1965).

Arteriosclerotic plaques have been markedly reduced and have even disappeared following the intra-arterial infusion of hydrogen peroxide (Finney et al, 1966).

The reversal of many types of shock has been achieved by infusion of hydrogen peroxide into the thoracic aorta (Urschel et al, 1964) (Urschel et al, 1965).

In summary, the following points of the Baylor group should be made:

1) **Dilute solutions of hydrogen peroxide can be used as an oxygen source to maintain or resuscitate the anoxic heart of small animals. This can be accomplished by either pericardial perfusion or coronary infusion via the retrograde catheterization of the right carotid artery and passing the catheter to the coronary ostia.**

2) **Pericardial perfusions of dilute solutions of hydrogen peroxide alone serve to maintain a functional heart in large animals.** By the Nitro BT staining technique, it was found that even during the pericardial perfusion of dilute solutions of hydrogen peroxide in large animals, the septum remained essential anoxic.

3) **By adding DMSO to the dilute hydrogen peroxide being perfused to the pericardium in large animals following coronary artery ligation, results indicate the maintenance of a functioning heart.** By the Nitro BT staining technique, it has been shown that DMSO may aid in the diffusion of oxygen into the thick myocardium, thus affording a higher degree of protection from anoxia.

Additional possibilities for increasing prooxidant status:

- Possibly study taking O_3 IV (autohemotherapy)
- Possibly study taking O_3 by rectal insufflation
- Possibly study iron (Fe++) and Vit. C orally (over the counter dosages) (Do not take iron simultaneously with oral hydrogen peroxide)

- Possibly study Ca++ orally (over the counter dosages)
- Possibly study copper supplementation (over the counter dosages)
- Consider avoiding diets high in antioxidants, other than vitamin C (which can act as a prooxidant at high levels or in the presence of iron)
- Consider avoiding general antioxidant supplements, other than vitamin C
- Possibly study NaOCl orally
- Possibly study NaOCl IV
- Possibly study taking, doctor supervised, high-dose vit. C 60,000 mg I.V. twice a week (Univ. Kansas & NIH)
- Possibly study taking redox cycler, such as ubiquinone, CoQ 10, can act as a prooxidant
- Possibly study taking EGCG supplement 315 mg BID or drink green tea (2 teabags)
- Possibly study Vancomycin (a chloramine) and H_2O_2 to produce $^1O_2$
- Possibly study vit. K (a quinone) redox cycler to produce $^1O_2$
- Possibly study redox cycler, such as doxycycline, 100 mg. per day
- Possibly consider ingesting ethanol daily in moderation only (avoid sugar, if treating cancer)
- Consider resveratrol (grape extract) wine ingredient (over counter dosage) acts as a prooxidant
- Possibly study consumption of caffeine or instant coffee (contains peroxide), if no problems with arrhythmias
- Possible study periodic hyperthermia (sauna, heating blankets, etc.) or systemic warming of patients, which will increase oxygen tension
- Consider eating prooxidant sulforaphane foods (broccoli, cauliflower, and Brussels sprouts) cruciferous veggies
- Possibly study chloroquine, tempol
- Consider red light phototherapy
- Consider doctor-supervised photodynamic therapy
- Consider doctor-supervised sonodynamic therapy
- Possibly study Bactrim or Spectra (cotrimaxazole)

- Consider studying low dose methylene blue (a photosensitizer)
- Possibly study chloramine T (N-chloro-p-toluene-sulfonamide)

Tempol, artemisinin, and chloroquine appear to demonstrate little cytotoxicity in the absence of preexisting oxidative stress, thus sparing normal cells. L-arginine and singlet oxygen therapy are other possibilities for future investigations.

Aminoglycosides such as gentamicin, tobramycin, alizarin and netilmicin are oxygen dependent for their antimicrobial activity. Vancomycin is another antibiotic that does not kill microorganisms well under low oxygen tensions. Sulfonamides antimicrobial effect is potentiated in hyperbaric oxygen. Similarly, many of the chemotherapeutic drugs are oxygen dependent.

Polymorphonuclear cells require oxygen to kill organism by producing superoxide, hydrogen peroxide, singlet oxygen and other products via the respiratory burst (Barbior. 1974). The PMN is protected by detoxifying free radicals with superoxide dismutase, catalase and glutathione.

It has been shown in numerous studies that the degree of polymorphonuclear cell function in killing of bacteria is directly dependent on oxygen tension (DeChatelet. 1975) (Hohn. 1977).

Two common antioxidant additives: BHT and BHA

Butylated Hydroxytoluene- BHT, and Butylated Hydroxyanisole-BHA are preservatives (antioxidants) for oil containing products due to their antioxidant properties. BHA is generally used to keep fats from becoming rancid and BHT is used to prevent oxidative rancidity of fats. BHT has been used since 1949 and despite it being a known carcinogen, it is still used today.

These two closely related chemicals can still be found in many foods and personal care products like, cosmetics, pharmaceuticals, personal ointments, meat, beer, butter, meats, cereals, chewing gum, baked goods, snack foods, dehydrated potatoes, rice products, dried soup, food packaging, animal feed and rubber and petroleum products.

Based on animal tests, a chemical that causes cancer in at least one organ in three different species indicates that it might be carcinogenic in humans. BHT has caused various disorders in animals such as cancer, reduced body weight, increased blood cholesterol levels, and it has been linked to birth defects in rats. That is why the **U.S. Department of Health and Human Services considers BHA to be "reasonably anticipated to be a human carcinogen"**. Nevertheless, the Food and Drug Administration still permits **BHA to be used in foods. Japan has banned the use of BHT and BHA and the U.K. and several European countries have severely restricted it's use all citing considerable safety risks**.

Serious concerns have been raised about the use of BHT in food products. BHT is a suspected mutagen and carcinogen. There have been cases in which some individuals have had difficulty metabolizing BHT, resulting in health and behavior changes.

BHT has been banned for use in food in Japan (1958), Romania, Sweden, and Australia. The US has barred it from being used in infant foods. However some food industries have eliminated it from their products including McDonald's as of 1986.

Some foods in which BHA is used include: butter, meats, cereals, chewing gum, baked goods, snack foods, dehydrated potatoes, and beer.

Butylated hydroxytoluene (BHT) is a fat-soluble organic compound primarily used as an antioxidant food additive (E number E321). It also used as an antioxidant in cosmetics, pharmaceutical drugs, jet fuels, rubber and petroleum products, and embalming fluid.

BHT is produced by the reaction of p-cresol with isobutylene. It was patented in 1947 and received approval of the Food and Drug Administration for use as a food additive and preservative in 1954. BHT reacts with free radicals, slowing the rate of autoxidation in food, preventing changes in the food's color, odor, and taste.

Antioxidants BHT and BHA can be carcinogenic and anti-carcinogenic

When administered prior to or at the time of carcinogen exposure, the phenolic antioxidants butylated hydroxyanisole (BHA) and butylated hydroxytoluene (BHT) are effective inhibitors of carcinogenesis in several target organs.

However, **chronic, post-carcinogen administration of BHT apparently enhances tumorigenesis in certain animal models for liver and lung cancer. The anti-carcinogenic activity of post-carcinogen administration of BHA and BHT in the mammary gland is in contrast to the apparent tumor-enhancing activity of BHT in the liver and lung** (McCormick DL, Major N and Moon RC. 1984).

More confusion: Yet, BHT has been tested extensively for toxicity and used widely for many years. It does not contain any ingredient designated as a known, probable, or suspected human carcinogen by IARC, NTP, ACGIH, or OSHA.

And still others claim: **BHA & BHT** are widely used as preservatives, stabilizers and antioxidants. **BHA is known to cause cancer in humans. Both BHA and BHT are toxic to the liver and kidneys.** BHT may react with other ingested substances to cause the formation of carcinogens. BHT is banned in England. http://www.healthyeatingadvisor.com/9cancer-causingchemicals.html accessed 8-9-09.

BHA has at least epigenetic carcinogenic activity and BHT causes hemorrhagic complications and alters offspring fed BHT. http://www.mindfully.org/Plastic/Antioxidants/BHA-BHT.htm (Madhavi et al, 1996).

There is evidence that certain persons may have difficulty metabolizing BHA and BHT, resulting in health and behavior changes.

BHA and BHT are tumor promoters

"...Specific toxic effects to the lung have only been observed with BHT. The other described toxic effects of BHA and BHT are less characteristic and often occur only after high dosage and long-term treatment.

However, BHA induces in animals tumors of the fore-stomach, which are dose dependent, whereas BHT induces liver tumors in long-term experiments. ... all published findings agree with the fact that **BHA and BHT are tumor promoters.** In contrast to BHA and BHT, vitamin E is not carcinogenic." (Kahl and Kappus. 1993).

The American Academy of Pediatrics (AAP) had real concerns about major drug additives: – **Sulfites, antioxidants** found in many anti-asthma drugs, have been known to induce "serious reactions" such as wheezing, breathing difficulties and chest tightening in asthmatic children. Sulfites are also found in some anti-inflammatories, antibiotics, and the anti-allergy drug epinephrine.

BPA (bisphenol A): a common harmful antioxidant

The antioxidant, BPA, is a common industrial and environmental pollutant. Recently, it garnered publicity for being a contaminant in plastic products used by babies, including feeding bottles. Infants and children are estimated to have the highest daily intake of BPA. It is used to make plastics and products containing bisphenol A-based plastics have been in commerce use since 1957 and at least 8 billion pounds of BPA are used by manufacturers yearly.

The phenolic antioxidants serve as polymer stabilizers.

Polycarbonate plastic, which is clear and nearly shatter-proof, is used to make a variety of common products including baby and water bottles, sports equipment, medical and dental devices, dental fillings and sealants, eyeglass lenses, CDs and DVDs, and household electronics. BPA is also used in the synthesis of polysulfones and polyether ketones, as **an antioxidant** in some plasticizers, and as a polymerization inhibitor in PVC.

Epoxy resins containing bisphenol A are used as coatings on the inside of almost all food and beverage cans. BPA-based products are also used in foundry castings and for lining water pipes.

In 2007, a consensus statement by 38 experts on bisphenol A concluded that average levels in people are above those that cause harm to many animals in laboratory experiments. A panel convened by the U.S. National Institutes of Health determined that there was "some concern" about BPA's effects on fetal and infant brain development and behavior. A 2007 review has concluded that BPA, like other **xenoestrogens**, should be considered as a player within the nervous system that can regulate or alter its functions through multiple pathways.

Investigators determined that in mice and rats, even nanomolar dosage could induce significant effects on memory processes. Bisphenol-A has been shown to bind to thyroid hormone receptor and perhaps have selective effects on its functions.

A 2009 review of available studies has concluded that "perinatal BPA exposure acts to exert persistent effects on body weight and adiposity," possibly leading to obesity.

A 2010 review at Tufts University Medical School concluded that Bisphenol A **may increase cancer risk**. A 2009 in vitro study has concluded that BPA is able to induce neoplastic transformation in human breast epithelial cells (Fernandez and Russo, 2009).

Another 2009 study concluded that maternal oral exposure to low concentrations of BPA during lactation increases mammary carcinogenesis in a rodent model (Jenkins et al, 2009).

BPA can promote the growth of neuroblastoma cells. A 2010 in vitro study has concluded that BPA potently promote invasion and metastasis of neuroblastoma cells.

A 2010 study on mice has concluded that perinatal exposure to 10 micrograms/mL of BPA in drinking water enhances allergic sensitization and bronchial inflammation and responsiveness in an animal model of asthma.

The first large study of health effects on humans associated with bisphenol A exposure was published in September 2008 by Iain Lang and colleagues in the *Journal of the American Medical Association*. The cross-sectional study of almost 1,500 people assessed exposure to bisphenol A by looking at levels of the chemical in urine. The authors found that **higher bisphenol A levels were significantly associated with heart disease, diabetes, and abnormally high levels of certain liver enzymes.**

A later similar study performed by the same group of scientists, published in January 2010, confirmed, despite of lower concentrations of BPA in the second study sample, **an associated increased risk for heart disease.**

A 2006 study in rats has shown that neonatal bisphenol A exposure at 10 µg/kg levels increases prostate gland susceptibility to adult-onset precancerous lesions and hormonal carcinogenesis and a 2009 study has found that newborn rats exposed to a low-dose of BPA (10 µg/kg) increased prostate cancer susceptibility when adults.

Teenagers carry 30 percent more I bisphenol A (BPA) in their bodies than older adults and a 2010 study that analyzed BPA urinary concentrations has concluded that **for people under 18 years of age BPA may negatively impact human immune function.**

A 2010 study of Austrian, Swiss and German population has suggested polycarbonate (PC) baby bottles as the most prominent role of exposure for infants, and canned food for adults and teenagers.

And so characteristic of antioxidants, a 2010 study has found that **BPA may reduce sensitivity to chemotherapy treatment of specific tumors** (Lapensee et al, 2010).

Dental sealants, BPA and danger

On January 2, 2011, the Chicago Tribune carried an article entitled, "Sealants worth the risk." Dental sealants are a popular plastic coating applied to the teeth, which can reduce tooth decay in children by 70 percent. However, they are made with bisphenol A (BPA), a controversial and ubiquitous synthetic antioxidant that in low doses has been associated with changes in behavior, prostate and urinary tract development and early onset of puberty.

Caution is raised but according to an article in the journal *Pediatrics*, there are gaping holes in the data, including the "quality and quantity of BPA absorption." Curiously, the American Dental Association says there is **no basis for health concerns relative to BPA exposure** from any dental material. As I recall, they once said the same thing about mercury in tooth filling amalgams….but, they were wrong.

At the same time, they caution pregnant women against exposure to dental sealants and composites (tooth colored materia used to treat cavities), which also contain BPA.

I am amazed by the similar harmful effects of BPA and the antioxidant vitamins A, C and E.

Synergistic carcinogenic effect of antioxidants

Once again, we see the harmful potential of common antioxidants. Cumulatively, they may combine to produce an overall weakened state with an EMOD insuffiency, which allows for the manifestation of a wide range of disease conditions.

The carcinogenicity of low dietary levels of the antioxidants butylated hydroxyanisole (BHA), caffeic acid, sesamol, 4-methoxyphenol (4-MP) and catechol, known to target the forestomach or glandular stomach, were examined alone or in combination in a 2-year long-term experiment and their modifying effects assessed in a medium-term multiorgan rat model. In the carcinogenicity study, slightly increased incidences of fore-stomach papillomas were found in the sesamol- (15.8%), caffeic acid- (14.8%), catechol- (3%) and 4-MP- (11.5%) treated groups as compared with basal diet (0%), and **a significant increase was observed with the five antioxidants in combination** (42.9%, $P < 0.001$). In the low dose case, the incidence of fore-stomach papillomas was significantly increased only in the combination group. The results indicate that **even at low dose levels phenolic compounds can exert additive/synergistic effect on carcinogenesis** (Hirose et al, 1998).

The synthetic antioxidant BHA was first found to exert carcinogenic potential in rat and hamster fore-stomach epithelium. Many antioxidants have been shown to modify carcinogenesis, and as a rule, they inhibit the initiation stage by reducing the interaction between carcinogen and DNA. However, both promotion and inhibition have been reported for second-stage carcinogenesis, depending on the organ site, species of animal, or initiating carcinogen (Ito and Hirose, 1989).

The anti-oxidant food additive, butylated hydroxytoluene (BHT) was fed to rats and BHT resulted in a significant increase in liver weight. The liver cells presented gradual vacuolization, cytoplasmic disintegration, "moth-eaten" appearance, ballooning degeneration, hepatocellular necrosis, aggregation of chromatin material around the periphery of the nuclear envelope, SER proliferation, RER clumping with broken cisternae, withered and autolyzed mitochondria, augmentation of lipid droplets and glycogen depletion (Safer and ak-Nughamish, 1999).

And lastly, since there is widespread use of antioxidants in the food processing industries, especially oil and oil based ones and since the ban on the further usage of butylated hydroxyanisole (BHA) and butylated hydroxytoluene (BHT) by the Food and Agriculture Organization of the United Nations (FAO) in 1980, there have been several reports indicating that BHA and BHT might have detrimental effects. BHT is more toxic than BHA and this rat study clearly indicates that at the concentrations of 0.75%, BHA and BHT are harmful to the blood (Jayalakshmi and Sharma, 1986).

Food (feed) antioxidants for animals and fish

Antioxidants prevent fat oxidation (rancidity). Rancidity creates off-flavors and off-odors which dramatically decrease palatability and food consumption. Antioxidants also prevent the destruction of several nutrients. They provide direct protection to a number of vitamins which are unstable to the effects of oxygen.

Natural antioxidants such as ascorbic acid (vitamin C) and vitamin E or other related tocopherols are effective antioxidants but are relatively short lived when compared to the chemical antioxidants. Due to the realities of the pet food distribution system and the relatively low volumes and slow use of exotic bird foods, the time interval between manufacturing a product and feeding it may be beyond the effective life of a natural antioxidant. If the product could be produced, refrigerated and consumed within a few months, natural antioxidants might be practical. But, since this time frame cannot be guaranteed, it seems prudent to manufacturers to use the more stable petro-chemical antioxidants for this critical function.

The commonly used chemical antioxidants, butylated hydroxyani-sol (BHA), butylated hydroxytoluene (BHT) and ethoxyquin, are all chemicals that research indicates could be potential carcinogens when fed to certain species at high levels. The use of antioxidants has been questioned by scientists, pet owners and retailers.

Some product ingredients sound more like rocket fuel than like food.

http://www.fao.org/docrep/x5738e/x5738e0b.htm. accessed 1-4-11.

The FAO is the Food and Agriculture Organization of the United Nations and it makes recommendation for additive amounts of anti-oxidants to animal and fish food supplies. Oxidation can affect feeds and feedstuffs, resulting in rancidity of fats, destruction of vitamins A, D, and E, pigmenters (carotenoids) and amino acids with resultant lowered biological energy values for the diet.

Care should be used to make certain that the ingredients included in the feeds provide adequate margins of safety of vitamins A, E, and other natural antioxidants; e.g., lecithin. The use of unstable fats and oils or other pro-oxidants in the feed should be minimized whenever possible.

Antioxidants have been used in commercial fish foods in the USA for over 20 years. Although hundreds of chemicals have been tested, only a few have shown the qualifications necessary to make them suitable for use in preventing undesirable oxidations in feedstuffs, in finished feeds, and in the guts and carcasses of animals. In order for an antioxidant to be useful in animal feeding, it must have the following qualifications:

(a) it must be effective in preserving animal and vegetable fats, vita-mins, and other feed qualities subject to oxidative destruction;

(b) it must be non-toxic to man and to farm animals (i.e., chickens, swine, fish, etc.);

(c) it should be effective at very low concentrations; and

(d) it must be low enough in cost to be economically practical.

COMMONLY USED FEED ANTIOXIDANTS

Of the chemical compounds that have been investigated thus far, three have been found to be outstandingly effective antioxidants for feeds and feed ingredients and can be used both efficiently and economically. They are:

(a) Ethoxyquin (generic term: 1,2-dihydro-6-ethoxy-2,2,4- trimethyl-quinoline)

(b) BHA (butylated hydroxyanisole);

(c) BHT (butylated hydroxytoluene)

Ethoxyquin, however, has been demonstrated to be the most efficacious, followed closely by BHT and BHA.

With the advent of rations containing a high level of animal and vegetable fats, the requirement for antioxidant protection has become very apparent. The majority of studies over the last few years has focused on ethoxyquin as a preservative or antioxidant. **Other chemical preservatives are: ascorbic acid, propionic acid, benzoic acid, citric acid and their various salts.** There are technological problems (i.e., moisture level, etc.) associated with the use of these preservatives. Economics, however, remain the most important consideration which limit their use in fish foods.

Commonly Used Chemical Preservatives Generally Recognized as Safe

Ascorbic acid

Ascorbyl palmitate

Benzoic acid

BHA

BHT

Calcium ascorbate

Calcium propionate

Calcium sorbate

Citrate acid

Dilauryl thiodipropionate

Distearyl thiodipropionate

Erythorbic acid

Ethoxyquin

Formic acid

Methylparaben

Potassium bisulphite

Potassium metabisulphite

Potassium sorbate

Propionic acid

Propul gallate

Propul paraben

Resin guaiae

Sodium ascorbate

Sodium benzoate

Sodium bisulphite

Sodium metabisulphite

Sodium nitrite

Sodium propionate

Sodium sorbate

Sodium sulphite

Sorbic acid

Stannous chloride

Sulphur dioxide

THBP - Trihydroxy-butyrophenone

TBHQ - Tertiary-butylhydroquinone

Thiodipinic acid

Tocopherols

Altogether too often, it is the practice to use levels of vitamin E far above the animals' nutrient requirement and the result is economically unfavorable. It has been shown in diets designed for chicken and turkey breeders that ethoxyquin has a vitamin E sparing effect.

Antioxidants prevent oxidative losses of vitamins A and E and pigmenters (oxy- and keto-cerotenoids) in stored mixed feeds. Antioxidants stabilize critical oxidation-susceptible nutrients that are naturally present in a fish feed composed of several feedstuffs so that losses are minimal from mixing and storing. If pigmenting substances are used, the anti-oxidants are definitely needed. The benefits of adequate, consistent use span all facets of fish production which include the processing and handling of feedstuffs, formulation, and fish cultural practices.

The U.S. Food and Drug Administration permits the following levels of antioxidant in finished feed:

(a) ethoxyquin (1,2 dihydro-6-ethoxy-2,2,4- trimethy quinoline): 150 ppm,
(b) BHT (butylated hydroxytoluene): 200 ppm, and
(c) BHA (butylated hydroxyanisole): 200 ppm.

A 2005 reassessment of inert ingredient tolerance of ethoxyquin was commissioned by the US Environmental Protection Agency (EPA). The reassessment states that "studies indicate that **ethoxyquin is toxic to aquatic invertebrates, and mildly toxic to fish" when ingested.**

Please realize that all of these antioxidants can contaminate animal products, such as eggs, milk, meat, etc. and the housing facilities or feed lots in which they are enclosed. Also, the antioxidant laced fish food is capable to contaminating the surrounding waters and ultimately getting into aquifers and municipal water supplies and create ecological disasters.

It is readily apparent that there are over 3 dozen antioxidants which may be added to feed stocks.

Flint River Ranch Pet Foods do not contain any of the following chemical preservatives, instead they use natural Vitamin E, a closely related fat-soluble compound known as Tocopherols. Their website states:

Ethoxyquin

- Promoted kidney carcinogenesis.
- Significantly increased incidence of stomach tumors.
- Enhanced bladder carcinogenesis.

BHA

- Enhanced stomach and urinary bladder carcinogenesis.
- Causes squamous-cell carcinomas in stomachs.

(Cancers of this type are among the most lethal and fastest acting, the swiftest effects being seen among animals with light colored fur.)

BHT

- Promoted urinary bladder carcinogenesis.
- Could be a promoter of thyroid carcinogenesis.

Studies have noted that BHA and other antioxidants, particularly Propyl Gallate and ethoxyquin, showed additional effects in inducing stomach hyperplasia and cytotoxicity.

BHA and BHT are used in human and pet foods to keep fats from going rancid. Both have been linked to cancer in laboratory animals; it's unknown whether they cause the same in people and dogs. There is evidence that certain people may have difficulty metabolizing BHA and BHT, resulting in health and behavior changes. Again, we don't know if the same is true for our dogs.

According to Dr. Wendell Belfield, DVM practicing veterinarian for some 26 years, both BHA and BHT are known to cause liver and kidney dysfunction and are banned in some European countries. He adds that ethoxyquin is suspected of causing cancer.

Ethoxyquin is listed and identified as a hazardous chemical by OSHA. It has a rating of 3 on a scale of 1 to 6, with 6 being super toxic requiring less than 7 drops to cause death. When manufactured by Monsanto, the containers are marked with the word POISON. **Monsanto makes no representations and will not be responsible for damages of any nature whatsoever.** The Department of Agriculture lists and controls Ethoxyquin as a pesticide.

In 1994, David A. Dzanis, D.V.M., Ph.D, said, "As Americans become more health conscious, they are reading food labels and choosing products more carefully. Many people are extending this scrutiny to food for their pets as well. Pet food labels are regulated by different rules than foods for human consumption, but reading and understanding a pet food label can help consumers make proper food choices for their pets, too.

According to a document produced by the Environmental Protection Agency (EPA), "Dogs are more susceptible to ethoxyquin toxicity than rats, with elevated liver enzymes and microscopic findings in the liver occurring at doses as low as 4 mg/kg/day over a 90-day feeding period."

The FDA and pet food industry officials defend the use of ethoxyquin, saying that ethoxyquin is safer than rancid fats. While this may be true, artificial preservatives are not the only way to prevent rancidity. In addition, if ethoxyquin is safe, why is it not permitted to be added to human foods (other than three spices), and why is the acceptable level for pet foods 50 times the residual amount allowed in human food?

How then can a consumer find out if their dog's food contains ethoxyquin, BHA, BHT, or other artificial preservatives? Unfortunately, there are no easy answers.

Antioxidants added to food

Prior to the Civil War, people raised most of the food they ate and processing was limited to spices, salt and smoke. After the Civil War, the food supply system changed, cities grew, factories flourished and food manufacturers popped up. Scientific knowledge of food chemistry or antioxidants was practically nonexistent.

Antioxidants have diverse applications. They are used to prevent degradation in polymers, weakening in rubber and plastics, autoxidation and gum formation in gasoline, and discoloration of synthetic and natural pigments. They are used in foods, beverages, and cosmetic products to inhibit deterioration and spoilage.

Chemicals to keep products looking good until they were sold or to hide signs of spoilage were used without much restraint. Dangerous adulteration of foods became commonplace, such as the use of copper sulfate to keep vegetables appearance fresh and green and salicylic acid, borax and formaldehyde were also used dangerously.

Dr. Harvey Washington Wiley, chief chemist for the USDA was the predecessor to the FDA and he cautioned that the American people were being steadily poisoned by the dangerous chemicals that were being added to food with reckless abandon. In 1927 the Food, Drug and Insecticide Administration was created and later became the FDA.

It was not until 1958 that legislation was adopted requiring food and chemical manufactureresto test their additives before they were submitted to the FDA. Today, manufacturers are responsible for demonstrating their Generally Recognized as Safe (GRAS) status and providing evidence (such as scientific literature) to support it. Approximately 100 new substances are presented to the FDA for GRAS certification every year.

Food preservatives are classified into two main groups: antioxidants and antimicrobials.

Enzymes called phenolases catalyze the oxidation of certain molecules (e.g., the amino acid tyrosine) when fruits and vegetables, such as apples, bananas, and potatoes, are cut or bruised. The product of these oxidation reactions, collectively known as enzymatic browning, is a dark pigment called melanin. Antioxidants that inhibit enzyme-catalyzed oxidation include agents that bind free oxygen (i.e., reducing agents), such as **ascorbic acid (vitamin C), and agents that inactivate the enzymes, such as citric acid and sulfites.**

Among antioxidants, the synthetic compounds **butylated hydroxyanisole (BHA), propyl gallate, ethoxyquin, and diphenylamine are commonly used as food additives**. Quercetin belongs to a large natural group of antioxidants, the flavonoid family, with more than 6000 known members.

Antioxidants are food additives used since about 1947 to stabilize foods that by their composition would otherwise undergo significant loss in quality in the presence of oxygen. Undesirable changes include rancidity of unsaturated fats resulting in off-odors and discoloration of pigments.

Antioxidants prevent, delay or minimize the oxidation of foods to which they are added.

Antioxidants are used in all **cooking oils**, and **exposed potato chips, all fried foods**, catfish, **Twinkies, doughnuts, chicken, French fries**, etc. **Citrus juice** beverages have an oil soluble flavor antioxidant added, a tocopherol antioxidant, other than alpha-tocopherol, added to a citrus juice beverage, such as orange juice, to preserve the flavor sensory attributes of stored juice.

Antioxidative compositions contain **quercetin, vitamin B1, vitamin B2, vitamin B3, vitamin B6, vitamin B12, vitamin C, caffeine, epigallocatechin gallate (EGCG), epicatechin, epicatechin gallate, epigallocatechin, and polypheron E.**

Frying processes utilizing cooking oil at elevated temperatures can cause various degradation effects in the oil including oxidation, hydrolysis and/or polymerization. Thus, antioxidants are added to nearly all cooking oils, unless specified otherwise. Deep **frying oils** combined with phytosterols are instrumental in deep-fried food products. The **deep frying** compositions have a phytosterol ester content of up to about 50 weight percent.

Some claim **olive oil** has the highest amount of heart-protective monounsaturated fats and polyphenols — antioxidants that have anti-inflammatory and anti-clotting properties. Others claim, "Rich in antioxidants, Heloi's rice bran oil is the healthiest cooking oil."

Gamma Oryzanol is a powerful antioxidant that can only be found in **rice bran oil**, not in any other vegetable oils.

Some cooking vessels have a means of adding antioxidants directly to the preparation to prevent spoilage or deterioration of the cooked food.

According to Sue Dengate and the Food Intolerance Network, **antioxidants 310-312 and 319-321, used to prevent rancidity in oils, can cause a full range of reactions from asthma to insomnia, depression, tiredness, learning difficulties and children's behavior problems**.

Her website states, "After battling with her son's behavior following such treats as supposedly additive-free fish and chips and ice cream cones, the winner, Jenny Savige from Warragul in Victoria, wrote: *"Antioxidants are secret unless you go to extreme lengths to ask the supplier of the food and then the manufacturer of the contents ... what hope have we got if such nasty additives are hidden in our foods?"*

Antioxidants are the most hidden of all additives. There are four ways consumers can be tripped up.

* manufacturer fails to list ingredient on the product label
* ingredient is unlisted under the 5% labeling loophole
* consumer hotline gives wrong information when contacted
* staff give incorrect information regarding unlabelled food, e.g. takeaways

The 5% labeling loophole

In Australia, antioxidants do not have to be listed if vegetable oil forms less than 5% of the final product. And, what are consumers to do when consumer hotlines say that their products are antioxidant free?

The 5% labeling loophole says, "If the amount of an ingredient in a food is less than 5% of the food (such as 4.5 per cent sunflower oil added to soymilk), a food additive (such as antioxidant TBHQ, 319) in that ingredient does not have to be included in the ingredients list on the label unless the food additive is performing a technological function in the final food."

With restaurants in general or eating out, **any oils used to cook your food will almost certainly contain at least one of these potentially harmful antioxidant additives**.

Check the ingredients of **margarine, dairy blends, crackers, biscuits, bread, baked goods, croissants, potato crisps, snack foods, muesli bars, crushed garlic in oil, soymilk and other processed foods** for likely antioxidant additives. But, they may not be labeled.

Harmful Antioxidants (310-312) (319-321)

310 - Propyl gallate; 311 - Octyl gallate; 312 - Dodecyl gallate; 319 - tert-Butylhydroquinone, tBHQ; 320 - Butylated hydroxyanisole, BHA; 321 - Butylated hydroxytoluene, BHT.

Alternative antioxidants

300 - Ascorbic acid (vitamin C); 301 - Sodium ascorbate; 302 - Calcium ascorbate; 303 - Potassium ascorbate; 304 - Ascorbyl palmitate; 306 - Mixed tocopherols (vitamin E); 307 - dl-a-Tocopherol; 308 - g-Tocopherol; 309 - d-Tocopherol.

The harmful antioxidant additives are found in cooking oils, margarines, lards and any other fats or oils. Nearly every processed food congtains some kind of fat or oil. It doesn't matter whether the ingredient label says vegetable oil, a specific oil like canola or sunflower, fats of vegetable origin, or beef tallow - unless they list some of the safe alternatives, they will probably contain one of these harmful additives.

TBHQ (tert-butylhydroquinone) is a common antioxidant and it keeps fats from becoming rancid, so it is an additive in lots of foods. TBHQ can be oxidized into all sorts of additional products, such as tert-butylquinone, which can be bad for the liver. some studies say that TBHQ can cause cancer in lab animals and other studies say it may have protective effects. The jury is still out.

Could antioxidants cause rise in allergies?

In Louisiana, many of us are plagued by seasonal allergies. Currently, maple, oak and pine trees are at their height for pollen production and sinuses are flaring up everywhere.

Yet, there is an unexplained increase in allergies of all kind around the globe and not just an increase in seasonal allergies. Common allergies are due to cat hair, dust and pollen and, according the National Institutes of Health, about 54 percent of Americans are sensitive to at least one allergy-inducing substance.

The rate of allergies more than doubled from the 1970s to the 1990s, which has resulted in increased sneezing, wheezing and itchy, watery eyes and a spike in sales of antihistamines. Strangely, food allergies in children also rose about 18 percent during this same time interval, according to the Centers for Disease Control and Prevention. This has resulted in peanut-free kindergarteners because of the high incidence of peanut allergies in today's kids.

Explanations for the allergy increases have ranged from the simple to the ridiculous, i.e., 1) Our "children are too clean" and not exposed to enough dirt to stimulate their developing immune systems (the hygiene hypothesis). Reportedly, children raised in day care centers and exposed to cross infections from other children have fewer allergies. 2) The "global warming crowd" has jumped into the fray and proposed that man-made warming has resulted in plants flowering earlier in the year and producing more over all pollen. 3) As opposed to the "we are too clean crowd" there is the "we are too dirty crowd", who argue that increasing smog and air pollution are making allergies worse, especially for asthmatics. And 4) There are those who explain the increase as simply an increase in more people being diagnosed with allergies.

A leading dermatologist said that, "Whereas before people were told you just have dry skin or a rash, now they're told, you have eczema." In short, we barely have a clue as to the real explanation for this increase in allergies.

The above "guesses" could be partially true or totally wrong but all experts admit that the real reason remains a mystery and the increase may be due to many factors, including the injudicious intake of antioxidants.

I believe that antioxidants, contained in everything from food to multivitamins, may be partially responsible for the curious rise in allergy and asthma cases, especially in children. (Please review the section on multivitamins.)

We realize that there is no good explanation for our increasing sniffles and sneezes. Good advise is to try to avoid outside conditions during the heavy pollen season and to wear a face mask if cutting the lawn or activities which stir up lots of dust. Ask your doctor about the proper antihistamine for you and the proper dosage. Try to avoid nasal sprays for prolonged periods because of "rebound." It is ironic that during one of the most beautiful times of the year, we have to try to avoid becoming its victim. It just isn't fair but who said life is fair.

Also, look out for those hidden sources (unlabeled) of antioxidants.

Antioxidant suppositories and inhalants

There are even antioxidant suppositories for radiation proctopathy and antioxidants to be used with nasal inhalers. There is a therapeutic nasal inhalant for using bioflavanoids and vitamin C as a topical antioxidant (United States Patent 6180663). Also, there is aromatherapy with antioxidants.

Also, the "Solutions to Aging" website says, "**ORAL SUPPLEMENTATION OF ALL FORMS OF GLUTATHIONE (an antioxidant) DOES NOT RAISE TISSUE LEVELS OF GLUTATHIONE.**" Therefore the only way one could truly raise the reduced glutathione levels in body was by undergoing costly direct intravenous administration of reduced glutathione. What makes this product truly revolutionary is that clinical case studies have demonstrated we are now able to raise tissue levels of reduced glutathione by our ability to combine pure pharmaceutical grade Reduced Glutathione into our proprietary patent pending **suppository base**, thus effectively allowing Reduced Glutathione in combination with N Acetyl Cysteine to be delivered directly into the blood stream effecting an elevation of the serum glutathione levels. Each Reduced Glutathione, TMG & Orotates suppository contains the following: Reduced Glutathione 250mg; N-Acetyl Cysteine 125mg Trimethylglycine 100mg; Ascorbyl Palmitate 75mg Calcium 400mg; Phosphotidylcholine; Phosphotidylserine and phosphotidylethanolamine. http://www.solutionstoaging.com/reducedglutathionesuppository.html (accessed 12-28-10).

The **Zetpil Melatonin Plus suppository** as developed after pharmacological research offered clear evidence that melatonin is best absorbed via the rectum. Accordingly, the scientist and development team at Zetpil have developed a formulation that combines melatonin, the precursors for reduced glutathione formation, **key**

antioxidants in a proprietary base that was specially developed to further enhance absorption of all the bioactive ingredients. Note melatonin has been shown in repeated studies not only to maintain the levels of the cellular antioxidant glutathione but to actually increase glutathione levels. This is especially important since individuals using classical antioxidants such as Vitamin C, Vitamin E actually deplete the cellular antioxidant rGSH.

The preceding are merely examples of the wide ranging sources that contain antioxidants.

Ginkgo biloba

Dietary supplements extol their wondrous claims everywhere. The Food and Drug Administration (FDA) estimates that there are 29,000 supplements on the market, with 1,000 new ones introduced annually.

Ginkgo supplements are among the best-selling herbal medications in the U.S. and Europe and it ranks as a top medicine prescribed in France and Germany.

There is no mandate for the FDA to screen or test the never-ending stream of supplements entering or on the market for either safety or effectiveness. However, investigators at University of Virginia School of Medicine and Wake Forest University Baptist Medical Center helped conduct the "Ginkgo biloba for the Evaluation of Memory (GEM)" study.

They evaluated the effects of ginkgo, an antioxidant, on the occurrence or prevention of dementia. Ginkgo is one of the world's most widely advertised herbal supplements claiming to improve memory and cognition.

The GEM study showed that 240 mg of ginkgo daily had no effect on the onset of dementia or development of Alzheimer's.

Chief study investigators said, "The results were disappointing and surprising." Unfortunately, ginkgo's widespread use, based on the belief that it helps memory function, does not hold up to scientific scrutiny. According to the National Institute on Aging, Alzheimer's affects nearly 4.5 million Americans and it will claim one in 10 baby boomers. Nearly a half-million new Alzheimer's cases will be diagnosed annually.

Even worse, with the three main drugs Aricept (donepezil), Exelon (rivastigmine) and Reminyl, Razadyne (galantamine), which are approved for use in mild-to-moderate Alzheimer's disease, not one of six clinical trials conducted by Italian researchers found that these drugs significantly reduced the rate of progression from mild cognitive impairment (MCI) to dementia.

Alzheimer's remains an incurable disease with a slowly progressive mild memory loss, which ends horribly with severe brain damage and death. Experts increasingly advise reliance on keeping mentally and physically active and not being taken in by false hopes of unproven supplements or drugs. With no cure available or in sight, we must push for more government sponsored research on all forms of dementia. Do it, before we forget to do it.

Ginkgo has been taken as a mental health supplement for hundreds of years, and is also said to benefit blood flow, and combat free radicals. Yet, according to a 2010 paper recently published in the Journal of the American Medical Association, ginkgo biloba had no discernible affect on the mental acuity of people as they aged.

This comes on the heels of a 2008 study by the same team that showed that ginkgo had no affect on Alzheimer's or dementia. The JAMA report is a blow to the reputation of the supplement and could prove potentially damaging to suppliers of the supplement who sell over $100 million in the US alone.

For those looking to boost their mental agility, or to simply keep it strong as they age, it looks like ginkgo biloba is no longer a good option.

The study was conducted by Dr. Steven DeKosky of the University of Virginia. 3000 people aged 72 to 96 were followed for an average of six years. Half took 120mg of ginkgo per day while the other half received a placebo. There was no measured difference in attention, memory, or cognitive capability.

DeKosky's research is part of the Ginkgo Evaluation of Memory (GEM) study funded by the National Center for Complementary and

Alternative Medicine and the National Institute for Aging. While there have been other studies suggesting the myriad efficacies of gingko, DeKosky's study is much larger and carries the approval of JAMA.

As disappointing as this news may be for gingko proponents, it's undoubtedly beneficial to those of us wanting to know the truth.

The antioxidant polyphenols have been found to contribute most of its antioxidant activity. A purified proanthocyanidin polymer accounted for 86.6% of the total proanthocyanidins, and for 37.7% of the total antioxidant activity of this leaf extract. (Qaadan et al, 2010).

Doxorubicin evokes oxidative stress and precipitates cell apoptosis in testicular tissues. Ginkgo biloba extract 761 (EGb), a widely used herbal medicine with potent anti-oxidant and anti-apoptotic properties, could protect testes from such doxorubicin injury. EGb protected against the oxidative and apoptotic actions of doxorubicin on testes. EGb may be a dangerous adjuvant therapy medicine, potentially protecting neoplastic lesions (Yeh et al, 2009).

EGb 761 was able to protect mitochondria from the attack of hydrogen peroxide, antimycin and Abeta. Furthermore, EGb 761 reduced ROS levels and ROS-induced apoptosis in lymphocytes from aged mice treated orally with EGb 761 for 2 weeks. Their data further emphasize neuroprotective properties of EGb 761, such as protection against Abeta-toxicity, and antiapoptotic properties (Eckert et al, 2003).

In short, advertising works but neither ginkgo nor the current medications have proven to be effective.

Common (NSAID) drugs increase heart attacks and strokes

There is a saying that "all medicines contain a little poison." That should be updated to say, "Many medicines contain significant amounts of poison and some medicines contain lots of poison." Even drugs which have been around for decades and taken by millions annually can cause serious adverse effects.

For example, the group of **antioxidants known as non-steroidal anti-inflammatory drugs (NSAIDs)** are being increasingly scrutinized as a cause of heart attacks and strokes. Coincidentally, **I have seen this same pattern of increased heart disease and stroke**

with the antioxidant vitamins A and E. NSAIDs include naproxen, ibuprofen, diclofenac, celecoxib, etoricoxib, rofecoxib (Vioxx), and lumiracoxib. Rofecoxib and lumiracoxib were associated with twice the risk of heart attack, while ibuprofen was associated with more than three times the risk of stroke.

When all "vascular events" - heart attacks, stroke, or vascular disease - were taken together, the risks increased by 40 per cent on these drugs. Ibuprofen can double the risk of suffering a heart attack and Vioxx was banned in the USA in 2004. To me, these numbers are shocking.

At the time, the medical profession was calling Vioxx a "wonder drug." Yet, consumers have heard so little regarding the dangers of these popular products. In 2005, a Texas court awarded Carol Ernst, the widow of Robert Ernst, who died aged 59 from a heart attack leading to his fatal arrhythmia, $253 million in damages against the Merck drug company. Doctors had reported 103 cases to which they suspected Vioxx contributed to death.

This may slow down doctors just a bit before they reach for their prescription pad. On the other hand, maybe not. If they have a patient who is painfully disabled by arthritis, logically, they are going to prescribe a NSAID to help him tolerate the disease and improve his quality of life.

This new study, by a team at Bern University, evaluated 31 studies involving over 116,000 patients who took the painkillers regularly, mostly for arthritis pain, and concluded, "The options for the treatment of chronic musculoskeletal pain are limited and patients and clinicians need to be aware that cardiovascular risk needs to be taken into account when prescribing these drugs." The use of other nonsteroidal anti-inflammatory drugs not covered by their analysis should be reconsidered, as well as the over the counter availability of nonsteroidal anti-inflammatory drugs. Of all of the NSAIDs, Naproxen, in particular, was considered quite safe.

We should follow the advice of "take the smallest dose for the shortest length of time possible." If you do not need a particular medicine, do not take it. If in doubt, do not hesitate to consult your physician. Stay safe.

Prof Randolph M. Howes MD, PhD

Medical Headlines, Spurious Associations and Junk Science

It is estimated that there are currently 25 thousand medical/scientific journals turning out over one million publications annually.

It is also estimated that 50% of these papers have reached the wrong conclusions.

Personally, I feel that the percentage of erroneous conclusions is higher than their estimate. I keep one computer file on "spurious (meaning not genuine, false, fake, etc.) associations" for medical/scientific papers. Large studies lend themselves to misinterpretation and misrepresentation of underlying facts.

Slick advertisers capitalize on these ludicrous false associations. So-called observational or epidemiological studies have especially been prone to drawing false conclusions, i.e. elderly people have gray hair; so, gray hair causes aging. This false conclusion is wrong and only shows an "association" of graying of the hair and aging.

Association is not causation. Strange things happen when statistical analysis is applied to medical science.

Some "headline" examples of recent spurious associations in the medical literature are as follows: "Large thighs may protect the heart," "Short legs linked to liver disease," "Short limbs linked with higher risk of memory loss," "Women eating one quarter grapefruit a day had 30% higher risk of breast cancer," "Rainfall autism theory suggested," "Autumn babies at greater risk of asthma," "Watching TV increases risk of autism," "Cell phones can affect sperm quality," "Hairspray linked to birth defects," and "Too much TV linked to higher asthma risk."

We must carefully evaluate all studies, apply good old common sense (in addition to scientific scrutiny) and avoid acceptance of unusual conclusions with blind faith or religious fervor. Studies that report a link between some new risk factor and disease are everywhere and frequently mean little or nothing.

Do not take the hook, remain somewhat skeptical and await actual proof, before adopting life style changes or swallowing the latest "magic pill."

214

Today, people will jump on the newest medical bandwagon faster than they leaped on the cash for clunkers program. This is exactly what happened with the subject of risk factors for heart disease. Hundreds of heart disease risk factors have been reported, the dangers of cholesterol oxidation was popularized as was fatty diets and we still do not have the answers, although currently inflammation is the leading "cause de jour."

Be wary of strange medical claims. We must remain enthusiastic concerning medical science but must also be dedicated to truthful reporting. It is ironic that accepting nonsense medical "headlines" may be your greatest medical risk factor for your overall well being.

Introduction of new terms

Perhaps, it is time to introduce a few new terms.

Hyper-antioxidosis - too much (cumulative) antioxidants in the system

Hyper-antioxinemia - too much (cumulative) antioxidants in the blood

Antioxidant hypervitaminosis - excessively high systemic levels of antioxidant vitamins; an over burden or overload of antioxidants

Antioxidant toxicity - the harmful effects of antioxidant overload, which can result in EMOD insufficiency and disease allowance

CONCLUSIONS

Radicophobes can ignore the truth or they can reject the truth but they can not change the magnificent truths regarding the crucial role of EMODs in the life process of all aerobes or the inherent splendor of oxygen.

R. M. Howes M.D., Ph.D.
1/26/09

My Way

I live in rural Louisiana on a cattle ranch and obsessively work on oxygen metabolism research via the internet. I work to bring better health care to the poor and rural citizens of Louisiana and to correct Louisiana's dismal health care rankings. I am blessed with a good family, adequate material assets and the industriousness to put out pathological levels of effort to search for discoveries and scientific truths.

I invented the triple lumen venous catheter, (The Arrow Howes catheter) which became the number one venous catheter in the world and has helped save the lives of over 20 million critically ill patients world wide. However, the potential of my work with EMODs will dwarf these past accomplishments. I must press forward. I must help reduce pain and suffering for all of our citizens. To that end, I continue the struggle. I continue the battle.

If You Want To Argue With Me

If you want to argue with me, you will have to prove to me that you take the associated risks seriously by actually reading as much research as I have and be able to discuss it with me and answer ALL of my questions to my satisfaction.

Denial of the harmful potential of antioxidant vitamins is one of the most dangerous conspiracy theories out there. This is not a case in which there is no scientific evidence. The studies have been done and the evidence is clear. There are more articles and studies that I could find, but I have found enough.

It appears that no matter how much research I do, no matter how many studies I have cited, many antioxidant vitamin proponents will NOT accept or even acknowledge them. If you believe that I am proffering fallacious arguments, please point them out and make a case as to why I am wrong so that earnest debate can take place. This is a debate with science on one side and profits or ignorance on the other.

After all, if there is a connection between common diseases and the antioxidant vitamins, manufacturers and marketers are looking at quite a hefty law suit. Ergo, an official admission of guilt from the pharmaceutical and dietary supplement industries will never occur as it could set a legal precedence for a massive class action lawsuit that could cost them billions of dollars.

Although I have presented over 250 studies showing non-effective or harmful effects of the antioxidant vitamins, let me give the 3 biggest pieces of evidence against their use:

1) **the cumulative data of 80 studies showing harm**

2) **the 170 other cases showing no effect or marginal effects**

3) **the 5 most prevalent antioxidants in the body, when in excess, cause known disease and death, i.e., cholesterol, uric acid, bilirubin, testosterone and estrogen.**

With so much contradictory and confusing information out there, it is no wonder that most people just throw up their hands and go on eating and living the way they've always done. It is often hard to discern from what we see and hear in the media exactly what course of action we should take to prevent cancer. We hear so much con-

218

tradictory advice from scientists and so-called experts that it's hard to know what to believe. And as scientists learn more about cancer, their advice changes.

Antioxidants Are Ganging Up On Us

Consider this: vitamin A, vitamin C, vitamin E, multivitamins, prenatal vitamins, bilirubin, estrogen, testosterone, cholesterol, uric acid, BPA, BHT, BHA, and over three dozen antioxidant food additives are having a cumulative affect, in that they are making it harder for our bodies to maintain adequate protective levels of EMODs. Thus, we see increasing diseases, such as allergies, asthma, diabetes, cancer, heart disease, etc.

However, this is a preventable situation and we must first acknowledge it and then act on it. Please review the harmful consequences of these antioxidants in this book. If that does not get your attention, nothing will!

Even McCormick's black pepper is getting in on the action, with advertisements stating in bold letters, "Introduce **ANTIOXIDANTS** to your morning scramble (eggs)." In fact, they refer to black pepper as a "super spice."

Not to be left behind, peddlers of CoQ10 run ads stating that, **"CoQ10 has been hailed as one of the most significant heart health discoveries in recent years."** Yet, microscript at the bottom of the advertisement states, "These statements have not been evaluated by the FDA. These products are not intended to diagnose, treat, cure or prevent any disease."

Lack of Safety of Vitamins and Antioxidants

Increasingly, investigational reports are showing that vitamins and antioxidant dietary supplements are failing to curtail or decrease the incidence of many of the diseases they were claimed to help prevent or to cure. In the USA, nutrient deficiencies are rare and over nutrition and over weight are rampant.

The exuberant fanfare, which followed the 1954 free radical theory of oxidative stress and aging, has quieted to a whimper. I have followed these studies for years and have accumulated study results on over eight million patients worldwide.

Basically, vitamins A, C, and E and their precursors of beta-carotene and alpha-tocopherol, have frequently failed to alter the occurrence or the course of cancer, heart disease, diabetes, arthritis or cataracts. Most alarming of all, some of the largest studies indicate that these vitamins and dietary supplements actually increase the incidence of cancer, strokes and overall mortality in certain groups of patients, especially smokers or those exposed to asbestos.

Major health organizations, such as the American College of Cardiology, the American Heart Association (AHA), the AHA Nutrition Committee, the US Preventive Services Task Force, the Institute of Medicine, and the American Heart Association Science Advisory statement, recommend against the taking of these vitamin and antioxidant supplements. Cancer patients who pop vitamins during chemotherapy and radiation therapy may unwittingly be sabotaging their own treatment, since many cancer treatment regimens rely upon the tumoricidal action of free radicals.

Sadly, many patients state that they will continue the consumption of these vitamins and antioxidants, even if they are shown to be scientifically ineffective. This demonstrates the significant power of media brainwashing and of unrestrained advertising and marketing.

Also, many common foods, such as breads, juices and cereals, are fortified with these same vitamins and antioxidants and this adds to the daily intake and dosage of these potentially harmful agents. Genetic engineers are altering fruits and vegetables (Franken-foods) to produce many times their normal content of antioxidants.

Unfortunately, many of today's dieticians and nutritionists advocate and encourage the use of vitamins and antioxidants, thus, repeating the "party line" as though it was gospel.

The vitamin and dietary supplement industry is a $27 billion business and over 150 million Americans are currently taking these products and over 1 million of our youth are taking sports-enhancing supplements. Many physicians are not only recommending and prescribing these agents but are also jumping on the multi-level marketing band-wagon to sell these products in their offices.

Major food and pharmaceutical companies own over 50% of the manu-facturing or distribution of these agents. Citizens and patients are be-coming increasingly confused by reports of the danger and harm caused by drugs, which they had been led to believe were safe, such as hormone replacement therapy, Vioxx, Celebrex, Prozac, Lipitor, Crestor, fen-phen, Accutane, Paxil and now, vitamins and antioxidant supplements.

Now, the number of deaths from legal drugs exceeds the number of deaths from illegal drugs and far exceeds the number of deaths from car accidents.

The current antioxidant "anti-aging" craze is taking on a carnival at-mosphere, even within traditional medical practices and 21st century snake-oil salesmen are currently more plentiful than they have ever been in the history of our planet. Fact: we do not know what causes or controls the aging process.

These subjects are discussed in detail in my books: *U.T.O.P.I.A., Unified Theory of Oxygen Participation in Aerobiosis* (767 pages) R.M. Howes, M.D., Ph.D. Free Radical Publishing Co., © 2004 and in my newest book: *The Medical and Scientific Significance of Oxygen Free Radical Metabolism* (931 pages) R.M. Howes, M.D., Ph.D. Free Radical Publishing Co. © 2005. Most of my books can be reviewed free of charge online at www.thepundit.com or www.iwillfindthecure.org.

I am an "oxy-addict"…. and so are you.

R. M. Howes, M.D., Ph.D.
6/5/10

I urge you to eat a well balanced diet, containing lots of fresh fruits and vegetables and to get moderate daily physical exercise, stop smoking, avoid stress, avoid taking unnecessary medications or supplements and keep weight under control. Avoid mental and physical stress. This approach makes both good common and scientific sense.

Yet, in today's society it is the norm to be taking some sort of drug or pill, ranging from regular antioxidant vitamin supplements to the more dangerous (and potentially lethal) legally prescribed drugs. My best advice for antioxidant vitamins is to avoid synthetics and rely on a balanced, nutritious diet with lots of fresh fruits and vegetables.

However, many people will not listen to this advice, even when their life depends on it.

In 2000, William A Pryor stated that, "**About one half of American cardiologists take supplemental vitamin E,** about the same number as take aspirin." I believe that will be changing.

Many Antioxidants Are Not Well Absorbed

Generally, processed foods contain fewer antioxidants than fresh and uncooked foods, since the preparation processes may expose the food to oxygen. (Henry and Heppell, 2002).

Many other antioxidants are not vitamins and are made in the body. For example, ubiquinol (coenzyme Q) is poorly absorbed from the gut and is made in humans through the mevalonate pathway. (Turnen et al, 2004). Polyphenols are poorly absorbed.

Also, there is glutathione, which is made from amino acids. As any glutathione in the gut is broken down to free cysteine, glycine and glutamic acid before being absorbed, even large oral doses have little effect on the concentration of glutathione in the body. (Witsche et al, 1992) (Flagg et al, 1994).

Although large amounts of sulfur-containing amino acids such as acetylcysteine can increase glutathione, no evidence exists that eating high levels of these glutathione precursors is beneficial for healthy adults. (van de Poll et al, 2006).

Maternal diet influences cord plasma levels of beta-carotene and vitamin C, but not vitamins A and E

The aim of the present study was to test the hypothesis that **maternal intake of antioxidant vitamins is associated with maternal and cord plasma levels at delivery. Women were recruited in early pregnancy** in Aberdeen Maternity Hospital and habitual diet during pregnancy was assessed by a food-frequency questionnaire mailed at 34 weeks gestation. Blood samples were taken at recruitment (n 1,149) and maternal (n 1,149) and cord blood samples (n 747) taken at delivery for analyses of **vitamins A, C, E and beta-carotene. Maternal plasma levels of vitamin E and beta-carotene at delivery were significantly higher than levels in early pregnancy while levels of vitamins A and C were significantly lower**. Positive correlations were observed for maternal levels of all the vitamins between early pregnancy and delivery. **At delivery, maternal plasma concentrations of vitamins A, E and beta-carotene were significantly higher than cord levels, while maternal levels of vitamin C were significantly lower**. There were significant correlations between maternal and cord plasma concentrations for beta-carotene and vitamin C but not for vitamins A or E. Maternal dietary intakes were positively correlated with maternal plasma levels of vitamins C, E and beta-carotene in early pregnancy, with maternal plasma levels of beta-carotene and vitamin C at delivery and with cord plasma levels of beta-carotene and vitamin C. The results from the present study show that, in this population, **maternal diet influences cord plasma levels of beta-carotene and vitamin C, but not vitamins A and E** (Scaife et al, 2006). **I believe that if the mother is getting excess antioxidants, so is the developing fetus and this can produce an EMOD insufficiency in the baby and allow for early disease manifestation, including asthma and allergies. Oxidation is essential as a signaling mechanism for gene activation and inactivation in the developing fetus.**

There is a powerful source of influence you may not have considered: your life as a fetus. The nutrition you received in the womb; the antioxidants, pollutants, drugs and infections you were exposed to during gestation; your mother's health and state of mind while she was pregnant with you - all these factors shaped you as a baby and continue to affect you to this day.

This is the provocative contention of a field known as "fetal origins," whose pioneers assert that the nine months of gestation constitute the most consequential period of our lives, permanently influencing the wiring of the brain and the functioning of organs such as the heart, liver and pancreas. There are references to the fetal origins of cancer, cardiovascular disease, allergies, asthma, hypertension, diabetes, obesity, mental illness.

I believe that antioxidants are going to figure prominently, and perhaps dangerously, in fetal origins. If mercury, ingested by the mother, can potentially cause autism and brain damage, what might antioxidants be responsible for, including autism and brain damage?

Antioxidant Status In Vegetarians Versus Omnivores

Every day, vegetarians consume many carbohydrate-rich plant foods such as fruits and vegetables, cereals, pulses, and nuts. As a consequence, **their diet contains more antioxidant vitamins (vitamin C, vitamin E, and beta-carotene) and copper than that of omnivores. Intake of zinc is generally comparable to that by omnivores.** However, **the bioavailability of zinc in vegetarian diets is generally lower than that of omnivores**. Dietary intake of selenium is variable in both groups and depends on the selenium content of the soil. **Measurements of antioxidant body levels in vegetarians show that a vegetarian diet maintains higher antioxidant vitamin status (vitamin C, vitamin E, beta-carotene)** but variable antioxidant trace element status as compared with an omnivorous diet. To evaluate the antioxidative potential of a vegetarian diet versus an omnivorous diet, more studies are needed in which the total antioxidant capacity is determined rather than the status of a single antioxidant nutrient (Rauma and Mykkanen, 2000).

Beta-carotene, vitamins C and E, zinc and selenium levels are influenced by sex, age, diet, smoking status, alcohol consumption and corpulence in adults.

Investigators assessed relationships between energy, nutrient and food intakes, alcohol consumption, smoking status and body mass index (BMI), and serum concentrations of beta-carotene, alpha-tocopherol, vitamin C, selenium and zinc.

METHODS: Data on health status, alcohol consumption, smoking habits, anthropometric data and biochemical measurements were obtained in **1,821 women aged 35-60 y and 1,307 men aged 45-60 y, participant to the SU.VI.MAX Study**. Data on dietary intake were available on a subsample who reported six 24-h dietary records during the first 18 months of the study.

RESULTS: **Women had higher baseline serum beta-carotene and vitamin C concentrations and lower concentration for serum vitamin E, zinc and selenium than men.**

In women, younger age was associated with lowered mean concentration of serum beta-carotene, vitamin E and selenium.

In men, only differences were observed for serum zinc, which was lower in older men. **Current smokers of both sexes had significantly lower concentrations of serum beta-carotene, vitamin C and selenium, and, only in women, of vitamin E, than nonsmokers.**

Alcohol consumers had lower concentrations of serum beta-carotene and higher selenium concentrations.

Serum beta-carotene and vitamin C concentrations were lower in obese subjects. There were positive associations of dietary beta-carotene, vitamin C and E with their serum concentrations. Age, nutrient and alcohol intakes, serum cholesterol, BMI and smoking status explained 15.2% of the variance of serum beta-carotene in men and 13.9% in women, and 10.8 and 10.0% for serum vitamin C, and 26.3 and 28.6% for serum vitamin E, respectively.

Conclusion: Serum antioxidant nutrient concentrations are primarily influenced by sex, age, obesity, tobacco smoking, alcohol consumption and especially dietary intake of those antioxidant nutrients (Galan et al, 2005).

Estimation of Antioxidant Intakes from Diet and Supplements in U.S. Adults:

These authors state that, "The importance of antioxidants in reducing risks of chronic diseases has been well established **(RMH Note:**

I disagree.); however, antioxidant intakes by a free-living population have not yet been estimated adequately." In this study, they aimed to estimate total antioxidant intakes from diets and supplement sources in the U.S. population. The USDA Flavonoid Database, food consumption data, and dietary supplement use data of 8809 U.S. adults aged 19 y and over in NHANES 1999–2000 and 2001–2002 were used in this study. Daily total antioxidant intake was **208 mg vitamin C** (46 and 54% from diets and supplements, respectively), **20 mg alpha-tocopherol** (36 and 64), **223 µg retinol activity equivalents carotenes** (86 and 14), **122 µg selenium** (89 and 11), and **210 mg flavonoids** (98 and 2). Antioxidant intakes differed among socio-demographic subgroups and lifestyle behaviors. Energy-adjusted dietary antioxidant intakes were higher in women, older adults, Caucasians, nonconsumers of alcohol (only for vitamin C and carotenes), nonsmokers (only for vitamin C, vitamin E, and carotenes), and in those with a higher income and exercise level (except for flavonoids) than in their counterparts ($P < 0.05$). **Consumption of fruits, vegetables, and whole grains may be a good strategy to increase antioxidant intake.** (Ock et al, 2010).

Prenatal Vitamins May Be Unnecessary And Dangerous

There is a little known danger to prenatal vitamins that goes largely unaddressed. This danger is with over doses of vitamin A. While it is a necessary vitamin for the proper development of the fetus, vitamin A can be extremely toxic in large doses and can cause major birth defects and liver toxicity as well as fetal death. Shockingly, many prenatal vitamins contain two, three, and sometimes four times what the government considers safe levels of the vitamin. During pregnancy, you only need about 2,500 IUs of vitamin A. Check your prenatals and make sure that they contain no more than 8,000 to 10,000 IUs of vitamin A but do not cut healthy foods such as carrots, eggs, and meat out of your diet.

Do not take prenatal vitamins "just in case," as this is unwise, as long as your intake of the B vitamins is adequate and you have no other deficiencies. Usually, prenatal vitamins are similar to other multivitamins except that they contain higher levels of folic acid, calcium and iron.

Fat-soluble vitamins A, D, E and K are stored in your liver and body fat, where, according to the American Pregnancy Association, toxic side effects of excess intake can begin to wreak havoc on you and your baby. Reportedly, water soluble vitamins such as C and B can be flushed from your body when taken in excess, but may lead to irritation of your digestive system.

The National Institutes of Health Office of Dietary Supplements warns that most dietary supplements have not been thoroughly tested for safety in pregnant women, nursing mothers or children. Discuss any prenatal vitamins you are taking or thinking about taking with your doctor.

Please remember that folic acid is the synthetic form of folate, a member of the family of B vitamins that is involved in regulating DNA synthesis and gene expression. Because of these crucial functions, folate plays an important role in fetal development - **folate is essential during pregnancy, especially early on in pregnancy, for the prevention of neural tube defects**. Folate is abundant in green vegetables like spinach, collards, bok choy, artichokes, and broccoli. Synthetic folic acid is not the same as getting it from vegetables.

The Shocking News With Folic Acid (contained in prenatal vitamins and multivitamins)

Observational studies provide only circumstantial evidence and credible evidence is obtained only by way of controlled trials.

Scientific studies have exposed the significant dangers to women and their children, from taking folic acid supplements:

Women who followed the typical recommendations to take folic acid during pregnancy and were followed by researchers for thirty years were twice as likely to die from breast cancer. (Charles et al, 2004).

Another study following women for ten years concluded that **those who took multivitamins containing folic acid increased their breast cancer risk by 20-30%.** (Stolzenberg-Solomen et al, 2006).

227

Folic acid in supplement form may contribute to producing a cancer-promoting environment in the body – in addition to breast cancer, **synthetic folic acid has been linked to dramatic increases in prostate and colorectal cancers, as well as overall cancer incidence.** (Fife et al, 2009) (Hirsch et al, 2009) (Figueiredo et al, 2009).

Folic acid supplementation by pregnant women has been associated with increased incidence of childhood asthma, infant respiratory tract infections, and cardiac birth defects. (Whitrow, 2009) (Haberg et al, 2009).

Last November, a study by researchers from Haukeland University Hospital in Bergen, Norway, found that patients with heart disease had an increased risk of cancer and death from any cause if they had received treatment with folic acid and vitamin B12. The findings are especially revealing because foods are not fortified with folic acid in Norway (unlike in countries including the US, where flour and grain products contain added folic acid to reduce birth defects).

Folic Acid Has Antioxidant Activity

The free radical scavenging properties and possible antioxidant activity of folic acid are reported. Pulse radiolysis technique is employed to study the one-electron oxidation of folic acid in homogeneous aqueous solution. The radicals used for this study are CCl_3O_2 (*), N_3(*), SO_4(*-), Br_2(*-), *OH, and O(*-). All these radicals react with folic acid under ambient condition at an almost diffusion-controlled rate producing two types of transients. Considering the chemical structure of folic acid, the absorption maximum at 430 nm has been assigned to a phenoxyl radical. The latter one is proposed to be a delocalized molecular radical. A permanent product has been observed in the oxidation of folic acid with CCl_3O_2(*) and N_3(*) radicals, with a broad absorption band around 370-400 nm. Folic acid is seen to scavenge these radicals very efficiently. In the reaction of thiyl radicals with folic acid, it has been observed that folic acid can not only scavenge thiyl radicals but can also repair these thiols at physiological pH. While carrying out the lipid peroxidation study, in spite of the fact that folic acid is considerably soluble in water,

we observed a significant inhibition property in microsomal lipid peroxidation. A suitable mechanism for oxidation of folic acid and repair of thiyl radicals by folic acid has been proposed (Joshi et al, 2001).

Safety Measures You Need To Practice:

- Think about what you are taking and why you are taking it. First, you should have a need to take an antioxidant vitamin, such as a verified vitamin deficiency or a metabolic problem which prevents you from absorbing or metabolizing vitamins. Otherwise, do not take synthetic antioxidant vitamins.
- Consider adverse interactions with other medicines or supplements that you are taking. When in doubt, consult your doctor or pharmacist (not a salesperson in a supplement store or a representative for supplement marketers or manufacturers).
- Be very careful concerning exaggerated claims on the internet, television or printed media regarding antioxidant vitamins.
- Look for the "USP Verified" mark. It indicates that the supplement manufacturer has voluntarily asked U.S. Pharmacopeia, a trusted nonprofit, private standards-setting authority, to verify the quality, purity, and potency of its raw ingredients or finished products. USP maintains a list of verified products on its website.
- Do not assume more is better. It is possible to overdose even on beneficial vitamins and minerals. Avoid any product that is claimed to contain "megadoses." Hypervitaminosis is a serious problem. Do not over supplement because many common food products are "antioxidant fortified."
- Report problems
  Let your doctor know if you experience any symptoms after you start taking a supplement. And if you end up with a serious side effect, ask your doctor or pharmacist to report it to the FDA, or do it yourself at *www.fda.gov/medwatch* or by calling 800-332-1088.

- Research in the right places
  Be skeptical about claims made for supplements in ads, on TV, and by sales staff. If a claim sounds too good to be true, it probably is. Instead, try these sources:
- The National Institutes of Health's Office of Dietary Supplements.
- The FDA, for alerts, advisories, and other actions.
- Consumer Reports Health's dietary supplements and natural health products information.

Please remember that three of the largest randomized, controlled trials (Alpha tocopherol, beta carotene trial, Beta carotene and retinol efficacy trial and Selenium and vitamin E cancer prevention trial) were shut down almost 21 months early by investigators because it would have been unethical and unwise to continue these studies in which harmful adverse effects were obviously endangering and harming participants.

$$H_2O_2WES' \quad H^1O_2LY \quad GR^1\Delta_gIL$$

I believe that the grail is oxygen and its various electronically modified derivatives.

My Parting Shot

Certainly, there are studies concluding that antioxidant vitamins and supplemental antioxidants may cure, prevent, or treat many diseases and aging. However, these studies lack consistency. In short, antioxidants have not been reliably or scientifically proven to cure, prevent or treat any disease or aging....NOT EVEN ONE!

Even the highly touted antioxidant loaded fruit and vegetables are being shown to make little difference in reducing your risk of developing cancer. The December 2010 issue of the British Journal of Cancer and work published in April, 2010 in the Journal of the National Cancer Institute, found that eating a lot of fruit and vegetables has only "a very modest" protective effect against cancer. That conclusion was

based on a decade of research on almost 500,000 people in 10 European countries.

For lung cancer, recent large prospective analyses with detailed adjustment for smoking have not shown a convincing association between fruit and vegetable intake and reduced risk. For other common cancers, including colorectal, breast and prostate cancer, epidemiological studies suggest little or no association between total fruit and vegetable consumption and risk.

My opponents, like some at the Pauling Institute, may argue that my studies "ignore the broad totality of evidence that comes to largely opposite conclusions," but that was an old, unsupported and untimely argument. Just read my books.

Also, please remember that our bodies need a limited supply of antioxidants to donate electrons to oxygen and thus bolster our prooxidant defenses. Ergo, I refer to antioxidants at these levels as being "pre-oxidants or co-oxidants."

The human body is a miraculous mixture of a biochemical gumbo. Prooxidants and a continually functional oxidative system protect us from pathogens, cancer and other diseases. The potential for disease manifestation is always there and if EMODs reach an insufficiency level, disease will appear. Resistance to diseases seems to decrease as our antioxidant burden increases. Reduced immunity and resistance can be seen with chronic granulomatous disease, AIDS, chronic steroid use, etc.

There appears to be a tripping point, which can be triggered by over dosing on antioxidants. We are currently participating in the largest global experiment in history by ingesting ever increasing quantities of antioxidants. Since there is profit involved, manufacturers are aggressively pushing sales of all things considered to be antioxidants.

Our bodies have to struggle to accommodate for these antioxidant over loads on a daily basis and the petro-chemical antioxidants, introduced in our food and our environment, last much longer than the natural ones found in fruits and vegetables. These antioxidants disrupt the natural oxidative chemistry of the body and make us more vulnerable to infections and cancer.

Hence, I look at it as death, a day at a time. It is slow and insidious....a day at a time.

The food industry strives for foods that look attractive, taste good and resist spoilage. Profit is the bottom line and health considerations are way down the priority list. Over 3,000 food additives are in the food we consume today and many of these are antioxidants. Our bodies are acting as chemical depositories or petro-chemical antioxidant waste bins.

For half a century, brominated oils have been added to fruit juice to maintain a long standing look of freshness but they have serious side effects, such as changes in heart tissue, enlargement of the thyroid, kidney damage and changes in the liver and testicles. Canada, Holland and Germany have banned brominated oils from bottled drinks but they can still be imported from other countries.

Regulations are slow and enforcement is even slower.

Heaven only knows the effects these additives can be having on a developing human fetus. We can not compromise safety for the sake of having an appealing look or good taste for our food and drink products.

You must be thinking, "How can all of this be true?," since we are living longer than ever and many people appear to be in good health. Remember, as you are aware, our bodies are miraculous and it has a keen ability to compensate for adversity but only up to certain limits. Yes, we now have antibiotics, insulin and effective surgical procedures to help us live longer but if we augment our prooxidant systems, we may live even longer and healthier lives.

We need to try to limit and avoid over loading on things that have been scientifically proven to be harmful, such as antioxidants.

Currently, our processed foods have antioxidants, preservatives, chemical flavors, buffers, hydrolyzers, hydrogenators, alkalizers, acidifiers, modifiers, emulsifiers, stabilizers, thickeners, clarifiers, disinfectants, anti-foaming agents, anti-caking agents and thousands of other additives. But, we must not let profit sacrifice safety.

The antioxidant vitamin craze was based on the free radical theory, which has been invalidated because of its repeated failures to meet the requirements of the scientific method. The old notions that EMODs are inherently deleterious and that they cause wanton damage have been proven to be blatantly wrong. In fact, they are crucial for normal metabolism. Yes, EMODs are essential.

Billions of post-mitotic cells (cells which have long lives and do not divide), such as those in the brain and heart, can survive for over a century in an EMOD-laden matrix without apparent harm. Thus, how toxic can EMODs be? EMODs are ubiquitous and omnipresent. Ergo, how toxic can EMODS be?

I have arduously and selectively accumulated over 250 studies showing the ineffectiveness and the harmful potential of the common antioxidant vitamins A, C and E. Multivitamins and many other antioxidant supplements are increasingly being scrutinized for safety.

We can neither deny this data nor should we ignore it.

Let me see if I can hit the nail on the head. My entire book is about human healthcare and the possibility that antioxidant overload or over burden can diminish our protective levels of EMODs, thus, allowing the manifestation of a wide range of diseases. This likely represent a huge, "preventable" source or cause for disease, pain and suffering. So, what are we going to do about it? Nothing?

The worst thing we can do is NOTHING, whereby ignorance prevails! In the end, science-based evidence must rule. Be informed and then decide if you wish to take supplemental antioxidants or if you wish to give them to your loved ones.

I liken antioxidant use to playing Russian roulette or smoking cigarettes, in that I definitely do not recommend either. But, if you are aware of the consequences and you chose to pull the trigger or puff away and inhale the smoke, then, so be it. The choice is yours.

This approach makes a lot of sense to me.

Stay smart and stay healthy.

REFERENCES FOR THE EDUCATED
CONSUMER - SECTION ONE

(Avenell et al. 2005) (Avenell A. et al. Effect of multivitamin and multimineral supplements on morbidity from infections in older people (MAVIS trial): Pragmatic, randomized, double blind, placebo controlled trial. BMJ 2005;331:324)

(Baader et al, 1994) (Baader, S. L., Bruchelt, G., Trautner, M. C., Boschert, H., and Niethammer, D. Uptake and cytotoxicity of ascorbic acid and dehydroascorbic acid in neuroblastoma (SK-N-SH) and neuroectodermal (SK-N-LO) cells. Anticancer Res., 14: 221–227, 1994)

(Bairati et al, 2005 Aug 20) (Bairati I, Meyer F, Gélinas M, Fortin A, Nabid A, Brochet F, Mercier JP, Têtu B, Harel F, Abdous B, Vigneault E, Vass S, Del Vecchio P, Roy J. Randomized trial of antioxidant vitamins to prevent acute adverse effects of radiation therapy in head and neck cancer patients. J Clin Oncol. 2005 Aug 20;23(24):5805-13)

(Bairati et al, 2006) (Bairati I, Meyer F, Jobin E, et al. Antioxidant vitamins supplementation and mortality: a randomized trial in head and neck cancer patients. Int J Cancer (2006) 119(9):2221–2224)

(Balla t al, 1964) (Balla, G.A., Finney, J.W., Aronoff, B.L., Byrd, D.L., Race, G.J., Mallams, J.T. and Davis, G. Use of intra-arterial hydrogen peroxide to promote wound healing: Part I: Regional intra-arterial therapy - technical surgical aspects. Part II: wound healing - clinical aspects. Amer J Surg 1964; 108: 621)

(Barbior. 1974) (Babior, B.M. Oxygen dependent microbial killing by phagocytes. N Engl J Med 1974; 298: 659-668, 721-726)

(Bardia et al, 2008) (Bardia A, Tleyjeh IM, Cerhan JR, Sood AK, Limburg PJ, Montori VM. "Efficacy of antioxidant supplementation in reducing primary cancer incidence and mortality: systematic review and meta-analysis." Mayo Clin Proc. 2008 83(1):23-34)

(Begona Ruiz-Larrea et al. 2000) (Begona Ruiz-Larrea M. et al. Antioxidant activities of estrogens against aqueous and lipophilic radicals;

differences between phenol and catechol estrogens. Chemistry and Physics of Lipids. Volume 105, Issue 2, April 2000, Pages 179-188)

(Bjelakovic et al, Cochrane Database Syst Rev. 2004) (Bjelakovic G, Nikolova D, Simonetti RG, Gluud C. Antioxidant supplements for preventing gastrointestinal cancers. Cochrane Database Syst Rev (2004) (4):CD004183)

(Bjelakovic et al, Lancet. 2004) (Bjelakovic G, Nikolova D, Simonetti RG, Gluud C. Antioxidant supplements for prevention of gastrointestinal cancers: a systematic review and meta-analysis. Lancet (2004) 364:1219–28)

(Bjelakovic et al., 2006) (Bjelakovic G, Nagorni A, Nikolova D, et al. Meta-analysis: antioxidant supplements for primary and secondary prevention of colorectal adenoma. Aliment Pharmacol Ther. 2006;24:281-91)

(Bjlakovic pp. 842-57 et al, 2007) (Bjlakovic G, Nikolova D, Gluud LL, Simonetti RG, Gluud C. "Mortality in randomized trials of antioxidant supplements for primary and secondary prevention: systematic review and meta-analysis." JAMA 2007 28;297(8):84-57)

(Bjelakovic et al, 2007) (Goran Bjelakovic, Dimitrinka Nikolova, Lise Lotte Gluud, Rosa G. Simonetti, and Christian Gluud. "Mortality in Randomized Trials of Antioxidant Supplements for Primary and Secondary Prevention; Systematic Review and Meta-analysis." JAMA 2007;297:842-857. Vol. 297 No. 8, February 28, 2007)

(Bradley et al, 1965) (Bradley, B.E., Jr., Vedros, N.A., Defalco, A.J., Lawson, D.W., Vineyard, G.C. and Urschel, H.C. The effect of intra-arterial hydrogen peroxide in rabbits infected with clostridum perfringens. J Trauma 1965; 6: 799)

(Buettner and Jurkiewicz, 1996) (Buettner GR. & Jurkiewicz BA, (1996) Catalytic metals, ascorbate and free radicals: combinations to avoid. Radiat. Res. 145, 532-541)

(Caraballoso et al., 2003) (Drugs for preventing lung cancer in healthy people. M. Caraballoso et al. Cochrane Database Syst Rev. 2003;(2):CD002141)

(Carr and Frei. 1999) (Carr A, Frei B (1 June 1999). "Does vitamin C act as a pro-oxidant under physiological conditions?". FASEB J. 13 (9): 1007–24)

(Charles et al, 2004) (Charles D et al. Taking folate in pregnancy and risk of maternal breast cancer. BMJ 2004;329:1375-6)

(Chen et al. 2005) (Chen Q, Espey MG, Krishna MC, Mitchell JB, Corpe CP, Buettner GR, Shacter E, and Levine L, Pharmacologic ascorbic acid concentrations selectively kill cancer cells: Action as a pro-drug to deliver hydrogen peroxide to tissues. PNAS. September 20, 2005. Vol. 102. No. 38. pp. 13604-13609)

(Chen et al. 2007) (Chen Q, Espey MG, Sun AY, Lee J, Krishna MC, Shacter E, Choyke P, Pooput C, Kirk KL, Buettner GR, and Levine M, Ascorbate in pharmacologic concentrations selectively generates ascorbate radical and hydrogen peroxide in extracellular fluid in vivo. PNAS. May 22, 2007. Vol. 104. No. 21. pp. 8749-8754)

(Chen et al. 2008) (Chen Q, Espey MG, Sun AY, Pooput C, Kirk KL, Krishna MC, Khosh DB, Drisko J, Levine M, Pharmacologic doses of ascorbate act as a prooxidant and decrease growth of aggressive tumor xenografts in mice. PNAS. August 12, 2008. Vol. 105. No. 32. pp. 11105-11109)

(Clark and Lambertson. 1971) (Clark, J.M., and Lambertson, C.J. Pulmonary oxygen toxicity: a review. Pharmacol Rev 1971; 23: 37-133)

(Dabbagh et al, 1997) (Dabbagh, A.J., Shwaery, G.T., Keaney, J.F. Jr. and Frei, B. Effect of iron overload and iron deficiency on atherosclerosis in the hypercholesterolemic rabbit. Arterioscler Thromb Vasc Biol 1997; 17(11): 2638-2645)

(Davidson, 1989) (Davidson, D.L.W. Hyperbaric oxygen therapy in the treatment of multiple sclerosis. Report from Action for Research into Multiple Sclerosis, London, England 1989)

(Davies et al, 2009) (Davies EC, et al. Adverse drug reactions in hospital in-patients: a prospective analysis of 3695 patient-episodes. PLoS One. 2009;4(2):e4439)

(DeChatelet. 1975) (DeChatelet, L.R. Oxidative bactericidal mechanisms of polymorphonuclear leukocytes. J Infect Dis 1975; 131: 295-303)

(De Luca, L. M. & Ross, S.A., 1996) (De Luca, L. M. & Ross, S.A. (1996) Beta-carotene increases lung cancer incidence in cigarette smokers. Nutr. Rev. 54:178-180)

(Demchenko et al, 2001) (Demchenko IT, Boso AE, Whorton AR, and Piantadosi CA. Nitric oxide production is enhanced in rat brain before oxygen-induced convulsions. Brain Res 917: 253-261, 2001)

(Demchenko et al, 2003) (Demchenko IT, Atochin DN, Boso AE, Astern J, Huang PL, and Piantadosi CA. Oxygen seizure latency and peroxynitrite formation in mice lacking neuronal or endothelial nitric oxide synthases. Neurosci Lett 344: 53-56, 2003)

(de Souza et al. 2007) (Multivitamins do not improve radiation therapy-related fatigue: results of a double-blind randomized crossover trial. de Souza et al. 2007. Am J Clin Oncol. 2007 Aug;30(4):432-6)

(Dickinson et al, 2009) (Dickinson A, Boyon N, Shao A. Physicians and nurses use and recommend dietary supplements: report of a survey. Nutr J. 2009 Jul 1;8:29)

(Dripps and Comroe. 1947) (Dripps RD and Comroe JH Jr. The effect of the inhalation of high and low oxygen concentration on respiration, pulse rate, ballistocardiogram and arterial oxygen saturation (oximeter) of normal individuals. J Physiol 149: 277-291, 1947)

(Drisko et al, 2003) (Drisko JA, Chapman J, Hunter VJ. The use of antioxidants with first-line chemotherapy in two cases of ovarian cancer. J Am Coll Nutr 2003;22:118–23)

(Duarte and Lunec. 2005) (Duarte TL, Lunec J (2005). "Review: When is an antioxidant not an antioxidant? A review of novel actions and reactions of vitamin C". Free Radic. Res. 39 (7): 671–86)

(Eckert et al, 2003) (Eckert A, et al. Effects of EGb 761 Ginkgo biloba extract on mitochondrial function and oxidative stress. Pharmacopsychiatry. 2003 Jun;36 Suppl 1:S15-23)

(Erdman et al, 2009) (Erdman JW Jr, Ford NA, Lindshield BL. Are the health attributes of lycopene related to its antioxidant function? Arch Biochem Biophys. 2009 Mar 15;483(2):229-35)

(FDA, 1995) (Food and Drug Administration. Prescription drug product labeling; medication guide requirements. *Federal Register* Vol. 60, No. 164, August 24, 1995)

(Fernandez and Russo, 2009) (Fernandez, S.V.; Russo, J. (2009). "Estrogen and Xenoestrogens in Breast Cancer". *Toxicologic Pathology* 38 (1): 110)

(Ferreira et al, 2004) (Ferreira PR, Fleck JF, Diehl A, et al. Protective effect of alpha-tocopherol in head and neck cancer radiation-induced mucositis: a double-blind randomized trial. Head Neck (2004) 26(4):313–321)

(Fife et al, 2009) (Fife, J et al. Folic Acid Supplementation and Colorectal Cancer Risk; A Meta-analysis. Colorectal Dis. 2009 Oct 27. [Epub ahead of print])

(Figueiredo et al, 2009) (Figueiredo JC et al. Folic acid and risk of prostate cancer: results from a randomized clinical trial. J Natl Cancer Inst. 2009 Mar 18;101(6):432-5)

(Finney et al, 1961) (Finney, J.W., Collier, R.E., Balla, G.A., Tomme, J.W., Wakley, J., Race, G.J., Urschel, H.C., D'Errico, A.D. and Mallams, J.T. The preferential localization of radioisotopes in malignant tissue by regional oxygenation. Nature 1961; 202: 1172)

(Finney et al, 1965) (Finney, J.W., Balla, G.A., Collier, R.E., Wakely, J., Urschel, H.C. and Mallams, J.T. Differential localization of isotopes in tumors through the use of intra-arterial hydrogen peroxide: Part 1: Basic science. Amer J Roentgen 1965; 94: 783)

(Finney et al, 1965; 16: 62) (Finney, J.W., Balla, G.A., Mallams, J.T. and Race, G.J. Peripheral blood changes in humans and experimental animals following the infusion of hydrogen peroxide into the internal carotid artery. Angiology 1965; 16: 62)

(Finney et al, 1966) (Finney, J.W., Balla, G.A., Jay, B.E., Race, G.J., Urschel, H.C., Greenlee, R.G. and Mallams, J.T. Removal of cholesterol and other lipids from human atheromatous arteries by dilute hydrogen peroxide. Angiology 1966; 17: 223)

(Flagg et al, 1994) (Flagg EW, Coates RJ, Eley JW (1994). "Dietary glutathione intake in humans and the relationship between intake and plasma total glutathione level". Nutr Cancer 21 (1): 33–46)

(Flaire et al, 2010) (Flaire E. et al, Effect of 6 Weeks of n-3 Fatty-Acid Supplementation on Oxidative Stress in Judo Athletes. Int J Sport Nutr Exerc Metab. 2010 Dec;20(6):496-506)

(Galan et al, 2005) (Galan P,Viteri FE, Bertrais S, Czernichow S, Faure H, Arnaud J, Ruffieux D, Chenal S, Arnault N, Favier A, Roussel AM, Hercberg S. Serum concentrations of beta-carotene, vitamins C and E, zinc and selenium are influenced by sex, age, diet, smoking status, alcohol consumption and corpulence in a general French adult population. Eur J Clin Nutr. 2005 Oct;59(10):1181-90)

(Goodman et al, 2004) (Goodman GE,Thornquist MD, Balmes J, Cullen MR, Meyskens Jr. FL, Omenn GS, et al. The Beta-Carotene and Retinol Efficacy Trial: Incidence of Lung Cancer and Cardiovascular Disease Mortality During 6-Year Follow-up After Stopping Beta-Carotene and Retinol Supplements. J Natl Cancer Inst 2004;96:1743-50)

(Gottlieb and Neubauer. 1988) (Gottlieb, S.R. and Neubauer, R.A. Multiple sclerosis: its etiology, pathogenesis, and therapeutics with emphasis on the controversial use of HBO. J Hyper Med 1988; 5: 143-164)

(Gottlieb. 1989) (Gottlieb, S.F. Proposed criteria for evaluating disease entities for inclusion in accepted indications category for hyperbaric oxygen treatment. J Hyper Med 1989; 4: 33-37)

(Haberg et al, 2009) (Haberg SE et al, Folic acid supplements in pregnancy and early childhood respiratory health. Arch Dis Child. 2009 Mar;94(3):180-4)

(Hail N, Cortes M, Drake EN, Spallholz JE, 2008) (Hail N, Cortes M, Drake EN, Spallholz JE (July 2008)."Cancer chemoprevention: a radical perspective". Free Radic. Biol. Med. 45 (2): 97–110)

(Halliwell, 1990) (Halliwell B, (1990) "How to characterize a biological antioxidant", Free Radical Res. Commun. 9, 1-32)

(Han et al, 2001) (Han H,Wang H, Long H, Nattel S,Wang Z. Oxidative preconditioning and apoptosis in L-cells. Roles of protein kinase B and mitogen-activated protein kinases. J Biol Chem. 2001;276:26357–26364)

(Heinonen et al, 1994) (Heinonen, O.P., J.K. Huttunen, D. Albanes & ATBC cancer prevention study group. 1994. The effect of vitamin E and beta carotene on the incidence of lung cancer and other cancers in male smokers. N. Engl. J. Med. 330:1029-1035)

(Henderson and Fingar. 1987) (Henderson, B.W. and Fingar, V.H. Relationship of tumor hypoxia and response to photodynamic treatment in an experimental mouse model. Cancer Res 1987; 47: 3110-3114)

(Henry and Heppell, 2002) (Henry C, Heppell N 2002. Nutritional losses and gains during processing: future problems and issues. Proc Nutr Soc 61;1:145-8)

(Hirose et al, 1998) (Hirose M, et al. Carcinogenicity of antioxidants BHA, caffeic acid, sesamol, 4-methoxyphenol and catechol at low doses, either alone or in combination, and modulation of their effects in a rat medium-term multi-organ carcinogenesis model. Carcinogenesis. 1998 Jan;19(1):207-12)

(Hirsch et al, 2009) (Hirsch S et al. Colon cancer in Chile before and after the start of the flour fortification program with folic acid. Eur J Gastroenterol Hepatol. 2009 Apr;21(4):436-9)

(Hohn. 1977) (Hohn, D.C. Oxygen and leukocyte microbial killing. Davis, J.C., Hunt, T.K. Eds. Hyperbaric Oxygen Therapy, Bethesday, Undersea Med Soc 1977; 101-110)

(Howes, 2004) (Howes, R. M. U.T.O.P.I.A. - Unified Theory of Oxygen Participation in Aerobiosis. © 2004. Free Radical Publishing Co. Kentwood, LA, available at www.iwillfindthecure.org.)

(Howes, 2005) (R.M. Howes. The Medical and Scientific Significance of Oxygen Free Radical Metabolism © Free Radical Publishing. 2005; 934 pages. available at: www.iwillfindthecure.org)

(Howes RM: "The Free Radical Fantasy," 2006) (Howes RM: "The Free Radical Fantasy," The Annals of New York Academy of Sciences, 2006, Vol. 1067, pp. 22-26)

(Howes RM. Hydrogen Peroxide Monograph. 2006) (R.M. Howes. Hydrogen Peroxide Monograph 1: Scientific, Medical and Biochemical Overview. Free Radical Publishing. © 2006; 200 pages. available at: www.iwillfindthecure.org)

(Howes RM. A, C & E: Equivocal Scientific Studies. 2006) (Howes RM. Hydrogen Peroxide Monograph. 2006) (R.M. Howes. Monograph 2: Antioxidant vitamins A, C & E: Equivocal Scientific Studies, Free Radical Publishing. © 2006; 171 pages. available at: www.iwillfindthecure. org)

(Howes, Cardiovascular Disease. 2006) (R. M. Howes. Cardiovascular Disease and Oxygen Free Radical Mythology, Free Radical Publishing. © 2006; 308 pages. available at: www.iwillfindthecure.org)

(Howes, Diabetes. 2006) (R. M. Howes. Diabetes and Oxygen Free Radical Sophistry, Free Radical Publishing. © 2006; 366 pages. available at: www.iwillfindthecure.org)

(Howes RM. 2007) (Howes RM, 2007. The Consequent Downfall of the Free Radical Theory. HILICA.COM Article number 75. Published on 22nd January, 2007)

(Howes, Cancer, Apoptosis. 2007) (R.M. Howes M.D., PhD., 2007. Cancer, Apoptosis and Reactive Oxygen Species: A New Paradigm. PHILICA.COM Article number 86. Published on 26th February, 2007)

(Howes, Death. 2007) (R.M. Howes M.D., PhD., 2007. Antioxidant Vitamins A, C & E; Death in Small Doses and Legal Liability? PHILICA. COM Article number 89. Published on 5th April, 2007)

(Howes, Harm. 2007) (R.M. Howes M.D., PhD., 2007. Antioxidant Vitamins A, C and E: Assessing Potential for Harm PHILICA.COM Article number 83. Published on 15th February, 2007)

(Howes, 2008) (R. M. Howes. Reactive Oxygen Species Insufficiency (ROSI) as the Basis for Disease Allowance and Coexistence: Extraordinary Support for an Extraordinary Theory. Free Radical Publishing. Vol I, II & III. © 2008; 1564 pages. available at: www.iwillfindthecure.org)

(Howes, Philica. Feb 7, 2009) (Howes M.D., PhD., R. (2009). Dangers of Antioxidants in Cancer Patients: A Review. PHILICA.COM Article number 153. Published 7th February, 2009)

(Howes R : Cancer Therapy, 2010) (Howes R : Cancer Therapy: A Review with Scientific Validation for the Role of Electronically Modified Oxygen Derivatives in Oncologic Treatment Modalities. The Internet Journal of Alternative Medicine. 2010 Volume 8 Number 1)

(Howes R : Hydrogen Peroxide: 2010) (Howes R : Hydrogen Peroxide: A review of a scientifically verifiable omnipresent ubiquitous essentiality of obligate, aerobic, carbon-based life forms. The Internet Journal of Plastic Surgery. 2010 Volume 7 Number 1)

(Howes RM. Death in Small Doses: Book One, 2010) (Howes RM. Death in Small Doses: Antioxidant Vitamins A, C & E in the 21st Century. Book One: A Health Impact Statement For The Layman. Trafford Publishing, Indianapolis, Indiana. 2010)

(Howes RM. Death in Small Doses: Book Two, 2010) (Howes RM. Antioxidant Vitamins are Making A Killing; Antioxidant Vitamins A, C & E in the 21st Century. Book Two: A Health Impact Statement For The Medical Scientist. Trafford Publishing, Indianapolis, Indiana. 2010)

(Howes RM. Reactive Oxygen Species vs. Antioxidants: 2010) (R.M. Howes. Reactive Oxygen Species vs. Antioxidants: "The Oxypocalypse" or "The war that never was" Free Radical Publishing. © 2010; 550 pages. available at: www.iwillfindthecure.org)

(Hu and Kitts, 2000) (Hu C, Kitts DD. Studies on the antioxidant activity of Echinacea root extract. J Agric Food Chem. 2000 May;48(5): 1466-72)

(Hunt and van Winkle. 1976) (Hunt, T.K. and van Winkle, W. Wound healing: normal repair. In Dunphy, J.E. (ed): Fundamental of Wound Management in Surgery. South Plainfield, New Jersey: Chirurgecom, Inc., 1976; pp. 1-68)

(Hunt. 1979) (Hunt, T.K. Disorders of repair and their management. In Hunt T.K. and Dunphy J.E. (Eds): Fundamentals of Wound Management. New York: Appleton-Century-Crofts, 1979; pp. 68-168)

(Hunt et al, 1969) (Hunt, T.K., Zederfeldt, B. and Goldstick, T.K. Oxygen and healing. Am J Surg 1969; 118: 521-525)

(Ito and Hirose, 1989) (Ito N, Hirose M. Antioxidants—carcinogenic and chemopreventive properties. Adv Cancer Res. 1989;53:247-302)

Prof Randolph M. Howes MD, PhD

(Jackson et al. 2006) (Jackson IL. et al. ROS production and angiogenic regulation by macrophages in response to heat therapy. Int J Hyperthermia. 2006 Jun;22(4):263-73).

(Jang JH, Surh YJ. 2001) (Jang JH , Surh YJ. Protective effects of resveratrol on hydrogen peroxide-induced apoptosis in rat pheochromocytoma (PC12) cells. Mutat Res (2001) 496: 181-90)

(Jason et al, 1998) (Jason Lazarou, MSc; Bruce H. Pomeranz, MD, PhD; Paul N. Corey, PhD. Incidence of Adverse Drug Reactions in Hospitalized Patients. JAMA 1998; 279: 1200-05)

(Jayalakshmi and Sharma, 1986) (Jayalakshmi CP, Sharma JD. Effect of butylated hydroxyanisole (BHA) and butylated hydroxytoluene (BHT) on rat erythrocytes. Environ Res. 1986 Oct;41(1):235-8)

(Jenkins et al, 2009) (Jenkins, S.; Raghuraman, N.; Eltoum, I.; Carpenter, M.; Russo, J.; Lamartiniere, C. A. (2009). "Oral Exposure to Bisphenol a Increases Dimethylbenzanthracene-Induced Mammary Cancer in Rats". *Environmental Health Perspectives* 117 (6): 910–915)

(Joshi et al, 2001) (Joshi R, Ashikari S, Patro BS, Chattopadhyay S, Mukherjee T. Free radical scavenging behavior of folic acid: evidence for possible antioxidant activity. Free Radic Biol Med. 2001 Jun 15;30(12):1390-9)

(Kahl and Kappus. 1993) (Toxicology of the synthetic antioxidants BHA and BHT in comparison with the natural antioxidant vitamin E. Kahl R, Kappus H, Z *Lebensm Unters Forsch* 1993 Apr;196(4):329-38)

(Kudchodkar et al, 2000) (Kudchodkar, B.J., Wilson, J., Lacko, A. and Dory, L. Hyperbaric oxygen reduces the progression and accelerates the regression of atherosclerosis in rabbits. Arterioscler Thromb Vasc Biol 2000; 20(6): 1637-1643)

(Langemann et al, 1989) (Langemann, H., Torhorst, J., Kabiersch, A., Krenger, W., and Honegger, C. G. Quantitative determination of water- and lipid-soluble antioxidants in neoplastic and non-neoplastic human breast tissue. Int. J. Cancer, 43: 1169–1173, 1989)

(Lapensee et al, 2010) (Lapensee, E. W.; Lapensee, C. R.; Fox, S.; Schwemberger, S.; Afton, S.; Ben-Jonathan, N. (2010). "Bisphenol a and estradiol are equipotent in antagonizing cisplatin-induced cytotoxicity in breast cancer cells". *Cancer Letters* 290 (2): 167)

244

(Lawenda et al, 2008) (Lawenda BD, Kelly KM, Ladas EJ, Sagar SM, Vickers A, Blumberg JB. "Should supplemental antioxidant administration be avoided during chemotherapy and radiation therapy?" J Natl Cancer Inst. 2008 4;100(11):773-83)

(Lesperance et al, 2002) (Lesperance ML, Olivotto IA, Forde N, et al. Mega-dose vitamins and minerals in the treatment of non-metastatic breast cancer: an historical cohort study. Breast Cancer Res Treat (2002) 76(2):137–143)

(Levine et al. 2008) (Levine M, Espey MG, and Chen Q, Losing and finding a way at C: New promise for pharmacologic ascorbate in cancer treatment. Free Radical Biology & Medicine. 47 (2008) pp. 27-29)

(Lippman et al, 2009) (Effect of selenium and vitamin E on risk of prostate cancer and other cancers: the Selenium and Vitamin E Cancer Prevention Trial (SELECT). Lippman, SM. JAMA. 2009 Jan 7;301(1):39-51. Epub 2008 Dec 9)

(Madhavi et al, 1996) (Butylated hydroxyanisole (BHA; *tert*-butyl-4-hydroxyanisole) and Butylated hydroxytoluene (BHT; 2,6-di-*tert*-butyl-p-cresol) in *Food Antioxidants: Technological, Toxicological, and Health Perspectives*. Edited by DL Madhavi, SS Deshpande, and DK Salunkhe / Dekker 1996).

(Mallams et al, 1965) (Mallams, J.T., Balla, G.A. and Finney, J.W. Regional oxygenation and irradiation in the treatment of malignant tumors. Prog Clin Cancer 1965; 1: 137)

(Matsuzawa and Ichijo, 2005) (Matsuzawa A, Ichijo H. Stress-responsive protein kinases in redox-regulated apoptosis signaling. Antioxid Redox Signal. 2005;7:472–481)

(McCormick DL, Major N and Moon RC. 1984) (McCormick DL, Major N and Moon RC. Inhibition of 7,12-Dimethylbenz(a)anthracene-induced Rat Mammary Carcinogenesis by Concomitant or Postcarcinogen Antioxidant Exposure. Cancer Research 44, 2858-2863, July 1, 1984)

(Nechuta et al, 2010) (Nechuta S, Lu W, Chen Z. et el. Vitamin supplement use during breast cancer treatment and survival: a prospective cohort study. Cancer Epidemiol Biomarkers Prev. 2010 Dec 21. [Epub ahead of print])

(Neubauer et al, 1989) (Neubauer, R.A., Kagan, R.L. and Gottlieb, S.F. Use of hyperbaric oxygen for the treatment of aseptic bone necrosis. J Hyper Med 1989; 4: 69-76)

(Neuhouser et al, 2009) (Multivitamin Use and Risk of Cancer and Cardiovascular Disease in the Women's Health Initiative Cohorts. Marian L. Neuhouser et al. Arch Intern Med. 2009;169(3):294-304)

(Nichols and Lambertsen. 1969) (Nichols, C.W. and Lambertsen, C.J. Effects of high oxygen pressures on the eye. N Engl J Med 1969; 291: 25-30)

(Niinikoski et al, 1972) (Niinikoski, J., Hunt, T.K. and Zederfeldt, B. Oxygen supply in healing tissue. Am J Surg 1972; 123: 247-253)

(Nylander et al, 1985) (Nylander, G., Lewis, D., Nordstrom, H. and Larson, J. Reduction of post-ischemic edema with hyperbaric oxygen. Plast Reconstr Surg 1985: 76: 595-603)

(Ock et al, 2010) (Ock K. Chun et al. Estimation of Antioxidant Intakes from Diet and Supplements in U.S. Adults. Journal of Nutrition. Vol. 140, No. 2, 317-324, February 2010)

(Omenn et al., 1996) (Risk factors for lung cancer and for intervention effects in CARET, the Beta-Carotene and Retinol Efficacy Trial. G.S. Omenn et al. J Natl Cancer Inst. 1996 Nov 6;88(21):1550-9)

(Palmquist et al, 1984) (Palmquist, B.M., Phillipson, B. and Barr, P.O. Nuclear cataract and myopia during hyperbaric oxygen therapy. Br J Ophthalmol 1984; 68: 113-117)

(Pellati et al, 2004) (Pellati F at al. Analysis of phenolic compounds and radical scavenging activity of Echinacea spp. J Pharm Biomed Anal. 2004 Apr 16;35(2):289-301)

(Perlman et al. 2010) (Multivitamin/Mineral supplementation does not affect standardized assessment of academic performance in elementary school children. Perlman et al. 2010. J Am Diet Assoc. 2010 Jul;110(7):1089-93)

(Qaadan et al, 2010) (Qaadan F et al, Polyphenols from Ginkgo biloba. Sci Pharm. 2010 Oct 28;78(4):897-907)

(Radasekaran et al, 2007) (Radasekaran NS, et al. Human αB-Crystallin Mutation Causes Oxido-Reductive Stress and Protein Aggregation Cardiomyopathy in Mice. Cell, Volume 130, Issue 3, 427-439, 10 August 2007)

(Rauma and Mykkanen, 2000) (Rauma AL, Mykkänen H. Antioxidant status in vegetarians versus omnivores. Nutrition. 2000 Feb;16(2): 111-9)

(Rigas and Sun, 2008) (Rigas B, Sun Y. Br J Cancer. Induction of oxidative stress as a mechanism of action of chemporeventive agents against cancer. 2008 Apr 8;98(7):1157-60)

(Rock, 2007) (Rock DL. Multivitamin-mineral supplements: who uses them? Am J Clin Nutr. 2007 Jan;85(1):277S-279S)

(Rothwell et al, 2010) (Rothwell P, et al "Long-term effect of aspirin on colorectal cancer incidence and mortality: 20-year follow-up of five randomized trials" Lancet 2010)

(Safer and ak-Nughamish, 1999) (Safer AM, ak-Nughamish AJ. Hepatotoxicity induced by the anti-oxidant food additive, butylated hydroxytoluene (BHT), in rats: an electron microscopical study. Histol Histopathol. 1999 Apr;14(2):391-406)

(Scaife et al, 2006) (Scaife AR, McNeill G, Campbell DM, Martindale S, Devereux G, Seaton A. Maternal intake of antioxidant vitamins in pregnancy in relation to maternal and fetal plasma levels at delivery. Br J Nutr. 2006 Apr;95(4):771-8)

(Scholl et al, 1992) (Scholl TO, Hediger ML, Fischer RL, Shearer JW. Anemia vs iron deficiency: increased risk of preterm delivery in a prospective study. Am J Clin Nutr. 1992 May;55(5):985–8)

(Schreiner. 1974) (Schreiner, A. Hyperbaric oxygen therapy in bactericides infections. Acta Chir Scand 1974; 140: 73-76)

(Sheffield. 1985) (Sheffield, P.J. Tissue oxygen measurements with respect to soft-tissue wound healing with normobaric and hyperbaric oxygen. HBO Review 1985; 6: 18-46)

(Skyhar et al, 1986) (Skyhar, M.J., Hargens, A.R., Strauss, M.B. et al. Hyperbaric oxygen reduces edema and necrosis of skeletal muscle in compartment syndromes associated with hemorrhagic hypotension J Bone Joint Surg 1986; 68A: 1218-1224)

(Spielholz et al. 1997) (Spielholz, C., Golde, D. W., Houghton, A. N., Nualart, F., and Vera, J. C. Increased facilitated transport of dehydro-ascorbic acid without changes in sodium-dependent ascorbate transport in human melanoma cells. Cancer Res., 57: 2529–2537, 1997)

(Starfield B. 2000) (Barbara Starfield, MD, MPH, Is US Health Really the Best in the World?, JAMA, Volume 284, No. 4, July 26, 2000)

(Stohs and Bagchi. 1995) (Stohs SJ, Bagchi D (1995). "Oxidative mechanisms in the toxicity of metal ions". Free Radic. Biol. Med. 18 (2): 321–36)

(Stolzenberg-Solomen et al, 2006) (Stolzenberg-Solomon RZ et al. Folate intake, alcohol use, and postmenopausal breast cancer risk in the Prostate, Lung, Colorectal, and Ovarian Cancer Screening Trial. Am J Clin Nutr. 2006 Apr;83(4):895-904)

(Strauss et al, 1983) (Strauss, M.B., Hargens, A.R., Gershuni, D.H., Greensberg, D.A., Crenshaw, A.G., Hart, G.B. and Akeson, W.H. Reductions of skeletal muscle necrosis using intermittent hyperbaric oxygen in a model compartment syndrome. J Bone Joint Surg 1983; 65A: 656-662)

(Strauss and Hart. 1984) (Strauss, M.B. and Hart, G.B. Crush injury and the role of hyperbaric oxygen. Top Emer Med 1984; 6: 9-24)

(Strauss et al, 1986) (Strauss, M.B., Hargens, A.R., Gershuni, D.H., Hart, G.B. and Akeson, W.H. Delayed use of hyperbaric oxygen for treatment of a model anterior compartment syndrome. J Ortho Res 1986; 4: 108-111)

(Strauss. 1987) (Strauss, M.B. Refractory osteomyelitis. J Hyper Med 1987; 2: 147-159)

(Strauss and Hart. 1989) (Strauss, M.B. and Hart, G.B. Hyperbaric oxygen and the skeletal-muscle compartment syndrome. Contemp Ortho 1989; 18: 167-174)

(Sukoff and Gottlieb. 1989) (Sukoff, M.H. and Gottlieb, S.F. Hyperbaric oxygen therapy. In Nussbaum E. (Ed): Pediatric Intensive Care 2nd ed. Mount Kisco, New York: Futura Publishing Inc. 1898; 483-507)

(Tibbles and Edelsberg. 1996) (Tibbles PM and Edelsberg JS. Hyperbaric-oxygen therapy. N Engl J Med 334: 1642-1648, 1996)

(Torbati et al, 1989) (Torbati D, Mokashi A, and Lahiri S. Effects of acute hyperbaric oxygenation on respiratory control in cats. J Appl Physiol 67: 2351-2356, 1989)

(Torbati et al, 1992) (Torbati D, Church DF, Keller JM, and Pryor WA. Free radical generation in the brain precedes hyperbaric oxygen-induced convulsions. Free Radic Biol Med 13: 101-106, 1992)

(Traber, 2006) (Traber, M.G. (2006). How much vitamin E? ... Just enough! American Journal of Clinical Nutrition, 84(5), 959-960)

(Turnen et al, 2004) (Turunen M, Olsson J, Dallner G (2004). "Metabolism and function of coenzyme Q". Biochim Biophys Acta 1660 (1 – 2): 171 – 99)

(Urschel et al, 1964) (Urschel, H.C., Jr., Finney, J.W., Morales, A.R., Balla, G.A., Mallams, J.T. and Race, G.J. Myocardial protection during aortic cross clamping with hydrogen peroxide [Abstract], Circulation 1964; 30: 172)

(Urschel et al, 1965) (Urschel, H.C., Jr., Finney, J.W., Balla, G.A., Race, G.J. and Mallams, J.T. Effects of hydrogen peroxide on the cardiovascular system. In Proceedings of the Third International Conference of Hyperbaric Medicine; 1965)

(Urschel et al, 1966) (Urschel, H.C., Jr., Morales, A.R., Finney, J.W., Balla, G.A., Race, G.J. and Mallams, J.T. Cardiac Resuscitation with Hydrogen Peroxide. 1966; 2(5): 665-682)

(Valko et al, 2007) (Valko M, Leibfritz D, Moncol J, Cronin MT, Mazur M, Telser J.Free radicals and antioxidants in normal physiological functions and human disease. Int J Biochem Cell Biol. 2007;39(1):44-84)

(van de Poll et al, 2006) (van de Poll MC, Dejong CH, Soeters PB (June 2006). "Adequate range for sulfur-containing amino acids and biomarkers for their excess: lessons from enteral and parenteral nutrition". J. Nutr. 136 (6 Suppl): 1694S–1700S)

(Velicer and Ulrich, 2008) (Velicer CM, Ulrich CM.Vitamin and Mineral Supplement Use Among US Adults After Cancer Diagnosis: A Systematic Review. Journal of Clinical Oncology, Vol 26, No 4 (February 1), 2008: pp. 665-673)

(Weingart et al, 2000) (Weingart SN, Wilson RM, Gibberd RW, Harrison B. Epidemiology of medical error. BMJ 2000;320:774-777)

(Wenisch et al. 1996) (Wenisch C. et al. Mild Intraoperative Hypothermia Reduces Production of Reactive Oxygen Intermediates by Polymorphonuclear Leukocytes. Anesth Analg 1996;82:810-6)

(Wester K. et al, 2008) (Wester K. et al. Incidence of fatal adverse drug reactions: a population based study. Br J Clin Pharmacol. 2008 Apr;65(4):573-9)

(Whitrow, 2009) (Whitrow MJ. Effect of Supplemental Folic Acid in Pregnancy on Childhood Asthma: A Prospective Birth Cohort Study. Am J Epidemiol. 2009 Oct 30. [Epub ahead of print])

(Williams, K.J. and Fisher, E.A., 2005) (Williams, K.J. and Fisher, E.A. Oxidation, lipoproteins, and atherosclerosis: which is wrong, the antioxidants or the theory? Current Opinion in Clinical Nutrition & Metabolic Care. 8(2):139-146, March 2005)

(Witsche et al, 1992) (Witschi A, Reddy S, Stofer B, Lauterburg B (1992). "The systemic availability of oral glutathione". Eur J Clin Pharmacol 43 (6): 667–9)

(Yeh et al, 2009) (Yeh YC et al. A standardized extract of Ginkgo biloba suppresses doxorubicin-induced oxidative stress and p53-mediated mitochondrial apoptosis in rat testes. Br J Pharmacol. 2009 Jan;156(1):48-61)

(Zabel et al, 1996) (Zabel DD, Hopf HW, Hunt TK. The role of nitric oxide in subcutaneous and transmural gut tissue oxygenation. Shock 1996;5:341–3)

(Zhai Z et al, 2007) (Zhai Z et al. Alcohol extracts of Echinacea inhibit production of nitric oxide and tumor necrosis factor-alpha by macrophages in vitro. Food Agric Immunol. 2007 Sep;18(3-4):221-236)

CHAPTER FIFTEEN

INTRODUCTION - ALTER EGO OF ANTI-OXIDANTS

I have searched for unifying mechanisms to explain cancer and heart disease causation and prevention. I have condensed the overall data into a few basic underlying mechanisms, contingent upon their association with EMODs. Those mechanisms deal with the antioxidants and prooxidants controlling widely divergent cellular biochemical pathways. Every biochemical pathway is in some sense connected to many other pathways and I have discussed some of the pathways specifically affected by the electronically modified oxygen derivatives (EMODs) and their role in modulating normal and abnormal cellular metabolic processes.

The Howes ratiocination of EMOD insufficiency and disease allowance.

EMODs do not cause wanton destruction to cells or within cells. They are part of a highly organized and compartmentalized system. Random events have little to do with any of it, until things go wrong.

Epidemiology teaches that every statistical association has only 3 possible explanations: a) bias, b) chance, and c) cause. However, I impugn this statement and would add to this 1) partial fabrication of data, 2) unscrupulous manipulation of data and 3) completely made up data, i.e., bald-faced liars.

Most antioxidants have a prooxidant alter ego

In actuality, free radicals perform many crucial roles in normal, healthy physiological processes, such as bolstering our immune system and promoting protective oxidations. It is important to realize that **many vitamins and supplements classified as antioxidants are actually *redox agents*, meaning that they act as antioxidants in some instances and pro-oxidants in others.**

Prooxidants and antioxidants are designed to exist in alternating redox and oxidative states. This markedly increases the difficulty of intrepreting redox data and is seldom addressed in the literature or considered in formulating so-called scientific theories or arriving at accurate conclusions.

As I have said before, "Antioxidants and prooxidants are flip sides of the same redox coin."

Unfortunately, many erroneously believed that correlation equals causation but they are allowing themselves to be misled and confused.

The continued non-acceptance of the null findings of over 181 clinical trials on vitamin and antioxidant supplements, presented in my last book (Death In Small Doses?), has **no scientific basis or biochemical plausibility**.

Normal redox homeostasis **may be pathologically disturbed by overzealous use of antioxidants. We may be unconsciously overdosing on antioxidants, since they are available from such wide ranging sources.**

Paracelsus stated, "Practice should not be based on speculative theory; theory should be derived from practice. Experience is the judge; if a thing stands the test of experience, it should be accepted; if it does not stand this test, it should be rejected." **RMH Note: This**

could well refer to the situation with antioxidants and the free radical theory. In theory, they should work but in practice, they do not. Ergo, they should be summarily rejected.

A comprehensive literature review shows that antioxidant therapies have enjoyed unjustified support in preclinical studies across disparate animal models, but have shown little or no benefit in human intervention studies or clinical trials. A total reassessment of the role of antioxidant vitamins in human health is in order.

My UTOPIA and EMOD insufficiency theories present a new perspective, more correctly based on the most contemporaneous experimental findings and the most reliable clinical studies.

For example, the ideal drug to treat cancer would not only be potent and highly selective for tumors but would also be broken down quickly into harmless compounds. This is exactly the manner that my cancer therapy method utilizing singlet oxygen delivery works!

The underlying principles of the free radical theory have been proven to be unsound hundreds of times. The free radical theory has been tested and it has failed the tests hundreds of times, as evidenced by the following data in Section Two.

SECTION TWO

FOR THE MEDICAL SCIENTIST

69 additional antioxidant studies added in 2011

This is a selective systematic over view of **69 additional interventional initial or follow up studies,** showing either marginal effect, negligible effect, or no effect at all **(making a grand total of such studies now at 250).**

Twenty **additional (20)** of these studies/reports showed harmful effects of the antioxidant vitamins **A** (beta carotene), **C** (ascorbic acid) or **E** (alpha tocopherol), multivitamins or combinations thereof **(making a grand total of such studies now at 80).**

Total number of participants for all of the above 69 studies is in excess of **600,000 subjects (grand total now approaching 9 million),** some of which may have been repeats in follow up or parallel studies. **Studies with multivitamins, which contain the antioxidant vitamins, were also included.**

This 2011 list of 69 studies is arranged as follows: Paper (study) number; Title of Study or Paper; Author reference; and Chronological Year; and Number of participants or trials in the respective study, if applicable.

1) **Lack of an association between serum vitamin E and myocardial infarction in a population with**

high vitamin E levels. (Hense et al. 1993) (#4,002 men and women).

2) Blood antioxidants and indices of lipid peroxidation in subjects with angina pectoris. (Duthie et al. 1994) (#25 subjects with stable angina pectoris with 200 matched controls).

3) Dietary factors and risk of prostate cancer: a case-control study in Ontario, Canada. (Rohan et al. 1995) (#414).

4) Energy, nutrient intake and prostate cancer risk: a population-based case-control study in Sweden. (Andersson et al. 1996) (#1,062).

5) No effect of supplementation with vitamin E, ascorbic acid, or coenzyme Q10 on oxidative DNA damage estimated by 8-oxo-7,8-dihydro-2'-deoxyguanosine excretion in smokers. (Priemé et al. 1997) (#142 smoking men).

6) Vitamin E Worsens Metabolic Parameters in Type 2 Diabetics. (Skrha et al. 1997) (#12).

7) Dietary intake of antioxidant (pro)-vitamins, respiratory symptoms and pulmonary function: the MORGEN study (Grievink et al. 1998) (#6,555 adults).

8) Antioxidant nutrient intake and diabetic retinopathy: the San Luis Valley Diabetes Study. (Mayer-Davis et al. 1998) (#387 participants with type 2 diabetes).

9) Prospective association between lipid soluble antioxidants and coronary heart disease in men.

The Multiple Risk Factor Intervention Trial. (Evans et al. 1998) (#743).

10) Oral vitamin C and endothelial function in smokers: short-term improvement, but no sustained beneficial effect. (Raitakari et al. 2000) (#20 healthy young adult smokers).

11) Effects of vitamin E on chronic and acute endothelial dysfunction in smokers. (Neunteufl et al, 2000) (#22 healthy male smokers).

12) Smoking characteristics, antioxidant vitamins, and carotid artery wall thickness among life-long smokers. (de Waart et al. 2000) (#158 male life-long cardiovascular disease (CVD)-free smokers).

13) Controlled trial of alpha-tocopherol and beta-carotene supplements on stroke incidence and mortality in male smokers. (Leppala et al. 2000) (#28,519 male cigarette smokers).

14) A controlled clinical trial of vitamin E supplementation in patients with congestive heart failure (Keith et al, 2001) (#56 with advanced heart failure).

15) Antioxidants to slow aging, facts and perspectives. (STUDY) (Bonnefoy et al. 2002) (#not applicable).

16) Selenium and vitamin E supplements for prostate cancer: evidence or embellishment? (Moyad et al. 2002) (#not applicable).

17) Vitamin E in cardiovascular disease: has the die been cast? (Yusoff. K. 2002) (#not applicable).

18) **Plasma carotenoids and tocopherols and risk of myocardial infarction in a low-risk population of US male physicians. (Hak et al. 2003) (#531 physicians diagnosed with MI).**

19) **No long-term effect of combined vitamins E and C on coronary and peripheral endothelial function (Kinlay et al. 2004) (#not applicable).**

20) **Age-related cataract in a randomized trial of beta-carotene in women. (Christen et al. 2004) (#39,876).**

21) **A review of the epidemiological evidence for the 'antioxidant hypothesis'. (The British Nutrition Foundation was recently commissioned by the Food Standards Agency) (an independent review of the scientific literature on the role of antioxidants in chronic disease prevention) (Stanner et al. 2004) (#not applicable).**

22) **Fruit, vegetable, and antioxidant intake and all-cause, cancer, and cardiovascular disease mortality in a community-dwelling population in Washington County, Maryland (CLUE) (Genkinger et al. 2004) (#6,151).**

23) **Vitamin E and beta-carotene supplementation and hospital-treated pneumonia incidence in male smokers. (Hemila et al, 2004) (#29,133 men aged 50 to 69 years, who smoked at least five cigarettes per day).**

24) **Early Infant Multivitamin Supplementation Is Associated With Increased Risk for Food Allergy and Asthma (Milner et al. 2004) (#over 8,000).**

25) Effects of vitamins C and E on oxidative stress markers and endothelial function in patients with systemic lupus erythematosus: a double blind, placebo controlled pilot study. (Tam et al. 2005) (#39 patients with SLE).

26) Antioxidants for preventing pre-eclampsia. (Rumbold et al, Apr 18, 2005. CD004072) (#35,812 women and 37,353 pregnancies).

27) Vitamin E in the primary prevention of cardiovascular disease and cancer: the Women's Health Study: a randomized controlled trial. (Lee et al. 2005) (#39,876 healthy women)

28) Vitamin E supplementation in pregnancy. (Rumbold et al, Apr 18, 2005. CD004072) (#566 women).

29) Antioxidant vitamin supplementation in the prevention of cardiovascular disease (they are not recommended). (Yuen et al. 2005).

30) Vitamin E in the primary prevention of cardiovascular disease and cancer: the Women's Health Study: a randomized controlled trial. (Lee et al. 2005) (#39,876 healthy women)

31) Effect of multivitamin and multimineral supplements on morbidity from infections in older people (MAVIS trial) (Avenell et al. 2005) (910 men and women 65 or over)

32) Dietary supplementation with different vitamin C doses: no effect on oxidative DNA damage in healthy people. (Herbert et al. 2006) (#160 volunteers).

33) Carotenoids and cardiovascular health American Journal of Clinical Nutrition (not recommended). (Voutilainen et al. 2006) (#not applicable).

34) Vitamins C and E and the risks of pre-eclampsia and perinatal complications (Rumbold et al, 2006) (1,877 randomly assigned).

35) Beta carotene supplementation and age-related maculopathy in a randomized trial of US physicians (Christen et al. 2007) (#22,071 apparently healthy US male physicians).

36) Atherosclerosis and oxidant stress: the end of the road for antioxidant vitamin treatment? (Thomson et al. 2007) (#not applicable).

37) Effects of antioxidant supplementation on the aging process. (Fusco et al. 2007) (#not applicable).

38) Effect of high-dose alpha-tocopherol supplementation on biomarkers of oxidative stress and inflammation and carotid atherosclerosis in patients with coronary artery disease. (Devaraj et al. 2007) (#90 patients with CAD).

39) Multivitamins do not improve radiation therapy-related fatigue: results of a double-blind randomized crossover trial. (de Souza et al. 2007) (randomized 40 patients to either placebo or Centrum Silver).

40) Combined vitamin C and E supplementation during pregnancy for preeclampsia prevention: a systematic review (Polyzos et al, 2007)

(randomized 4680 pregnant women to either the combination of vitamin C and vitamin E or placebo).

41) Antioxidant therapy to prevent pre-eclampsia: a randomized controlled trial (Spinnato et al. 2007) (707 of 739 randomly assigned patients).

42) The effect of vitamin E on blood pressure in individuals with type 2 diabetes: a randomized, double-blind, placebo-controlled trial (Ward et al, 2007) (#58 with type 2 diabetes randomized).

43) National Institutes of Health State-of-the-Science Conference Statement: Multivitamin/Mineral Supplements and Chronic Disease Prevention (NIH State-of-the Science Panel. 2007).

44) High maternal plasma antioxidant concentrations associated with preterm delivery. (Joshi et al. 2008) (#140 normotensive pregnant women).

45) Vitamin E and age-related cataract in a randomized trial of women. (Christen et al. 2008) (#39,876).

46) Antioxidants in cardiovascular health and disease: key lessons from epidemiologic studies. (Icox et al. 2008) (#not applicable).

47) Observational studies on the effect of dietary antioxidants on asthma: a meta-analysis. (Gao et al. 2008) (#13,653).

48) Dietary antioxidants and the long-term incidence of age-related macular degeneration: the Blue Mountains Eye Study (Tan et al. 2008) (#Of 3,654 baseline (1992-1994) participants initially

49 years or older, 2,454 were reexamined after 5 years, 10 years, or both).

49) Effect of eicosapentaenoic and docosahexaenoic acid on resting and exercise-induced inflammatory and oxidative stress biomarkers: a randomized, placebo controlled, cross-over study (Bloomer et al, 2009).

50) Concentrations of antioxidant vitamins in maternal and cord serum and their effect on birth outcomes. (Wang et al. 2009) (#143 mother-neonate pairs).

51) Does antioxidant vitamin supplementation protect against muscle damage? (McGinley et al. 2009) (#not applicable).

52) WHO Vitamin C and Vitamin E trial group. World Health Organisation multicentre randomised trial of supplementation with vitamins C and E among pregnant women at high risk for pre-eclampsia in populations of low nutritional status from developing countries. (Villar et al, 2009) (#687 women).

53) Vitamin and mineral use and risk of prostate cancer: the case-control surveillance study. (Zhang et al. 2009) (#1,706 prostate cancer cases and 2,404 matched controls, total 4,111).

54) "Is the oxidative stress theory of aging dead?" (STUDY) (Pérez et al. 2009) (#not applicable).

55) The oxidative stress menace to coronary vasculature: any place for antioxidants? (Briasoulis et al. 2009) (#not applicable).

56) Oral antioxidant supplementation does not prevent acute mountain sickenss: Double blind, randomized placebo-controlled trial. (Baillie et al. 2009) (#83).

57) Total dietary antioxidant index and survival in patients with glioblastoma multiforme. (Il'yasova et al. 2009) (#814 glioblastoma multiforme cases).

58) Associations between alpha-tocopherol, beta-carotene, and retinol and prostate cancer survival (Watters et al. 2009) (#29,133).

59) Antioxidant Supplementation and Risk of Incident Melanomas. Results of a Large Prospective Cohort Study. (Asgari et al, 2009) (#69,671 men and women).

60) Antioxidants do not prevent post exercise peroxidation and may delay muscle recovery (Teixeira et al. 2009) (#20).

61) The response of gamma vitamin E to varying dosages of alpha vitamin E plus vitamin C (Guiterrez et al, 2009).

62) Vitamin E and age-related macular degeneration in a randomized trial of women. (Christen et al. 2010) (#39,876).

63) Vitamins C and E for prevention of pre-eclampsia in women with type I diabetes (DAPIT) (McCance et al. 2010) (#762 women).

64) Daily intake of antioxidants in relation to survival among adult patients diagnosed with malignant glioma. (DeLorenze et al. 2010) (#not applicable).

65) **Effects of vitamin on stroke subtypes: meta-analysis of randomized controlled trials. (Schurks et al. 2010) (#118,765).**

66) **Multivitamin/Mineral supplementation does not affect standardized assessment of academic performance in elementary school children (Perlman et al. 2010) (#students in grades three through six, approximate age range=8 to 12 years old).**

67) **Differential effects of concomitant use of vitamins C and E on trophoblast apoptosis and autophagy between normoxia and hypoxia-reoxygenation (Hung et al, 2010).**

68) **Is vitamin C supplementation beneficial? Lessons learned from randomised controlled trials (Lyddesfeldt and Poulsen, 2010).**

69) **Bioactive Dietary Polyphenols Decrease Heme Iron Absorption by Decreasing Basolateral Iron Release in Human Intestinal Caco-2 cells (Ma et al. 2010).**

Total as of 1-3-11 is the previous 181, plus the new 69, for an overall total of 250 studies showing negligible effects.

2 ANIMAL STUDIES

1. **Administration of large doses of vitamin C does not decrease oxidant-induced lung lipid peroxidation caused by bacterial-**

independent acute peritonitis Inflammation. (Demling et al. 2002).

2. Life-long vitamin C supplementation does
not affect oxidative damage or lifespan in
mice, but decreases expression of antioxidant protection genes. (Selman et al. 2006)
(MICE study).

20 STUDIES SHOWING HARMFUL EFFECTS

Italics indicates harmful adverse effects

1) Energy, nutrient intake and prostate cancer risk: a population-based case-control study in Sweden. (Andersson et al. 1996) (#1,062)

A total of **526 patients with newly diagnosed prostate cancer and 536 controls, (total 1,062) randomly** selected from the population register. *In age-adjusted analyses, there were positive associations of prostate cancer (all stages combined) risk with total energy intake as well as intake of total fat (saturated and monounsaturated), protein, retinol and zinc.* The positive association with energy intake was stronger for advanced cancer, with an excess risk of 70% for the highest quartile vs. the lowest. *After adjustment for energy intake, there was no apparent association of prostate cancers (all stages combined) with any of the investigated nutrients. However, a weak positive association between intake of retinol and advanced cancer was observed.* They concluded that our results provide some evidence that **total energy intake is a risk factor for prostate cancer**.

2) Vitamin E Worsens Metabolic Parameters in Type 2 Diabetics. (Skrha et al. 1997) (#12).

The influence of either short-term fasting or vitamin E administration on insulin action was studied in two groups of obese Type 2 diabetic patients. **Twelve patients** underwent 7 days of fasting (group A), whereas 600 mg of vitamin E was administered daily during 3 months in 9 diabetic patients (group B). Insulin action was examined by using hyperinsulinemic isoglycemic clamps (insulin infusion rate, 1.0 mU/kg/min) and insulin receptors on erythrocytes before and after respective regimens. An increase of glucose disposal rate and an increase of metabolic clearance rate of glucose were observed in group A after fasting. **On the contrary, *decreases of glucose disposal rate, metabolic clearance rate of glucose, and insulin receptor number were found after vitamin E administration as compared with pretreated values*.** A worsening of diabetes control as observed by an increase of HbA1C was present in the latter group. In summary, they found an improvement of insulin action after short-term fasting in contrast with the *worsening of metabolic parameters after vitamin E administration in obese Type 2 diabetic patients*.

3) Dietary intake of antioxidant (pro)-vitamins, respiratory symptoms and pulmonary function: the MORGEN study (Grievink et al. 1998) (#6,555 adults)

A study was undertaken to investigate the relationships between the intake of the antioxidant (pro)-vitamins C, E and beta-carotene and the presence of respiratory symptoms and lung function. METHODS: Complete data were collected in a cross sectional study in a random sample of the Dutch population on **6,555 adults** during 1994 and 1995. Antioxidant intake was assessed by a semi-quantitative food frequency questionnaire and respiratory symptoms (cough, phlegm, productive cough, wheeze, shortness of breath) were assessed by a self-administered questionnaire. Prevalence odds ratios for symptoms were calculated using logistic regression analysis. Linear regression analysis was used for forced expiratory volume in one second (FEV1) and forced vital capacity (FVC). The results are presented as a comparison between the 90th and 10th percentiles of antioxidant intake. RESULTS: **Vitamin C intake was not associated with most symptoms but was inversely related with cough**. Subjects with a high intake of vitamin C had a 53 ml higher FEV1 and 79 ml higher FVC than those with a low vitamin C intake. *Vitamin E intake showed no association with most symptoms and lung function, but had a positive association with productive cough. The intake of beta-carotene was not associated with most symptoms but had a positive association*

Prof Randolph M. Howes MD, PhD

with wheeze. However, subjects with a high intake of beta-caro-tene had a 60 ml higher FEV1 and 75 ml higher FVC than those with a low intake of beta-carotene.

CONCLUSIONS: The results of this study suggest that **a high in-take of vitamin C or beta-carotene is protective for FEV1 and FVC compared with a low intake, but not for respiratory symptoms.**

4) Antioxidant nutrient intake and diabetic retinopathy: the San Luis Valley Diabetes Study. (Mayer-Davis et al. 1998) (#387 partici-pants with type 2 diabetes). Diabetic retinopathy

(DR) is a major cause of visual impairment and blindness in adults. Antioxidant nutrients, such as vitamins C and E and beta-carotene, may be protective of some eye disorders, such as cataract and age-related macular degeneration, but a relationship between these nu-trients and DR has yet to be defined. The purpose of this study was to examine the relation between dietary and supplement intakes of vitamins C, E, and beta-carotene and the risk of DR. DESIGN: Both cross-sectional and longitudinal data were collected from participants in the San Luis Valley Diabetes Study, including non-Hispanic white and Hispanic adults in southern Colorado. PARTICIPANTS: A total of **387 participants with type 2 diabetes** completed at least 1 complete retinal examination and 24-hour dietary recall (including vi-tamin supplement use). MAIN OUTCOME MEASURES: Type 2 diabe-tes was defined according to World Health Organization criteria. DR was assessed by retinal photographs, using the Airlie House criteria to classify DR as none, background, preproliferative, or proliferative. Data for both eyes, from up to three clinic visits per participant, were used for analysis. Ordinal logistic regression analysis was used, taking advantage of multiple clinic visits by individual participants and obser-vations from both eyes, to assess the risk for increased DR severity over time as a function of changes in intake of vitamin C, vitamin E, and beta-carotene. Six categories of intake for each nutrient (first to fourth quintiles and ninth and tenth deciles) were considered to ascertain any potential threshold effect. Analyses accounted for age, duration of diabetes, insulin use, ethnicity, glycated hemoglobin, hy-

268

pertension, gender, and caloric intake. RESULTS: *An increase over time in vitamin C intake from the first to ninth deciles was associated with a risk for increased severity of Dia-betic retinopathy (DR)*, although excess risk was not observed for the tenth decile or the second through fourth quintiles compared to the first quintile. *Increased intake of vitamin E was associated with increased severity of Diabetic retinopathy (DR) among those not taking insulin.* Among those taking insulin, increased intake of beta-carotene was associated with a risk for severity of Diabetic retinopathy (DR).* CONCLUSIONS: **No protective effect was observed between antioxidant nutrients and Diabetic retinopathy (DR).** *Depending on insulin use, there appeared to be a potential for deleterious effects of nutrient antioxidants.* Further research is needed to confirm associations of nutrient antioxidant intake and DR.

5) Controlled trial of alpha-tocopherol and beta-carotene supplements on stroke incidence and mortality in male smokers. (Leppala et al. 2000) (#28,519 male cigarette smokers). Observational data suggest that diets rich in fruits and vegetables and with high serum levels of antioxidants are associated with decreased incidence and mortality of stroke. We studied the effects of alpha-tocopherol and beta-carotene supplementation. The incidence and mortality of stroke were examined in **28,519 male cigarette smokers aged 50 to 69 years without history of stroke who participated in the Alpha-Tocopherol, Beta-Carotene Cancer Prevention Study (ATBC Study).** The daily supplementation was 50 mg alpha-tocopherol, 20 mg beta-carotene, both, or placebo. The median follow-up was 6.0 years. A total of 1,057 men suffered from incident stroke: 85 men had subarachnoid hemorrhage; 112, intracerebral hemorrhage; 807, cerebral infarction; and 53, unspecified stroke. Deaths due to stroke within 3 months numbered 38, 50, 65, and 7, respectively (total 160). *alpha-Tocopherol supplementation increased the risk*

of subarachnoid hemorrhage 50% but decreased that of cerebral infarction 14%, whereas *beta-carotene supplementation increased the risk of intracerebral hemorrhage 62%. alpha-Tocopherol supplementation also increased the risk of fatal subarachnoid hemorrhage 181%.* The overall net effects of either supplementation on the incidence and mortality from total stroke were nonsignificant. *alpha-Tocopherol supplementation increases the risk of fatal hemorrhagic strokes* but prevents cerebral infarction. The effects may be due to the antiplatelet actions of alpha-tocopherol. *beta-Carotene supplementation increases the risk of intracerebral hemorrhage*, but no obvious mechanism is available. (Leppala et al. 2000).

6) Selenium and vitamin E supplements for prostate cancer: evidence or embellishment? (Moyad et al. 2002) (#not applicable).

Selenium and vitamin E are probably 2 of the most popular dietary supplements considered for use in the reduction of prostate cancer risk. This enthusiasm is reflected in the initiation of the Selenium and Vitamin E Chemoprevention Trial (SELECT). Is there sufficient evidence to support the use of these supplements in a large-scale prospective trial for patients who want to reduce the risk of prostate cancer? Results from numerous laboratory and observational studies support the use of these supplements, and data from recent prospective trials also add partial support. However, a closer analysis of the data reveals some interesting and unique associations. **Selenium supplements provided a benefit only for those individuals who had lower levels of baseline plasma selenium. *Other subjects, with normal or higher selenium levels, did not benefit and may have an increased risk for prostate cancer.*** The concept that supplements reduce prostate cancer risk only in those at a higher risk and/or those with lower plasma levels of these compounds is supported by trials examining beta-carotene supplements. Smokers may be the only individuals who benefit, as has also been shown with vitamin E supplementation. In 4 recent prospective studies, vitamin E was found to reduce the risk of prostate cancer in past/recent and current smokers and those with low levels of this vitamin. *Vitamin E supplements in higher doses (> or = 100 IU) were also associated with a higher risk of aggressive or fatal prostate cancer in nonsmokers from a past prospective study.* The dose of vitamin E in the SELECT trial (400 IU/day) is 8 times higher than what has been suggested to be effective (50 IU/day) by the largest randomized prospective trial in which the incidence rate of prostate cancer was used as an endpoint. Recent research also suggests that dietary vitamin E may be associated with a lower risk of prostate cancer than the vitamin E supplement. Additionally, **recent results from all past cardiovascular prospective, randomized trials suggest that vitamin E shows little benefit for cardiovascular disease risk, especially at the dose being used in the SELECT trial**. Other intriguing positive findings from past prospective studies of supplements suggest that aspirin and other nonsteroidal anti-inflammatory drugs have a role in reducing the risk of prostate cancer or other types of cancer (eg, colon cancer). It may be time to conduct a large costly trial to reconsider the use of selenium and vitamin E supplements for the reduction of prostate cancer risk. Some evidence for the use of these supplements exists, but **serious embellishment of study findings may be leading to an inappropriate use of these supplements in a clinical setting**.

7) Plasma carotenoids and tocopherols and risk of myocardial infarction in a low-risk population of US male physicians. (Hak et al. 2003) (#531 physicians diagnosed with MI).

One of the two available studies even suggests a higher risk for MI with higher gamma-tocopherol concentrations. Results from the prospective nested case-control Physicians' Health Study published by Hak et al. showed in a multivariate analysis that *men with high plasma gamma-tocopherol levels*

271

tended to have an increased risk of nonfatal and fatal MI - **Health's Professional Study, which included 39,910 U.S. male physicians.**

8) Early Infant Multivitamin Supplementation Is Associated With Increased Risk for Food Allergy and Asthma (Milner et al. 2004)

(#over 8,000) Dietary vitamins have potent immunomodulating effects in vitro. Individual vitamins have been shown to skew T cells toward either T-helper 1 or T-helper 2 phenotypic classes, suggesting that they may participate in inflammatory or allergic disease. With the exception of antioxidant protection, there has been little study on the effect of early vitamin supplementation on the subsequent risk for asthma and allergic disease. The objective of this study was to determine whether early vitamin supplementation during infancy affects the risk for asthma and allergic disease during early childhood. Methods. Cohort data were analyzed from the National Center for Health Statistics 1988 National Maternal-Infant Health Survey, which followed pregnant women and their newborns, and the 1991 Longitudinal Follow-up of the same patients, which measured health and disease outcomes. Patients were stratified by race and breastfeeding status. Factors that are known to be associated with alteration of risk for asthma or food allergies were identified using univariate logistic regression. Those factors were then analyzed in multivariate logistic regression models. Early vitamin supplementation was defined as vitamin use within the first 6 months. Results. There were >8000 total patients in the study. The overall incidence of asthma was 10.5% and of food allergy was 4.9%. In univariate analysis, male gender, smoker in the household, child care, prematurity (<37 weeks), being black, no history of breastfeeding, lower income, and lower education were associated with higher risk for asthma. Child care, higher levels of education, income, and history of breastfeeding were associated with a higher risk for food allergies. *In multivariate logistic analyses, a history of vitamin use within the first 6 months of life was associated with a higher risk for asthma in black infants. Early vitamin use was also associated with a higher risk for food allergies in the exclusively formula-fed population. Vitamin use at 3 years of* *age was associated with increased risk for food allergies* but not asthma in both breastfed and exclusively formula-fed infants. Conclusions. *Early vitamin supplementation is associated with increased risk for asthma in black children and food allergies in exclusively formula-fed children.* Additional study is warranted to examine which components most strongly contribute to this risk.

9) Antioxidants for preventing pre-eclampsia. (Rumbold et al, Apr 18, 2005. CD004072) (#35,812 women and 37,353 pregnancies) No

difference was seen between women taking any vitamins compared with controls for total fetal loss, early or late miscarriage or stillbirth and most of the other primary outcomes. *Women supplemented with vitamin C alone or combined with other supplements were at increased risk of giving birth preterm.* Taking vitamin supplements, alone or in combination with other vitamins, prior to pregnancy or in early pregnancy, does not prevent women experiencing miscarriage or stillbirth.

10) Vitamin E in the primary prevention of cardiovascular disease and cancer: the Women's Health Study: a randomized controlled trial. (Lee et al. 2005) (#39,876 healthy women)

Basic research provides plausible mechanisms and observational studies suggest that apparently healthy persons, who self-select for high intakes of vitamin E through diet or supplements, have decreased risks of cardiovascular disease and cancer. Randomized trials do not generally support benefits of vitamin E, but there are few trials of long duration among initially healthy persons. Objective To test whether vitamin E supplementation decreases risks of cardiovascular disease and cancer among healthy women. Design, Setting, and Participants In the Women's Health Study conducted between 1992 and 2004, **39,876 apparently healthy US women aged at least 45 years were randomly assigned to receive vitamin E or placebo and**

aspirin or placebo, using a 2 x 2 factorial design, and were followed up for an average of 10.1 years. Intervention Administration of 600 IU of natural-source vitamin E on alternate days. Main Outcome Measures Primary outcomes were a composite end point of first major cardiovascular event (nonfatal myocardial infarction, nonfatal stroke, or cardiovascular death) and total invasive cancer. Results During follow-up, there were 482 major cardiovascular events in the vitamin E group and 517 in the placebo group, a nonsignificant 7% risk reduction. There were no significant effects on the incidences of myocardial infarction or stroke, as well as ischemic or hemorrhagic stroke. For cardiovascular death, there was a significant 24% reduction. There was no significant effect on the incidences of total cancer (1437 cases in the vitamin E group and 1428 in the placebo group; or breast, lung , or colon cancers. Cancer deaths also did not differ significantly between groups. There was no significant effect of vitamin E on total mortality (636 in the vitamin E group and 615 in the placebo group). The Women's Health Study particularly focused on bleeding at multiple sites, and found no overall increased rate of bleeding **but *a small significantly increased risk for epistaxis among patients treated with vitamin E*** (relative risk 1.06 (95% confidence interval 1.01 to 1.11), P=0.02). Conclusions The data from this large trial indicated that 600 IU of natural-source vitamin E taken every other day provided no overall benefit for major cardiovascular events or cancer, did not affect total mortality, and decreased cardiovascular mortality in healthy women. These data do not support recommending vitamin E supplementation for cardiovascular disease or cancer prevention among healthy women. (Lee et al. 2005).

11) Antioxidant therapy to prevent pre-eclampsia: a randomized controlled trial (Spinnato et al. 2007) (707 of 739 randomly assigned patients)
Investigators studied whether antioxidant supplementation will reduce the incidence of pre-eclampsia among patients at increased risk. METHODS: A **randomized, placebo-controlled, double-blind clinical trial** was conducted at four Brazilian sites. Women between 12 0/7 weeks and 19 6/7 weeks of gestation and diagnosed to have chronic hypertension or a prior his-

tory of pre-eclampsia were randomly assigned to daily treatment with both vitamin C (1,000 mg) and vitamin E (400 International Units) or placebo. Analyses were adjusted for clinical site and risk group (prior preeclampsia, chronic hypertension, or both). A sample size of 734 would provide 80% power to detect a 40% reduction in the risk of pre-eclampsia, assuming a placebo group rate of 21% and alpha=.05. The alpha level for the final analysis, adjusted for interim looks, was 0.0458. RESULTS: **Outcome data for 707 of 739 randomly assigned patients revealed no significant reduction in the rate of preeclampsia,** adjusted risk ratio 0.87. **There were no differences in mean gestational age at delivery or rates of perinatal mortality, abruptio placentae, preterm delivery, and small for gestational age or low birth weight infants.** *Among patients without chronic hypertension, there was a slightly higher rate of severe pre-eclampsia in the study group.* CONCLUSION: **This trial failed to demonstrate a benefit of antioxidant supplementation in reducing the rate of pre-eclampsia among patients with chronic hypertension and/or prior pre-eclampsia.**

12) The effect of vitamin E on blood pressure in individuals with type 2 diabetes: a randomized, double-blind, placebo-controlled trial. (Ward et al, 2007) (#58).

Oxidative stress has been suggested to play a role in the development of diabetes, hypertension and vascular dysfunction. Vitamin E, a major lipid-soluble dietary antioxidant, has two major dietary forms, alpha-tocopherol and gamma-tocopherol. The potential importance of gamma-tocopherol has largely been overlooked. Our aim was to investigate the effect of alpha-tocopherol and gamma-tocopherol supplementation on 24-h ambulatory blood pressure (BP) and heart rate, vascular function and oxidative stress in individuals with type 2 diabetes. METHOD: **Fifty-eight individuals with type 2 diabetes were randomized in a double-blind, placebo-controlled trial. Participants were randomized to a daily dose of 500 mg/day RRR-alpha-tocopherol, 500 mg/day mixed tocopherols (60% gamma-**

tocopherol) or placebo for 6 weeks. Primary endpoints were 24-h ambulatory BP and heart rate, endothelium-dependent and independent vasodilation and plasma and urinary F2-isoprostanes. RESULTS: *Treatment with **alpha-tocopherol significantly increased systolic BP, diastolic BP, pulse pressure and heart rate versus placebo. Treatment with mixed tocopherols significantly increased systolic BP, diastolic BP, pulse pressure and heart rate versus placebo. Treatment with alpha-tocopherol or mixed tocopherols significantly reduced plasma F2-isoprostanes versus placebo***, but had no effect on urinary F2-isoprostanes. Endothelium-dependent and independent vasodilation was not affected by either treatment.

CONCLUSION: **In contrast to our initial hypothesis, *treatment with either alpha- or mixed tocopherols significantly increased BP, pulse pressure and heart rate in individuals with type 2 diabetes*.**

13) National Institutes of Health State-of-the-Science Conference Statement: Multivitamin/Mineral Supplements and Chronic Disease Prevention (NIH State-of-the Science Panel. 2007).

At least half of American adults take a dietary supplement, the majority of which are multivitamin/multimineral (MVM) supplements. As more and more Americans seek strategies for maintaining good health and preventing disease, and as the marketplace offers an increasing number of products to fulfill that desire, it is important that consumers have the best possible information to make their choices. Assessing the available scientific evidence on the benefits of MVM supplement use for chronic disease prevention, identifying the gaps in the evidence, and recommending an appropriate research agenda to meet the shortfalls are subjects considered in this report.

Most people assume that the ingredients in MVM supplements are safe. There is evidence, however, that certain ingredients in MVM supplements can produce adverse effects, including reports from RCTs that noted excess lung cancer occurring in asbestos workers and smokers consuming β-carotene. In addition, *esophageal cancer excess was found with long-term follow-up of older Chinese patients* (the Linxian study by Blot et al.) treated with selenium, β-carotene, and vitamin E supplements (Blot et al, 1993) (Blot WJ, Li JY, Taylor PR, Guo W, Dawsey S, Wang GQ, et al. Nutrition intervention trials in Linxian, China: supplementation with specific vitamin/mineral combinations, cancer incidence, and disease-specific mortality in the general population. J Natl Cancer Inst. 1993;85:1483–92) (NIH State-of-the Science Panel. 2007).

14) High maternal plasma antioxidant concentrations associated with preterm delivery. (Joshi et al. 2008) (#140 normotensive pregnant women). Our earlier study has shown that **increased maternal oxidative stress and reduced antioxidants like vitamin E and C play an important role in fetal growth in preeclampsia**. However, the role of antioxidants and their effects on gestation and birth outcome in normotensive pregnancies are not conclusive. The present study examined plasma malondialdehyde as a marker of oxidative stress and antioxidant concentrations (vitamins E and C) in maternal as well as in cord blood samples in normotensive women who delivered both preterm and at term. METHODS: **140 normotensive pregnant women** were recruited at Bharati Medical Hospital, Pune, India, during the year 2007. Maternal and cord samples were examined for oxidative stress levels and vitamin C and E concentrations in women who delivered preterm (n=40) and at term (n=100). Mean values were compared with those of women delivering at term using the t test. RESULTS: Increased ($p < 0.05$) oxidative stress was seen in preterm mothers as well as in cord samples. *Preterm mothers had higher vitamin C concentrations* ($p < 0.05$), **and these were positively associated with oxidative stress** ($p = 0.02$). **Vitamin E levels were comparable between groups**. CONCLUSIONS: Increased maternal circulating vitamin C concentrations and increased oxidative stress are associated with preterm delivery. **I believe that the increased vitamin C level**

in preterm (mothers) deliveries is significant and a cause of problems in the newborns.

15) Dietary antioxidants and the long-term incidence of age-related macular degeneration: the Blue Mountains Eye Study (Tan et al. 2008) (#Of 3,654 baseline (1992-1994) participants initially 49 years of older, 2,454 were reexamined after 5 years, 10 years, or both).

Investigators assessed the relationship between baseline dietary and supplement intakes of antioxidants and the long-term risk of incident age-related macular degeneration (AMD). DESIGN: Australian population-based cohort study. PARTICIPANTS: Of **3654 baseline (1992-1994) participants initially 49 years of older, 2454 were reexamined after 5 years, 10 years, or both**. METHODS: Stereoscopic retinal photographs were graded using the Wisconsin Grading System. Data on potential risk factors were collected. Energy-adjusted intakes of alpha-carotene; beta-carotene; beta-cryptoxanthin; lutein and zeaxanthin; lycopene; vitamins A, C, and E; and iron and zinc were the study factors. Discrete logistic models assessed AMD risk. Risk ratios (RRs) and 95% confidence intervals (CIs) were calculated after adjusting for age, gender, smoking, and other risk factors. MAIN OUTCOME MEASURES: Incident early, late, and any AMD. RESULTS: For dietary **lutein and zeaxanthin, participants in the top tertile of intake had a reduced risk of incident neovascular AMD**, and those with above median intakes had a reduced risk of indistinct soft or reticular drusen. For total zinc intake the RR comparing the top decile intake with the remaining population was 0.56 for any AMD and 0.54 for early AMD. The highest compared with the lowest tertile of total beta-carotene intake predicted incident neovascular AMD. Similarly, beta-carotene intake from diet alone predicted neovascular AMD. This association was evident in both ever and never smokers. Higher intakes of total vitamin E predicted late AMD. CONCLUSIONS: In this population-based cohort study, higher dietary lutein and zeaxanthin intake reduced the risk of long-term incident AMD. This study confirmed the Age-Related Eye Disease Study finding of protective influences from zinc against AMD. *Higher beta-*

carotene intake was associated with an increased risk of age-related macular degeneration (AMD).

16) Vitamins E and C in the prevention of cardiovascular disease in men: the Physicians' Health Study II randomized controlled trial (Sesso et al, 2008) (#14,641 US male physicians).

A randomized, double-blind, placebo-controlled factorial trial of vitamin E and vitamin C that began in 1997 and continued until its scheduled completion on August 31, 2007. CONCLUSIONS: In this large, long-term trial of male physicians, **neither vitamin E nor vitamin C supplementation reduced the risk of major cardiovascular events. These data provide no support for the use of these supplements (vitamins E and C) for the prevention of cardiovascular disease in middle-aged and older men. Neither vitamin E nor vitamin C had a significant effect on total mortality** but *vitamin E was associated with an increased risk of hemorrhagic stroke*.

17) Does antioxidant vitamin supplementation protect against muscle damage? (McGinley et al. 2009).

The antioxidant vitamins C (ascorbic acid) and E (tocopherol) are among the most commonly used sport supplements, and are often taken in large doses by athletes and other sportspersons because of their potential protective effect against muscle damage. Although there is some evidence to show that both antioxidants can reduce indices of oxidative stress, there is little evidence to support a role for vitamin C and/or vitamin E in protecting against muscle damage. Indeed, *antioxidant supplementation may actually interfere with the cellular signalling functions of ROS, thereby adversely affecting muscle performance. Since the potential for long-term harm does exist, the casual use of high doses of antioxidants by athletes and others should perhaps be curtailed.*

18) Vitamin and mineral use and risk of prostate cancer: the case-control surveillance study. (Zhang et al. 2009) (#1,706 prostate cancer cases and 2,404 matched controls).
Men who used zinc for ten years or more, either in a multivitamin or as a supplement, had an approximately two-fold increased risk of prostate cancer. The finding that long-term zinc intake from multivitamins or single supplements was associated with a doubling in risk of prostate cancer adds to the growing evidence for an unfavorable effect of zinc on prostate cancer carcinogenesis.

19) Effects of vitamin on stroke subtypes: meta-analysis of randomized controlled trials. (Schurks et al. 2010) (#118,765) Systematic review and meta-analysis of randomized, placebo controlled trials published until January 2010. **Data sources** Electronic databases (Medline, Embase, Cochrane Central Register of Controlled Trials) and reference lists of trial reports. **Selection criteria** Randomized, placebo controlled trials with ≥1 year of follow-up investigating the effect of vitamin E on stroke. **Review methods and data extraction** Two investigators independently assessed eligibility of identified trials. Disagreements were resolved by consensus. Two different investigators independently extracted data. Risk ratios (and 95% confidence intervals) were calculated for each trial based on the number of cases and non-cases randomized to vitamin E or placebo. Pooled effect estimates were then calculated. **Results** Nine trials investigating the effect of vitamin E on incident stroke were included, **totalling 118,765 participants (59,357 randomized to vitamin E and 59,408 to placebo).** Among those, seven trials reported data for total stroke and five trials each for hemorrhagic and ischemic stroke. Vitamin E had no effect on the risk for total stroke (pooled relative risk 0.98. In contrast, the risk for hemorrhagic stroke was increased (pooled relative risk 1.22, while the risk of ischemic stroke was reduced (pooled relative risk 0.90. There

was little evidence for heterogeneity among studies. Meta-regression did not identify blinding strategy, vitamin E dose, or morbidity status of participants as sources of heterogeneity. In terms of absolute risk, this translates into one additional hemorrhagic stroke for every 1250 individuals taking vitamin E, in contrast to one ischemic stroke prevented per 476 individuals taking vitamin E. **Conclusion** In this meta-analysis, *vitamin E increased the risk for hemorrhagic stroke by 22% and reduced the risk of ischemic stroke by 10%.* This differential risk pattern is obscured when looking at total stroke. Given the relatively small risk reduction of ischemic stroke and the generally more severe outcome of hemorrhagic stroke, *indiscriminate widespread use of vitamin E should be cautioned against.*

20) Differential effects of concomitant use of vitamins C and E on trophoblast apoptosis and autophagy between normoxia and hypoxia-reoxygenation

Concomitant supplementation of vitamins C and E during pregnancy has been reportedly associated with low birth weight, the premature rupture of membranes and fetal loss or perinatal death in women at risk for preeclampsia; however, the cause is unknown. They surmise that hypoxia-reoxygenation (HR) within the intervillous space due to abnormal placentation is the mechanism and hypothesize that concomitant administration of aforementioned vitamin antioxidants detrimentally affects trophoblast cells during HR. METHODOLOGY/ PRINCIPAL FINDINGS: Using villous explants, concomitant administration of 50 microM of vitamins C and E was observed to reduce apoptotic and autophagic changes in the trophoblast layer at normoxia (8% oxygen) but to cause more prominent apoptosis and autophagy during HR. Furthermore, increased levels of Bcl-2 and Bcl-xL in association with a decrease in the autophagy-related protein LC3-II were noted in cytotrophoblastic cells treated with vitamins C and E under standard culture conditions. In contrast, vitamin treatment decreased Bcl-2 and Bcl-xL as well as increased mitochondrial Bak and cytosolic LC3-II in cytotrophoblasts subjected to HR.

CONCLUSIONS/SIGNIFICANCE: **Our results indicate that concomitant administration of vitamins C and E has differential effects on the changes of apoptosis, autophagy and the expression of Bcl-2 family of proteins in the trophoblasts between normoxia and HR.** *These changes may probably lead to the impairment of placental function and suboptimal growth of the fetus* (Hung et al, 2010).

Note: This study is included but not counted because it was referenced in *Death In Small Doses*.

Antioxidant Supplementation and Risk of Incident Melanomas. Results of a Large Prospective Cohort Study. (Asgari et al, 2009) (#69 671 men and women) Objective: To examine whether *antioxidant supplement use is associated with melanoma risk in light of recently published data from the Supplementation in Vitamins and Mineral Antioxidants (SUVIMAX) study, which reported a 4-fold higher melanoma risk in women* randomized to receive a supplement with nutritionally appropriate doses of antioxidants. This specific study did not show an increased risk for melanoma.

The previous 60 studies, plus this 20, totals 80 studies showing adverse effects as of 1-5-11

SUMMARY OF ADVERSE EFFECTS

20 ADDITIONAL Antioxidant Vitamin Studies/ Reports

STUDIES SHOWING HARMFUL AFFECTS: (SYNOPSIS)

- *In age-adjusted analyses, there were positive associations of prostate cancer (all stages combined) risk with total energy intake as well as intake of total fat (saturated and monounsaturated), protein, retinol and zinc. After adjustment for energy intake, there was no apparent association of prostate cancers (all stages combined) with any of the investigated nutrients. However, a weak positive association between intake of retinol and advanced cancer was observed.* (Andersson et al. 1996).

- *Decreases of glucose disposal rate, metabolic clearance rate of glucose, and insulin receptor number were found after vitamin E administration as compared with pretreated values. There was a worsening of metabolic parameters after vitamin E administration in obese Type 2 diabetic patients.* (Skrha et al. 1997).

- *Vitamin E intake showed no association with most symptoms and lung function, but had a positive association with productive cough. The intake of beta-carotene was not associated with most symptoms but had a positive association with wheeze.* (Grievink et al. 1998).

- *Depending on insulin use, there appeared to be a potential for deleterious effects of nutrient antioxidants. An increase over time in vitamin C intake from the first to ninth deciles was associated with a risk for increased severity of* Diabetic retinopathy (DR). *Increased intake of vitamin E was associated with increased severity of* Diabetic retinopathy (DR) *among those not taking insulin.).* *Among those taking insulin, increased intake of* beta-carotene was associated with a risk for severity of Diabetic retinopathy (DR.). (Mayer-Davis et al. 1998).

- **Alpha-Tocopherol supplementation increased the risk of subarachnoid hemorrhage 50%** but decreased that of cerebral infarction 14%, whereas **beta-carotene supplementation increased the risk of intracerebral hemorrhage 62%. alpha-Tocopherol supplementation also increased the risk of fatal subarachnoid hemorrhage 181%.** *alpha-Tocopherol supplementation increases the risk of fatal hemorrhagic strokes* but prevents cerebral infarction. *beta-Carotene supplementation increases the risk of intracerebral hemorrhage.* (Leppala et al. 2000).

- *Other subjects, with normal or higher selenium levels, did not benefit and may have an increased risk for prostate cancer. Vitamin E supplements in higher doses (> or =100 IU) were also associated with a higher risk of aggressive or fatal prostate cancer in nonsmokers from a past prospective study.* (Moyad et al. 2002).

- *Men with high plasma gamma-tocopherol levels tended to have an increased risk of nonfatal and fatal myocardial infarction (MI).* (Hak et al. 2003).

- *Early vitamin supplementation is associated with increased risk for asthma in black children and food allergies in exclusively formula-fed children* (Milner et al. 2004).

- *Women supplemented with vitamin C alone or combined with other supplements were at increased risk of giving birth preterm.* (Rumbold et al, Apr 18, 2005. CD004072).

- The Women's Health Study particularly focused on bleeding at multiple sites, and found no overall increased rate of bleeding but *a small significantly increased risk for epistaxis among patients treated with vitamin E.* (Lee et al. 2005).

- *Among patients without chronic hypertension, there was a slightly higher rate of severe pre-eclampsia in the study group.* (Spinnato et al. 2007).

- *Treatment with either alpha- or mixed tocopherols significantly increased BP, pulse pressure and heart rate in individuals with type 2 diabetes* (Ward et al, 2007).

- *esophageal cancer excess was found with long-term follow-up of older Chinese patients* (the Linxian study by Blot et al.) *treated with selenium, β-carotene, and vitamin E supplements* (Blot et al, 1993) (NIH State-of-the Science Panel. 2007).

- *Preterm mothers had higher vitamin C concentrations.* (Joshi et al. 2008).

- *Higher beta-carotene intake was associated with an increased risk of age-related macular degeneration (AMD).* (Tan et al. 2008).

- *Antioxidant supplement use is associated with melanoma risk in light of recently published data from the Supplementation in Vitamins and Mineral Antioxidants (SUVIMAX) study, which reported a 4-fold higher melanoma risk in women.* (Asgari et al, 2009) referred to data from the SUVIMAX study and not Asgari's study.

- *Antioxidant supplementation may actually interfere with the cellular signalling functions of ROS, thereby adversely affecting muscle performance. Since the potential for long-term harm does exist, the casual use of high doses of antioxidants by athletes and others should perhaps be curtailed.* (McGinley et al. 2009).

- *Men who used zinc for ten years or more, either in a multivitamin or as a supplement, had an approximately two-fold increased risk of prostate cancer. The finding that long-term zinc intake from multivitamins or single supplements was associated with a doubling in risk of prostate cancer adds to the growing evidence for an unfavorable effect of zinc on prostate cancer carcinogenesis.* (Zhang et al. 2009).

- *The estimated probability of being diagnosed with prostate cancer over a 10-year period was 9.7% in the folic acid group and 3.3% in the placebo group.* (Figueiredo et al, 2009).

- *Vitamin E increased the risk for hemorrhagic stroke by 22%* and reduced the risk of ischemic stroke by 10%. *(indiscriminate widespread use of vitamin E should be cautioned against)* (Schurks et al. 2010).

- *Concomitant supplementation of vitamins C and E during pregnancy has been reportedly associated with low birth weight, the premature rupture of membranes and fetal loss or perinatal death in women at risk for preeclampsia. These changes may probably lead to the impairment of placental function and suboptimal growth of the fetus* (Hung et al, 2010).

- *Polyphenols bind to iron in the intestinal cells, forming a non-transportable complex.* This iron-polyphenol complex cannot enter the blood stream. Instead, it is excreted in the feces when cells are sloughed off and replaced. (Ma et al. 2010).

SHORTENED VERSION OF HARMFUL EFFECTS
(20 studies):

- **Positive association between retinol, zinc and prostate cancer.** (Anderssen et al. 1996)
- **Vitamin E associated with prediabetic changes in glucose metabolism** (Skrha et al. 1997)
- **Vitamin E positively associated with productive cough. Beta carotene associated with wheezing** (Grievink et al. 1998)
- **Vitamin C associated with increased severity of diabetic retinopathy. For those taking insulin, beta carotene and vitamin E was associated with increased severity of diabetic retinopathy** (Mayer-Davis et al. 1998)
- **Alpha tocopherol increased risk of subarachnoid hemorrhage 50% and beta carotene increased risk of intracerebral hemorrhage 62% and alpha tocopherol increased risk of fatal subarachnoid hemorrhage 181%** (Leppala et al. 2000)
- **Subjects with normal or higher selenium levels may have an increased risk for prostate cancer** (Moyad et al. 2002)
- **Men with high plasma gamma-tocopherol levels had an increased risk of nonfatal and fatal myocardial infarction (MI).** (Hak et al. 2003)
- **Early vitamin supplementation (multivitamins) is associated with increased risk for asthma in black children and food allergies in exclusively formula-fed children** (Milner et al. 2004)
- **Women supplemented with vitamin C alone or combined with other supplements were at increased risk of giving birth preterm.** (Rumbold et al, Apr 18, 2005. CD004072)
- **Vitamin E increased the risk of epistaxis** (Lee et al. 2005)
- **Among patients without chronic hypertension, there was a slightly higher rate of severe preeclampsia in the study (vitamin C and E) group.** (Spinnato et al. 2007)

- **Treatment with either alpha- or mixed tocopherols significantly increased BP, pulse pressure and heart rate in individuals with type 2 diabetes** (Ward et al, 2007).
- **Esophageal cancer excess was found with long-term follow-up of older Chinese patients treated with selenium, β-carotene, and vitamin E supplements** (Blot et al, 1993) (NIH State-of-the Science Panel. 2007).
- **Preterm mothers had higher vitamin C concentrations.** (Joshi et al. 2008)
- **Higher beta-carotene intake was associated with an increased risk of age-related macular degeneration (AMD).** (Tan et al. 2008)
- **Antioxidant supplement use is associated with melanoma risk in light of recently published data from the Supplementation in Vitamins and Mineral Antioxidants (SUVIMAX) study, which reported a 4-fold higher melanoma risk in women.** (Asgari et al, 2009) referred to data from the SUVIMAX study and not Asgari's study.
- **Antioxidant supplementation may actually interfere with the cellular signaling functions of ROS, thereby adversely affecting muscle performance.** (McGinley et al. 2009)
- **Men who used zinc for ten years or more, either in a multivitamin or as a supplement, had an approximately two-fold increased risk of prostate cancer.** (Zhang et al. 2009)
- **Prostate cancer over a 10-year period was 9.7% in the folic acid group and 3.3% in the placebo group.** (Figueiredo et al, 2009).
- **Vitamin E increased the risk for hemorrhagic stroke by 22%** and reduced the risk of ischemic stroke by 10%. (*indiscriminate widespread use of vitamin E should be cautioned against*) (Schurks et al. 2010)
- **Concomitant supplementation of vitamins C and E during pregnancy has been reportedly associated with low birth weight, the premature rupture of membranes and fetal loss or perinatal death in**

women at risk for pre-eclampsia. These changes may probably lead to the impairment of placental function and suboptimal growth of the fetus (Hung et al, 2010).

- **Polyphenols bind to iron in the intestinal cells, forming a non-transportable complex.** This iron-polyphenol complex cannot enter the blood stream. Instead, it is excreted in the feces when cells are sloughed off and replaced (Ma et al. 2010).

Chronological list of 69 additional studies added in 2011

CIRCA 1993

Lack of an association between serum vitamin E and myocardial infarction in a population with high vitamin E levels. (Hense et al. 1993) (#4,002 men and women)

The antioxidant effects of vitamin E may protect low density lipoproteins from peroxidation and thus inhibit the development of arteriosclerosis. Inverse associations between vitamin E levels and coronary heart disease have been reported from cross-sectional and ecologic studies. In the population-based **MONICA Augsburg cohort (2023 men, 1999 women, total 4,022, age 25-64 years at baseline in 1984, 93% of whom were reexamined in 1987/88)** we investigated the relationship between serum vitamin E concentrations and the risk of subsequent myocardial infarction (MI). Between 1984 and 1991, 46 cases of fatal and non-fatal myocardial infarction from this cohort were recruited for a nested case-control study. Four controls were sampled from the cohort for each case of MI with matching for age, sex, and total cholesterol. **There were no marked differences between cases and their matched controls in the means of vitamin E concentrations**

(33.9 mumol/l vs. 32.8 mumol/l, P = 0.37) or in the mean vitamin E/total cholesterol ratios (4.89 mumol/mmol vs. 4.82 mumol/mmol, P = 0.75). The covariate adjusted relative risk (RR) for fatal plus non-fatal MI in the lowest tertile of vitamin E relative to the upper two tertiles was 0.72 (90% confidence interval: 0.33-1.57). Likewise, for the lowest tertile of the ratio (vitamin E/total cholesterol) the RR was 0.81 (0.42-1.56). The association was not modified by history of previous coronary heart disease, fatality of MI, temporal distance of MI onset from vitamin E determinations, or season.

CIRCA 1994

Blood antioxidants and indices of lipid peroxidation in subjects with angina pectoris. (Duthie et al. 1994) (#25 subjects with stable angina pectoris with 200 matched controls)

They tested the antioxidant hypothesis of coronary heart disease (CHD) by comparing blood antioxidants, indices of lipid peroxidation and classic (CHD) risk factors of 25 subjects with stable angina pectoris with 200 matched controls. Angina subjects had significantly increased plasma concentrations of total cholesterol, low density lipoproteins and triglycerides although body mass index, plasma cotinine concentration and blood pressure were similar to those of the control group. **Plasma concentrations of vitamin A, vitamin C and cholesterol- adjusted vitamin E did not differ between the groups** although **subjects with angina had significantly decreased plasma uric acid concentrations and elevated indices of lipid peroxidation.** Although the results are compatible with the antioxidant hypothesis, **it is unclear whether the increased oxidative stress in angina sufferers is a cause or consequence of the disease.**

CIRCA 1995

Dietary factors and risk of prostate cancer: a case-control study in Ontario, Canada. (Rohan et al. 1995) (#414)

The relationship between risk of prostate cancer and dietary intake of energy, fat, vitamin A, and other nutrients was investigated in a case-control study conducted in Ontario, Canada. Cases were men with a recent, histologically confirmed diagnosis of adenocarcinoma of the prostate notified to the Ontario Cancer Registry between April 1990 and April 1992. Controls were selected randomly from assessment lists maintained by the Ontario Ministry of Revenue, and were frequency-matched to the cases on age. The study included **207 cases (51.4 percent of those eligible) and 207 controls** (39.4 percent of those eligible), and information on dietary intake was collected from them by means of a quantitative diet history. There was a positive association between energy intake and risk of prostate cancer, such that men at the uppermost quartile level of energy intake had a 75 percent increase in risk. In contrast, there was no clear association between the non-energy effects of total fat and monounsaturated fat intake and prostate cancer risk. There was some evidence for an inverse association with saturated fat intake, although the dose-response pattern was irregular. There was a weak (statistically nonsignificant) positive association between polyunsaturated fat intake and risk of prostate cancer. Relatively high levels of retinol intake were associated with reduced risk, but **there was essentially no association between dietary beta-carotene intake and risk. There was no alteration in risk in association with dietary fiber, cholesterol, and vitamins C and E.** Although these patterns were evident both overall and within age-strata, and persisted after adjustment for a number of potential confounding factors, **they could reflect (in particular) the effect of nonrespondent bias**.

CIRCA 1996

Energy, nutrient intake and prostate cancer risk: a population-based case-control study in Sweden. (Andersson et al. 1996) (#1,062)

The role of diet in the etiology of prostate cancer remains unclear, because results from several case-control and cohort studies on fat intake and risk of prostate cancer have been inconsistent; few of the studies have adjusted the results for caloric intake. To examine the relationship between energy, intake of several nutrients and risk of prostate cancer (all stages combined and advanced stages separately), we conducted a population-based case-control study in Orebro County, Sweden, from 1989 through 1994. A total of **526 patients with newly diagnosed prostate cancer and 536 controls, (total 1,062) randomly** selected from the population register and frequency-matched by age, were included in the analyses. Information about dietary intake was obtained from a self-administered semi-quantitative food frequency questionnaire. Odds ratios with 95% confidence intervals were estimated by unconditional logistic regression. *In age-adjusted analyses, there were positive associations of prostate cancer (all stages combined) risk with total energy intake as well as intake of total fat (saturated and monounsaturated), protein, retinol and zinc.* The positive association with energy intake was stronger for advanced cancer, with an excess risk of 70% for the highest quartile vs. the lowest. *After adjustment for energy intake, there was no apparent association of prostate cancers (all stages combined) with any of the investigated nutrients. However, a weak positive association between intake of retinol and advanced cancer was observed.* We conclude that our results provide some evidence that **total energy intake is a risk factor for prostate cancer.**

CIRCA 1997

No effect of supplementation with vitamin E, ascorbic acid, or coenzyme Q10 on oxidative DNA damage estimated by 8-oxo-7,8-dihydro-2'-deoxyguanosine excretion in smokers. (Priemé et al. 1997) (#142 smoking men).

The protective effect of fruit and vegetables against cancer has been related to their high antioxidant content. However, **results from intervention trials have not been conclusive on the protective effect of antioxidant supplementation.** In a randomized placebo-controlled trial we investigated the effect of dietary supplementation with antioxidants on a biomarker of oxidative DNA damage with mechanistic relation to carcinogenesis. One hundred forty-two smoking men aged 35-65 y were randomly assigned to one of the following seven treatments for 2 mo: 100 mg D-alpha-tocopheryl acetate plus 250 mg slow-release ascorbic acid twice a day (n = 20), 100 mg D-alpha-tocopheryl acetate twice a day (n = 20), 250 mg ascorbic acid twice a day (n = 21), 250 mg slow-release ascorbic acid twice a day (n = 21), 30 mg coenzyme Q10 in oil three times a day (n = 20), 30 mg coenzyme Q10 as granulate three times a day (n = 20), or placebo twice a day (n = 20). The trial outcome was the urinary excretion rate of 8-oxo-7,8-dihydro-2'-deoxyguanosine (8-oxodG)-a repair product of oxidative DNA damage. **Two months of supplementation did not result in significant changes in the urinary excretion rate of 8-oxodG in any group. The lack of effect of antioxidant supplementation on the excretion rate of 8-oxodG, despite substantial increases in plasma antioxidant concentrations, agrees with the results from recent large intervention studies with cancer as an endpoint. The cancer-protective effect of fruit and vegetables seems to rely not on the effect of single antioxidants but rather on other anticarcinogenic compounds or on a concerted action of several micronutrients present in these**

foods (Priemé H, Loft S, Nyyssönen K, Salonen JT, Poulsen HE. No effect of supplementation with vitamin E, ascorbic acid, or coenzyme Q10 on oxidative DNA damage estimated by 8-oxo-7,8-dihydro-2'-deoxyguanosine excretion in smokers. Am J Clin Nutr. 1997 Feb;65(2): 503-7).

Vitamin E Worsens Metabolic Parameters in Type 2 Diabetics. (Skrha et al. 1997) (#12)

The influence of either short-term fasting or vitamin E administration on insulin action was studied in two groups of obese Type 2 diabetic patients. Twelve patients underwent 7 days of fasting (group A), whereas 600 mg of vitamin E was administered daily during 3 months in 9 diabetic patients (group B). Insulin action was examined by using hyperinsulinemic isoglycemic clamps (insulin infusion rate, 1.0 mU/kg/min) and insulin receptors on erythrocytes before and after respective regimens. An increase of glucose disposal rate and an increase of metabolic clearance rate of glucose were observed in group A after fasting. On the contrary, **decreases of glucose disposal rate, metabolic clearance rate of glucose, and insulin receptor number were found after vitamin E administration as compared with pretreated values.** A worsening of diabetes control as observed by an increase of HbA1C was present in the latter group. In summary, they found an improvement of insulin action after short-term fasting in contrast with the worsening of metabolic parameters after vitamin E administration in obese Type 2 diabetic patients.

CIRCA 1998

Dietary intake of antioxidant (pro)-vitamins, respiratory symptoms and pulmonary function: the MORGEN study (Grievink et al. 1998) (#6,555 adults)

A study was undertaken to investigate the relationships between the intake of the antioxidant (pro)-vitamins C, E and beta-carotene and the presence of respiratory symptoms and lung function. METHODS: Complete data were collected in a cross sectional study in a random sample of the Dutch population on **6555 adults** during 1994 and 1995. Antioxidant intake was assessed by a semi-quantitative food frequency questionnaire and respiratory symptoms (cough, phlegm, productive cough, wheeze, shortness of breath) were assessed by a self-administered questionnaire. Prevalence odds ratios for symptoms were calculated using logistic regression analysis. Linear regression analysis was used for forced expiratory volume in one second (FEV1) and forced vital capacity (FVC). The results are presented as a comparison between the 90th and 10th percentiles of antioxidant intake.

RESULTS: **Vitamin C intake was not associated with most symptoms but was inversely related with cough**. Subjects with a high intake of vitamin C had a 53 ml higher FEV1 and 79 ml higher FVC than those with a low vitamin C intake. *Vitamin E intake showed no association with most symptoms and lung function, but had a positive association with productive cough. The intake of beta-carotene was not associated with most symptoms but had a positive association with wheeze.* However, subjects with a high intake of beta-carotene had a 60 ml higher FEV1 and 75 ml higher FVC than those with a low intake of beta-carotene.

CONCLUSIONS: The results of this study suggest that **a high intake of vitamin C or beta-carotene is protective for FEV1 and FVC compared with a low intake, but not for respiratory symptoms**.

Antioxidant nutrient intake and diabetic retinopathy: the San Luis Valley Diabetes Study. (Mayer-Davis et al. 1998) (#387 participants with type 2 diabetes) Diabetic retinopathy (DR) is a major cause of visual impairment and blindness in adults. Antioxidant nutrients, such as vitamins C and E and beta-carotene, may be protective of some eye disorders, such as cataract and age-related macular degeneration, but a relationship between these nutrients and DR has yet to be defined. The purpose of this study was to examine the relation between dietary and supplement intakes of vitamins C, E, and

beta-carotene and the risk of DR. DESIGN: Both cross-sectional and longitudinal data were collected from participants in the San Luis Valley Diabetes Study, including non-Hispanic white and Hispanic adults in southern Colorado. PARTICIPANTS: A total of **387 participants with type 2 diabetes** completed at least 1 complete retinal examination and 24-hour dietary recall (including vitamin supplement use). MAIN OUTCOME MEASURES: Type 2 diabetes was defined according to World Health Organization criteria. DR was assessed by retinal photographs, using the Airlie House criteria to classify DR as none, background, preproliferative, or proliferative. Data for both eyes, from up to three clinic visits per participant, were used for analysis. Ordinal logistic regression analysis was used, taking advantage of multiple clinic visits by individual participants and observations from both eyes, to assess the risk for increased DR severity over time as a function of changes in intake of vitamin C, vitamin E, and beta-carotene. Six categories of intake for each nutrient (first to fourth quintiles and ninth and tenth deciles) were considered to ascertain any potential threshold effect. Analyses accounted for age, duration of diabetes, insulin use, ethnicity, glycated hemoglobin, hypertension, gender, and caloric intake. RESULTS: *An increase over time in vitamin C intake from the first to ninth deciles was associated with a risk for increased severity of Diabetic retinopathy (DR)*, although excess risk was not observed for the tenth decile or the second through fourth quintiles compared to the first quintile. *Increased intake of vitamin E was associated with increased severity of DR among those not taking insulin. Among those taking insulin, increased intake of beta-carotene was associated with a risk for severity of Diabetic retinopathy (DR).*

CONCLUSIONS: **No protective effect was observed between antioxidant nutrients and Diabetic retinopathy (DR).** *Depending on insulin use, there appeared to be a potential for deleterious effects of nutrient antioxidants.* Further research is needed to confirm associations of nutrient antioxidant intake and DR.

Prospective association between lipid soluble antioxidants and coronary heart disease in men. The Multiple Risk Factor Intervention Trial. (Evans et al. 1998) (#743)

A nested case-control study was performed using participants enrolled in the **Multiple Risk Factor Intervention Trial (MRFIT)**. The cases involved nonfatal myocardial infarction or death from coronary heart disease. Serum samples (*n* = **734**) obtained at baseline and frozen for approximately 20 years were analyzed for the antioxidants, carotenoids, retinol, and α-, γ-, and total tocopherol. The concentrations of antioxidants were in the expected range and their association with low density lipoprotein (LDL) cholesterol reflected their absorption and transport mechanisms. Among nonsmokers, the odds ratios for quartile IV versus quartile I were 1.40 (0.40–4.89), for retinol, total carotenoids, and α-, γ-, and total tocopherol, respectively. The equivalent odds ratios (95% CI) for smokers were 0.90, and 0.52, respectively. **This analysis of antioxidant concentrations by quartiles indicated no significant association of antioxidant levels with the risk of coronary disease death or nonfatal myocardial infarction.**

CIRCA 2000

Oral vitamin C and endothelial function in smokers: short-term improvement, but no sustained beneficial effect (Raitakari et al, 2000) (20 healthy young adult smokers)

Investigators tested the hypothesis that antioxidant therapy would improve endothelial function in smokers. BACKGROUND: Several studies have documented a beneficial effect of short-term oral or parenteral vitamin C on endothelial physiology in subjects with early arterial dysfunction. Possible long-term effects of vitamin C on endothelial function, however, are not known. METHODS: they studied the effects of short- and long-term oral vitamin C therapy on endothelial function in **20 healthy young adult smokers** (age 36 +/- 6 years, 8 male subjects, 21 +/- 10 pack-years). Each subject was studied at baseline, 2 h after a single dose of 2 g vitamin C and 8 weeks after taking 1 g vitamin C daily, and after placebo, in a **randomized double-blind crossover study**. Blood samples were analyzed for plasma ascorbate levels and endothelial function was measured as flow-mediated dilation of the brachial artery, using high resolution ultrasound. Nitroglycerin-mediated dilation (endothelium-independent) was also measured at each visit. RESULTS: At baseline, plasma ascorbate level was low in the smokers, increased with vitamin C therapy after 2 h to 120 +/- 54 micromol/liter (p < 0.001) and remained elevated after eight weeks of supplementation at 92 +/- 32 micromol/liter. Flow-mediated dilation, however, increased at 2 h, but **there was no sustained beneficial effect after eight weeks**. Nitroglycerin-mediated dilation was unchanged throughout. CONCLUSION: **Oral vitamin C therapy improves endothelial dysfunction in the short term in healthy young smokers, but it has no beneficial long-term effect, despite sustained elevation of plasma ascorbate levels.**

Effects of vitamin E on chronic and acute endothelial dysfunction in smokers. (Neunteufl et al, 2000) (#22 healthy male smokers).

The aims of this study were to determine whether chronic or acute impairment of flow mediated vasodilation (FMD) in the brachial artery of smokers can be restored or preserved by the antioxidant vitamin E. BACKGROUND: Transient impairment of endothelial function after heavy cigarette smoking and chronic endothelial dysfunction in smokers result at least in part from increased oxidative stress. METHODS: We studied **22 healthy male smokers** (mean +/- SD, 23 +/- 9 cigarettes per day) randomly assigned to receive either 600 IU vitamin E per day (n = 11, age 28 +/- 6 years) or placebo (n = 11, age 27 +/- 6 years) for four weeks and 11 age-matched healthy male nonsmokers. Flow mediated vasodilation and endothelium-independent, nitroglycerin-induced dilation were assessed in the brachial artery using high resolution ultrasound (7.5 MHz) at baseline and after therapy. Subjects stopped smoking 2 h before the ultrasound examinations. At the end of the treatment period, a third scan was obtained 20 min after smoking a cigarette (0.6 mg nicotine, 7 mg tar) to estimate transient impairment of FMD. RESULTS: Flow mediated vasodilation at baseline was abnormal in the vitamin E and in the placebo group compared with nonsmoking controls. Using a two-way repeated measures analysis of variance (ANOVA) to examine the effects of vitamin E on FMD, we found no effect for the grouping factor (p = 0.5834) in the ANOVA over time but a highly significant difference with respect to time (p = 0.0065). The interaction of the time factor and the grouping factor also proved to be significant (p = 0.0318). Flow mediated vasodilation values remained similar after treatment for four weeks in both groups but declined faster after smoking a cigarette in subjects taking placebo compared with those receiving vitamin E. The transient attenuation of FMD (calculated as the percent change in FMD) was related to the improvement of the antioxidant status, estimated as percent changes in thiobarbituric acid-reactive substances. Nitroglycerin-induced dilation did not differ between study groups at baseline or after therapy. CONCLUSIONS: **These results demonstrate that oral supplementation of vitamin E can attenuate transient impairment of endothelial function after heavy smoking due to an improvement of the oxidative status but cannot restore chronic endothelial dysfunction within four weeks in healthy male smokers.**

Smoking characteristics, antioxidant vitamins, and carotid artery wall thickness among life-long smokers. (de Waart et al. 2000) (#158 male life-long cardiovascular disease (CVD)-free smokers)

They studied the associations between the common carotid-intima-media thickness (IMT), as a marker of atherosclerosis, and smoking characteristics and antioxidant vitamins among **158 male life-long cardiovascular disease (CVD)-free smokers.** An "increased" carotid IMT was defined as the upper 25%.

The prevalence of increased IMT was 2.5 times higher among smokers inhaling smoke deeply into the lungs than among moderate and non-inhalers. This association decreased when adjusted for other CVD risk factors. **Smokers with an increased carotid IMT did not differ significantly in mean antioxidant vitamin intake and status with the remaining group.** However, classical CVD risk factors contributed importantly to increased carotid IMT. In our study, depth of inhalation was the only smoking characteristic associated with carotid IMT although attenuated after adjustment for traditional risk factors for CVD. Furthermore, **in these life-long smokers not using any vitamin supplements, no associations were found for antioxidant vitamins.**

Controlled trial of alpha-tocopherol and beta-carotene supplements on stroke incidence and mortality in male smokers. (Leppala et al. 2000) (#28,519 male cigarette smokers).

Observational data suggest that diets rich in fruits and vegetables and with high serum levels of antioxidants are associated with decreased incidence and mortality of stroke. We studied the effects of alpha-tocopherol and beta-carotene supplementation. The incidence and mortality of stroke were examined in **28,519 male cigarette smokers aged 50 to 69 years without history of stroke who participated in the Alpha-Tocopherol, Beta-Carotene Cancer Prevention Study (ATBC Study).** The daily supplementation was 50 mg alpha-tocopherol, 20 mg beta-carotene, both, or placebo. The median follow-up was 6.0 years. A total of 1,057 men suffered from incident stroke: 85 men had subarachnoid hemorrhage; 112, intracerebral hemorrhage; 807, cerebral infarction; and 53, unspecified stroke. Deaths due to stroke within 3 months numbered 38, 50, 65, and 7, respectively (total 160). *alpha-Tocopherol supplementation increased the risk of subarachnoid hemorrhage 50%* but decreased that of cerebral infarction 14%, whereas *beta-carotene supplementation increased the risk of intracerebral hemorrhage 62%. alpha-Tocopherol supplementation also increased the risk of fatal sub-*

arachnoid hemorrhage 181%. The overall net effects of either supplementation on the incidence and mortality from total stroke were nonsignificant. *alpha-Tocopherol supplementation increases the risk of fatal hemorrhagic strokes* but prevents cerebral infarction. The effects may be due to the antiplatelet actions of alpha-tocopherol. *beta-Carotene supplementation increases the risk of intracerebral hemorrhage*, but no obvious mechanism is available. (Leppala et al. 2000).

CIRCA 2001

Antioxidant vitamins and prevention of cardiovascular disease: epidemiological and clinical trial data. (Marchioli et al. 2001) (#not available)

Naturally occurring antioxidants such as vitamin E, beta-carotene, and vitamin C can inhibit the oxidative modification of low density lipoproteins. This action could positively influence the atherosclerotic process and, as a consequence, the progression of coronary heart disease. A wealth of experimental studies provide a sound biological rationale for the mechanisms of action of antioxidants, whereas epidemiologic studies strongly sustain the "antioxidant hypothesis." **To date, however, clinical trials with beta-carotene supplements have been disappointing, and their use as a preventive intervention for cancer and coronary heart disease should be discouraged**. Only scanty data from clinical trials are available for vitamin C. As to vitamin E, discrepant results have been obtained by the Alpha-Tocopherol, Beta Carotene Cancer Prevention Study with a low-dose vitamin E supplementation (50 mg/d) and the Cambridge Heart Antioxidant Study (400-800 mg/d). The results of the GISSI-Prevenzione (300 mg/d) and HOPE (400 mg/d) trials suggest the absence of relevant clinical effects of vitamin E on the risk of cardiovascular events. Currently ongoing are several large-scale clinical trials that will help in clarifying the role of vitamin E in association with other antioxidants in the prevention of atherosclerotic coronary disease.

A controlled clinical trial of vitamin E supplementation in patients with congestive heart failure (Keith et al, 2001) (#56 with advanced heart failure).

Oxidative stress is increased in patients with congestive heart failure and can contribute to the progressive deterioration observed in these patients. Increased oxidative stress is the result of either an increased production of free radicals or a depletion of endogenous antioxidants, such as vitamin E. OBJECTIVE: They aimed to determine whether vitamin E supplementation of patients with advanced heart failure would modify levels of oxidative stress, thereby preventing or delaying the deterioration associated with free radical injury. DESIGN: **Fifty-six outpatients with advanced heart failure** (New York Heart Association functional class III or IV) were enrolled in **a double-blind randomized controlled trial for 12 wk.** At a baseline visit and at 2 follow-up visits, blood and breath samples were collected for the measurement of indexes of heart function and disease state, including malondialdehyde, isoprostanes, and breath pentane and ethane. Quality of life was also assessed at baseline and after 12 wk of treatment. RESULTS: Vitamin E treatment significantly increased plasma concentrations of alpha-tocopherol in the treatment group but **failed to significantly affect any other marker of oxidative stress or quality of life**. In addition, concentrations of atrial natriuretic peptide (a humoral marker of ventricular dysfunction), neurohormonal-cytokine markers of prognosis, tumor necrosis factor, epinephrine, and norepinephrine were unchanged with treatment and were not significantly different from those in the control group. CONCLUSION: **Supplementation with vitamin E did not result in any significant improvements in prognostic or functional indexes of heart failure or in the quality of life of patients with advanced heart failure.**

CIRCA 2002

Antioxidants to slow aging, facts and perspectives. (Bonnefoy et al. 2002) (#not applicable).

FREE RADICALS AND THE THEORY OF AGING: Severe oxidative stress progressively leads to cell dysfunction and ultimately cell death. Oxidative stress is defined as an imbalance between pro-oxidants and/or free radicals on the one hand, and anti-oxidizing systems on the other. The oxygen required for living may indirectly be responsible for negative effects; these deleterious effects are due to the production of free radicals, which are toxic for the cells (superoxide anions, hydroxyl radicals, peroxyl radicals, hydrogen peroxide, hydroperoxides and peroxinitrite anions). Free radical attacks are responsible for cell damage and the targeted cells are represented by the cell membranes, which are particularly rich in unsaturated fatty acids, sensitive to oxidation reactions; DNA is also the target of severe attacks by these reactive oxygen species (ROS). THE DEFENSE SYSTEMS: These are represented by the enzymes and free radical captors. The latter are readily oxidizable composites. **The free radical captor or neutralization systems of these ROS use a collection of mechanisms, vitamins (E and C), enzymes [superoxide dismutase (SOD), glutathion peroxidase (GPx) and others], and glutathion reductase (GSH), capable of neutralizing peroxinitrite.** The efficacy of this system is dependent on the genome for the enzymatic defence systems, and on nutrition for the vitamins. Some strategies aimed at reducing oxidative stress-related alterations have been performed in animals. However, **only a few can be used and are efficient in humans,** such as avoidance of unfavourable environmental conditions (radiation, dietary carcinogens, smoking...) and antioxidant dietary supplementation. DIETARY SUPPLEMENTATION: Epidemiological data suggests that antioxidants may have a beneficial effect on many age-related diseases: atherosclerosis, cancer, some neurodegenerative and ocular diseases. However, **the widespread use of supplements is hampered by several factors: the lack of prospective and controlled studies; insufficient knowledge on the pro-oxidant,**

oxidant and ant-oxidant properties of the various supplements; growing evidence that free radicals are not only by-products, but also play an important role in cell signal transduction, apoptosis and infection control. RECOMMENDATIONS: Although current data indicate that antioxidants cannot prolong maximal life span, the beneficial impact of antioxidants on various age-related degenerative diseases may forecast an improvement in life span and enhance quality of life. **The current lack of sufficient data does not permit the systematic recommendation of antioxidants.** Nevertheless, antioxidant-rich diets with fruit and vegetables should be recommended.

Selenium and vitamin E supplements for prostate cancer: evidence or embellishment? (Moyad et al. 2002) (# not available)

Selenium and vitamin E are probably 2 of the most popular dietary supplements considered for use in the reduction of prostate cancer risk. This enthusiasm is reflected in the initiation of the **Selenium and Vitamin E Chemoprevention Trial (SELECT).** Is there sufficient evidence to support the use of these supplements in a large-scale prospective trial for patients who want to reduce the risk of prostate cancer? Results from numerous laboratory and observational studies support the use of these supplements, and data from recent prospective trials also add partial support. However, a closer analysis of the data reveals some interesting and unique associations. **Selenium supplements provided a benefit only for those individuals who had lower levels of baseline plasma selenium.** *Other subjects, with normal or higher levels, did not benefit and may have an increased risk for prostate cancer.* The concept that supplements reduce prostate cancer risk only in those at a higher risk and/or those with lower plasma levels of these compounds is supported by trials examining beta-carotene supplements. Smokers may be the only individuals who benefit, as has also been shown with vitamin E supplementation. In 4 recent prospective studies, vitamin

E was found to reduce the risk of prostate cancer in past/recent and current smokers and those with low levels of this vitamin. ***Vitamin E supplements in higher doses (> or =100 IU) were also associated with a higher risk of aggressive or fatal prostate cancer in nonsmokers from a past prospective study.*** The dose of vitamin E in the SELECT trial (400 IU/day) is 8 times higher than what has been suggested to be effective (50 IU/day) by the largest randomized prospective trial in which the incidence rate of prostate cancer was used as an endpoint. Recent research also suggests that dietary vitamin E may be associated with a lower risk of prostate cancer than the vitamin E supplement. Additionally, **recent results from all past cardiovascular prospective, randomized trials suggest that vitamin E shows little benefit for cardiovascular disease risk, especially at the dose being used in the SELECT trial**. Other intriguing positive findings from past prospective studies of supplements suggest that aspirin and other nonsteroidal anti-inflammatory drugs have a role in reducing the risk of prostate cancer or other types of cancer (eg, colon cancer). It may be time to conduct a large costly trial to reconsider the use of selenium and vitamin E supplements for the reduction of prostate cancer risk. Some evidence for the use of these supplements exists, but **serious embellishment of study findings may be leading to an inappropriate use of these supplements in a clinical setting**.

Vitamin E in cardiovascular disease: has the die been cast? (Yusoff. K. 2002) (#not applicable)

Cardiovascular disease, in particular coronary artery disease (CAD), remains the most important cause of morbidity and mortality in developed countries and, in the near future, more so in the developing world. Atherosclerotic plaque formation is the underlying basis for CAD. Growth of the plaque leads to coronary stenosis, causing a progressive decrease in blood flow that results in angina pectoris. Acute myocardial infarction and unstable angina were recently recognised as related to plaque rupture, not progressive coronary stenosis. Acute thrombus formation causes an abrupt coronary occlusion. The characteristics of the fibrin cap, contents of the plaque, rheological factors and active inflammation within the plaque contribute to plaque rupture. Oxidative processes are important in plaque formation. Oxidized low density lipoproteins (LDL) but not unoxidized LDL is engulfed by resident intimal macrophages, transforming them into foam cells which develop into fatty streaks, the precursors of the atherosclerotic plaque. Inflammation is important both in plaque formation and rupture. Animal studies have shown that antioxidants reduce plaque formation and lead to plaque stabilization. In humans, high intakes of antioxidants are associated with lower incidence of CAD, despite high serum cholesterol levels. This observation suggests a role for inflammation in CAD and that reducing inflammation using antioxidants may ameliorate these processes. Men and women with high intakes of vitamin E were found to have less CAD. Vitamin E supplementation was associated with a significant reduction in myocardial infarction and cardiovascular events in the incidence of recurrent myocardial infarction. **In the hierarchy of evidence in evidence-based medicine, data from large placebo-controlled clinical trials is considered necessary. Results from various mega-trials have not shown benefits (nor adverse effects) conferred by vitamin E supplementation, suggesting that vitamin E has no role in the treatment of CAD. These results do not seem to confirm, at the clinical level, the effect of antioxidants against active inflammation during plaque rupture.** However, a closer examination of these studies showed a number of limitations, rendering them inconclusive in addressing the role of vitamin E in CAD prevention and treatment. Further studies that specifically address the issue of vitamin E in the pathogenesis of atherosclerosis and in the treatment of CAD need be performed. These studies should use the more potent antioxidant property of alpha-tocotrienol vitamin E.

CIRCA 2003

Plasma carotenoids and tocopherols and risk of myocardial infarction in a low-risk population of US male physicians. (Hak et al. 2003) (#531 physicians diagnosed with MI) One of the two available studies even suggests a higher risk for MI with higher gamma-tocopherol concentrations. Results from the prospective nested case-control Physicians' Health Study published by Hak et al. showed in a multivariate analysis that *men with high plasma γ-tocopherol levels tended to have an increased risk of nonfatal and fatal MI.* - Health's Professional Study, which included 39,910 U.S. male physicians. (*Circulation.* 2003;108:802.) Increased intake of carotenoids and vitamin E may protect against myocardial infarction (MI). However, prospective data on blood levels of carotenoids other than beta-carotene and vitamin E (tocopherol) and risk of MI are sparse. *Methods and Results*— We conducted a prospective, nested case-control analysis among male physicians without prior history of cardiovascular disease who were followed for up to 13 years in the Physicians' Health Study. Samples from **531 physicians diagnosed with MI** were analyzed together with samples from paired control subjects, matched for age and smoking, for 5 major carotenoids (alpha- and beta-carotene, beta-cryptoxanthin, lutein, and lycopene), retinol, and alpha- and gamma-tocopherol. **Overall, we found no evidence for a protective effect against MI for higher baseline plasma levels of retinol or any of the carotenoids measured.** Among current and former smokers but not among never-smokers, higher baseline plasma levels of beta-carotene tended to be associated with lower. **Men with higher plasma levels of gamma-tocopherol tended to have an increased risk of MI.** *Conclusions*— These prospective data do not support an overall protective relation between plasma carotenoids or

tocopherols and future MI risk among men without a history of prior cardiovascular disease.

CIRCA 2004

No long-term effect of combined vitamins E and C on coronary and peripheral endothelial function (Kinlay et al. 2004) (#30). They tested whether long-term administration of antioxidant vitamins C and E improves coronary and brachial artery endothelial function in patients with coronary artery disease (CAD). BACKGROUND: Endothelial function is a sensitive indicator of vascular health. Oxidant stress and oxidized low-density lipoprotein (LDL) impair endothelial function by reducing nitric oxide bioavailability in the artery wall. METHODS: They **randomly assigned 30 subjects with CAD to combined vitamin E (800 IU per day) and C (1000 mg per day)** or to placebos in a double-blind trial. Coronary artery endothelial function was measured as the change in coronary artery diameter to acetylcholine infusions (n = 18 patients), and brachial artery endothelial function was assessed by flow-mediated dilation (n = 25 patients) at baseline and six months. Plasma markers of oxidant stress (oxidized LDL and autoantibodies) were also measured.

RESULTS: Plasma alpha-tocopherol and ascorbic acid increased with active therapy. Compared to placebo, there was no improvement in coronary and brachial endothelial vasomotor function over six months. **Although vitamins C and E tended to reduce F2-isoprostanes, they failed to alter oxidized LDL or autoantibodies to oxidized LDL.** CONCLUSIONS: **Long-term oral vitamins C and E do not improve key mechanisms in the biology of atherosclerosis or endothelial dysfunction, or reduce LDL oxidation in vivo.**

Age-related cataract in a randomized trial of beta-carotene in women. (Christen et al.

2004) (#39,876). Investigators examined the development of age-related cataract in a trial of beta-carotene supplementation in women.

METHODS: The **Women's Health Study** is a randomized, double-masked, placebo-controlled trial originally designed to test the balance of benefits and risks of beta-carotene (50 mg on alternate days), vitamin E, and aspirin in the primary prevention of cancer and cardiovascular disease among **39,876 female health professionals** aged 45 years or older. The beta-carotene component of the trial was terminated early after a median treatment duration of 2.1 years. Main outcome measures were visually-significant cataract and cataract extraction, based on self-report confirmed by medical record review.

RESULTS: There were 129 cataracts in the beta-carotene group and 133 in the placebo group. For cataract extraction, there were 94 cases in the beta-carotene group and 89 cases in the placebo group. Subgroup analyses suggested a possible beneficial effect of beta-carotene in smokers. **CONCLUSIONS:** These **randomized trial data from a large population of apparently healthy female health professionals indicate that two years of beta-carotene treatment has no large beneficial or harmful effect on the development of cataract during the treatment period.**

A review of the epidemiological evidence for the 'antioxidant hypothesis'. (The British Nutrition Foundation was recently commissioned by the Food Standards Agency) (an independent review of the scientific literature on the role of antioxidants in chronic disease prevention) (Stanner et al. 2004). Although scientific rationale and observational studies have been convincing, randomized primary and secondary intervention trials have failed to show any consistent benefit from the use of antioxidant supplements on cardiovascular disease or cancer risk, with some trials even suggesting possible harm in certain subgroups. **The suggestion that antioxidant supplements can prevent chronic diseases has not been proved or consistently supported by the findings of published intervention trials.**

Fruit, vegetable, and antioxidant intake and all-cause, cancer, and cardiovascular disease mortality in a community-dwelling population in Washington County, Maryland (CLUE) (Genkinger et al. 2004) (#6,151).

Higher intake of fruits, vegetables, and antioxidants may help protect against oxidative damage, thus lowering cancer and cardiovascular disease risk. This Washington County, Maryland, prospective study examined the association of fruit, vegetable, and antioxidant intake with all-cause, cancer, and cardiovascular disease death. CLUE participants who donated a blood sample in 1974 and 1989 and completed a food frequency questionnaire in 1989 (N = 6,151) were included in the analysis. Participants were followed to date of death or January 1, 2002. Compared with those in the bottom fifth, participants in the highest fifth of fruit and vegetable intake had a lower risk of all-cause, cancer, and cardiovascular disease mortality. Higher intake of cruciferous vegetables was associated with lower risk of all-cause mortality. **No statistically significant associations were observed between dietary vitamin C, vitamin E, and beta-carotene intake and mortality.** Overall, **greater intake of fruits and vegetables was associated with lower risk of all-cause, cancer, and cardiovascular disease death.** These findings support the general health recommendation to consume multiple servings of fruits and vegetables (5-9/day).

Vitamin E and beta-carotene supplementation and hospital-treated pneumonia incidence in male smokers. (Hemila et al, 2004) (#29,133 men aged 50 to 69 years, who smoked at least five cigarettes per day)

Vitamin E and beta-carotene affect various measures of immune function and accordingly might influence the predisposition of humans to infections. However, only few controlled trials have tested this hypothesis. OBJECTIVE: To examine whether vitamin E or beta-carotene supplementation affects the risk of pneumonia in a controlled trial. DESIGN: The Alpha-Tocopherol Beta-Carotene Cancer Prevention (ATBC) study, a randomized, double-blind, placebo-controlled trial that examined the effects of vitamin E, 50 mg/d, and beta-carotene, 20 mg/d, on lung cancer using a 2 x 2 factorial design. The trial was conducted in the general community in southwestern Finland in 1985 to 1993; the intervention lasted for 6.1 years (median). The hypothesis being tested in the present study was formulated after the trial was closed. PARTICIPANTS: **ATBC study cohort of 29,133 men aged 50 to 69 years, who smoked at least five cigarettes per day**, at baseline. OUTCOME: The first occurrence of hospital-treated pneumonia was retrieved from the national hospital discharge register (898 cases). RESULTS: **Vitamin E supplementation had no overall effect on the incidence of pneumonia nor had beta-carotene supplementation.** Nevertheless, the age of smoking initiation was a highly significant modifying factor. **Among subjects who had initiated smoking at a later age** (> or =21 years; n = 7,469 with 196 pneumonia cases), **vitamin E supplementation decreased the risk of pneumonia**, whereas **beta-carotene supplementation increased the risk**. CONCLUSIONS: Data from this large controlled trial suggest that **vitamin E and beta-carotene supplementation have no overall effect on the risk of hospital-treated pneumonia in older male smokers**, but our subgroup finding that vitamin E seemed to benefit subjects who initiated smoking at a later age warrants further investigation.

Early Infant Multivitamin Supplementation Is Associated With Increased Risk for Food Allergy and Asthma (Milner et al. 2004) (#over 8,000)

Dietary vitamins have potent immunomodulating effects in vitro. Individual vitamins have been shown to skew T cells toward either T-helper 1 or T-helper 2 phenotypic classes, suggesting that they may participate in inflammatory or allergic disease. With the exception of antioxidant protection, there has been little study on the effect of early vitamin supplementation on the subsequent risk for asthma and allergic disease. The objective of this study was to determine whether early vitamin supplementation during infancy affects the risk for asthma and allergic disease during early childhood. Methods: Cohort data were analyzed from the National Center for Health Statistics 1988 National Maternal-Infant Health Survey, which followed pregnant women and their newborns, and the 1991 Longitudinal Follow-up of the same patients, which measured health and disease outcomes. Patients were stratified by race and breastfeeding status. Factors that are known to be associated with alteration of risk for asthma or food allergies were identified using univariate logistic regression. Those factors were then analyzed in multivariate logistic regression models. Early vitamin supplementation was defined as vitamin use within the first 6 months. Results. There were >8000 total patients in the study. The overall incidence of asthma was 10.5% and of food allergy was 4.9%. In univariate analysis, male gender, smoker in the household, child care, prematurity (<37 weeks), being black, no history of breastfeeding, lower income, and lower education were associated with higher risk for asthma. Child care, higher levels of education, income, and history of breastfeeding were associated with a higher risk for food allergies. *In multivariate logistic analyses, a history of vitamin use within the first 6 months of life was associated with a higher risk for asthma in black infants. Early vitamin use was also associated with a higher risk for food allergies* in the exclusively formula-fed population. *Vitamin use at 3 years of age was associated with increased risk for food allergies* but not asthma in both breastfed and exclusively formula-fed infants. Conclusions. **Early vitamin supplementation is associated with increased risk for asthma in black children and food allergies in exclusively formula-fed children.** Additional study is warranted to examine which components most strongly contribute to this risk.

CIRCA 2005

Effects of vitamins C and E on oxidative stress markers and endothelial function in patients with systemic lupus erythematosus: a double blind, placebo controlled pilot study. (Tam et al. 2005) (#39 patients with SLE).

Effects of vitamins C and E on oxidative stress markers and endothelial function in patients with systemic lupus erythematosus: a double blind, placebo controlled pilot study. Patients with systemic lupus erythematosus **(SLE) experience excess morbidity and mortality due to coronary artery disease** (CAD) that cannot be fully explained by the classical CAD risk factors. Among emerging CAD risk factors, oxidative stress is currently being emphasized. They evaluated the effects of long term antioxidant vitamins on markers of oxidative stress and antioxidant defense and endothelial function in **39 patients with SLE.** METHODS: Patients were **randomized** to receive either placebo or vitamins (**500 mg vitamin C and 800 IU vitamin E daily**) for 12 weeks. Markers of oxidative stress included malondialdehyde (MDA) and allantoin. Antioxidants measured included erythrocyte superoxide dismutase and glutathione peroxidase, plasma total antioxidant power (as FRAP value), and ascorbic acid and vitamin E concentrations. Endothelial function was assessed by flow-mediated dilatation (FMD) of the brachial artery and plasma concentration of von Willebrand factor (vWF) and plasminogen activator inhibitor type 1 (PAI-1). Primary outcome of the study included the change in lipid peroxidation as revealed by MDA levels. Secondary outcomes included changes in allantoin and antioxidant levels and change in endothelial function. RESULTS: After treatment, plasma ascorbic acid and alpha-tocopherol concentrations were significantly increased only in the vitamin-treated group, associated with a significant decrease in plasma MDA. Other oxidative stress markers and antioxidant levels remained unchanged in both groups. FMD and vWF and PAI-1 levels remained unchanged in both groups. CONCLUSION: **Combined administration of** vitamins **C** and **E** was associated with decreased lipid peroxidation, but did not affect endothelial function in patients with **SLE** after 3 months of therapy.

Antioxidants for preventing pre-eclampsia. (Rumbold et al, Apr 18, 2005. CD004072) (#35,812 women and 37,353 pregnancies) No difference was seen between women taking any vitamins compared with controls for total fetal loss, early or late miscarriage or stillbirth and most of the other primary outcomes. *Women supplemented with vitamin C alone or combined with other supplements were at increased risk of giving birth preterm.* Taking vitamin supplements, alone or in combination with other vitamins, prior to pregnancy or in early pregnancy, does not prevent women experiencing miscarriage or stillbirth.

Vitamin E supplementation in pregnancy. (Rumbold et al, Apr 18, 2005. CD004072) (#566 women). No difference was found between women supplemented with vitamin E in combination with other supplements during pregnancy compared with placebo for the risk of stillbirth, neonatal death, perinatal death, preterm birth, intrauterine growth restriction or birthweight, using fixed-effect models. **The data are too few to say if vitamin E supplementation either alone or in combination with other supplements is beneficial during pregnancy.**

Antioxidant vitamin supplementation in the prevention of cardiovascular disease (they are not recommended). (Yuen et al. 2005). Oxidative stress, in particular oxidative modification of LDL-cholesterol, appears to be of great importance in the pathogenesis of atherosclerosis. Various observational epidemiological studies have suggested that antioxidant vitamin intake is associated with reduced cardiovascular morbidity and mortality. Also, experimental studies in animals have demonstrated that antioxidant vitamins slow the progression of atherosclerosis. However, **prospective controlled clinical trials have failed to demonstrate a benefit of antioxidant vitamin supplementation in primary or secondary prevention of cardiovascular disease.** Thus, **the use of antioxidants and vitamin supplements as a preventive or therapeutic intervention can not be recommended**.

Vitamin E in the primary prevention of cardiovascular disease and cancer: the Women's Health Study: a randomized controlled trial. (Lee et al. 2005) (#39,876 healthy women)

Basic research provides plausible mechanisms and observational studies suggest that apparently healthy persons, who self-select for high intakes of vitamin E through diet or supplements, have decreased risks of cardiovascular disease and cancer. Randomized trials do not generally support benefits of vitamin E, but there are few trials of long duration among initially healthy persons. Objective: To test whether vitamin E supplementation decreases risks of cardiovascular disease and cancer among healthy women. Design, Setting, and Participants In the Women's Health Study conducted between 1992 and 2004, 39,876 apparently healthy US women aged at least 45 years were randomly assigned to receive vitamin E or placebo and aspirin or placebo, using a 2 x 2 factorial design, and were followed up for an average of 10.1 years. Intervention: Administration of 600 IU of natural-source vitamin E on alternate days. Main Outcome Measures: Primary outcomes were a composite end point of first major cardiovascular event (nonfatal myocardial infarction, nonfatal stroke, or cardiovascular death) and total invasive cancer. Results: During follow-up, there were 482 major cardiovascular events in the vitamin E group and 517 in the placebo group, a nonsignificant 7% risk reduction. **There were no significant effects on the incidences of myocardial infarction, as well as ischemic or hemorrhagic stroke. For cardiovascular** death, there was a significant 24% reduction. There was no significant effect on the incidences of total cancer (1437 cases in the vitamin E group and 1428 in the placebo group); or breast, lung, or colon cancers. Cancer deaths also did not differ significantly between groups. There was no significant effect of vitamin E on total mortality. The Women's Health Study particularly focused on bleeding at multiple sites, and found no overall increased rate of bleeding *but a small significantly increased risk for epistaxis among patients treated with vitamin E*. Conclusions The data from this large trial indicated that 600 IU of natural-source vitamin E taken every other day provided no overall benefit for major cardiovascular events or cancer, did not affect total mortality, and decreased cardiovascular mortality in healthy women. **These data do not support recommending vitamin E supplementation for cardiovascular disease or cancer prevention among healthy women.**

Effect of multivitamin and multimineral supplements on morbidity from infections in older people (MAVIS trial) (Avenell et al. 2005) (910 men and women 65 or over)

To examine whether supplementation with multivitamins and multiminerals influences self reported days of infection, use of health services, and quality of life in people aged 65 or over. **Design** Randomized, placebo controlled trial, with blinding of participants, outcome assessors, and investigators. **Setting** Communities associated with six general practices in Grampian, Scotland. **Participants 910 men and women** aged 65 or over who did not take vitamins or minerals. **Interventions** Daily multivitamin and multimineral supplementation or placebo for one year. **Main outcome measures** Primary outcomes were contacts with primary care for infections, self reported days of infection, and quality of life. Secondary outcomes included antibiotic prescriptions, hospital admissions, adverse events, and compliance. **Results** Supplementation did not significantly affect contacts with primary care and days of infection per person. Quality of life was not affected by supplementation. No statistically significant findings were found for secondary outcomes or subgroups. **Conclu-**

sion. Multivitamins offered no protection from infection for patients 65 and older. Routine multivitamin and multimineral supplementation of older people living at home does not affect self reported infection related morbidity.

CIRCA 2006

Dietary supplementation with different vitamin C doses: no effect on oxidative DNA damage in healthy people. (Herbert et al. 2006) (#160 volunteers). Antioxidants are believed to prevent many types of disease. Some previous studies suggest that dietary supplementation with vitamin C results in a decrease in the level of one of the markers of oxidative damage-8-oxoguanine in the DNA of peripheral blood mononuclear cells (PBMC). AIM OF TRIAL: To investigate the effect of different dose levels of dietary supplementation with vitamin C on oxidative DNA damage. METHODS: A randomized double-blind placebo-controlled trial was carried out using three different levels (80, 200 and 400 mg) of dietary vitamin C supplementation in a healthy population of 160 volunteers; supplementation was for a period of 15 weeks followed by a 10 week washout period. Peripheral blood samples were obtained every 5 weeks from baseline to 25 weeks.

RESULTS: An increase in PBMC vitamin C levels was not observed following supplementation in healthy volunteers. There was no effect found on 8-oxoguanine measured using HPLC with electrochemical detection for any of the three supplemented groups compared to placebo. 8-oxoadenine levels were below the limit of detection of the HPLC system used here. CONCLUSIONS: Supplementation with vitamin C had little effect on cellular levels in this group of healthy individuals, suggesting their diets were replete in vitamin C. The dose range of vitamin C used did not affect oxidative damage in PBMC DNA.

Carotenoids and cardiovascular health American Journal of Clinical Nutrition. (Voutilainen et al. 2006) (#not applicable)

Cardiovascular disease (CVD) is the main cause of death in Western countries. Nutrition has a significant role in the prevention of many chronic diseases such as CVD, cancers, and degenerative brain diseases. The major risk and protective factors in the diet are well recognized, but interesting new candidates continue to appear. It is well known that a greater intake of fruit and vegetables can help prevent heart diseases and mortality. **Because fruit, berries, and vegetables are chemically complex foods, it is difficult to pinpoint any single nutrient that contributes the most to the cardioprotective effects.** Several potential components that are found in fruit, berries, and vegetables are probably involved in the protective effects against CVD. Potential beneficial substances include antioxidant vitamins, folate, fiber, and potassium. Antioxidant compounds found in fruit and vegetables, such as vitamin C, carotenoids, and flavonoids, may influence the risk of CVD by preventing the oxidation of cholesterol in arteries. In this review, the role of main dietary carotenoids, ie, lycopene, beta-carotene, alpha-carotene, beta-cryptoxanthin, lutein, and zeaxanthin, in the prevention of heart diseases is discussed. Although it is clear that a higher intake of fruit and vegetables can help prevent the morbidity and mortality associated with heart diseases, **more information is needed to ascertain the association between the intake of single nutrients, such as carotenoids, and the risk of CVD. Currently, the consumption of carotenoids in pharmaceutical forms for the treatment or prevention of heart diseases cannot be recommended.**

Vitamins C and E and the risks of preeclampsia and perinatal complications (Rumbold et al, 2006) (#1,877) Supplementation with antioxidant vitamins has been proposed to reduce the risk of preeclampsia and

perinatal complications, but the effects of this intervention are uncertain. METHODS: They conducted a multicenter, **randomized trial of nulliparous women between 14 and 22 weeks of gestation**. Women were assigned to daily supplementation with 1000 mg of vitamin C and 400 IU of vitamin E or placebo (microcrystalline cellulose) until delivery. Primary outcomes were the risks of maternal preeclampsia, death or serious outcomes in the infants (on the basis of definitions used by the Australian and New Zealand Neonatal Network), and delivering an infant whose birth weight was below the 10th percentile for gestational age. RESULTS: Of the **1,877 women enrolled in the study, 935 were randomly assigned to the vitamin group and 942 to the placebo group (total - 1,877)**. Baseline characteristics of the two groups were similar. **There were no significant differences between the vitamin and placebo groups in the risk of preeclampsia, death or serious outcomes in the infant, or having an infant with a birth weight below the 10th percentile for gestational age.**

CONCLUSIONS: **Supplementation with vitamins C and E during pregnancy does not reduce the risk of preeclampsia in nulliparous women, the risk of intrauterine growth restriction, or the risk of death or other serious outcomes in their infants.**

CIRCA 2007

Beta carotene supplementation and age-related maculopathy in a randomized trial of US physicians (#22,071 apparently healthy US male physicians) (Christen et al. 2007). Investigators tested whether beta carotene supplementation affects the incidence of age-related maculopathy (ARM) in a large-scale randomized trial. **DESIGN:** Randomized, double-masked, placebo-controlled trial among **22,071 apparently healthy US male physicians** aged 40 to 84 years. Participants were randomly assigned to receive beta carotene (50 mg every other day) or placebo. Main Outcome Measure: Incident ARM responsible for a reduction in best-corrected visual acuity to 20/30 or worse. **RESULTS:** After 12 years of treatment and follow-up, there were 162 cases of ARM in the beta carotene group vs 170 cases in the placebo group. The results were similar for the secondary end points of ARM with or without vision loss and advanced ARM. **CONCLUSIONS:** These randomized data relative to 12 years of treatment among a large population of **apparently healthy men indicate that beta carotene supplementation has no beneficial or harmful effect on the incidence of ARM. Long-term supplemental use of beta carotene neither decreases nor increases the risk of ARM.**

Atherosclerosis and oxidant stress: the end of the road for antioxidant vitamin treatment? (Thomson et al. 2007)

Experimental data, however, have not translated into clinical benefit: most antioxidant vitamin trials have failed to reduce cardiovascular morbidity and mortality. Moreover, recent clinical trials have suggested that **mono-therapy with certain antioxidant vitamins like vitamin E may, in fact, be detrimental.** As a result of the disappointing outcome of 'antioxidant' vitamin trials, some authors have questioned both the utility of 'antioxidant' treatment in CVD and the supposedly central role of oxidative stress in atherogenesis. **The clinical promise of antioxidant vitamins has failed to translate into clinical benefit.**

Effects of antioxidant supplementation on the aging process. (Fusco et al. 2007).

Even if antioxidant supplementation is receiving growing attention and is increasingly adopted in Western countries, supporting evidence is still scarce and equivocal.

Effect of high-dose alpha-tocopherol supplementation on biomarkers of oxidative stress and inflammation and carotid atherosclerosis in patients with coronary artery disease. (Devaraj et al. 2007) (#90 patients with CAD).

Oxidative stress and inflammation are crucial in atherogenesis. alpha-Tocopherol is both an antioxidant and an antiinflammatory agent. OBJECTIVE: They evaluated the effect of RRR-alpha-tocopherol supplementation on carotid atherosclerosis in patients with stable coronary artery disease (CAD) on drug therapy. DESIGN: **Randomized, controlled, double-blind trial** compared RRR-alpha-tocopherol (1200 IU/d for 2 y) with placebo in **90 patients with CAD**. Intimal medial thickness (IMT) of both carotid arteries was measured by high-resolution B-mode ultrasonography at 0, 1, 1.5, and 2 y. At 6-mo intervals, plasma alpha-tocopherol concentrations, C-reactive protein (CRP), LDL oxidation, monocyte function (superoxide anion release, cytokine release, and adhesion to endothelium), and urinary $F_{(2)}$-isoprostanes were measured. RESULTS: alpha-Tocopherol concentrations were significantly higher in the alpha-tocopherol group but not in the placebo group. High-sensitivity CRP concentrations were significantly lowered with alpha-tocopherol supplementation than with placebo. alpha-Tocopherol supplementation significantly reduced urinary $F_{(2)}$-isoprostanes and monocyte superoxide anion and tumor necrosis factor release compared with baseline and placebo. **No significant difference was observed in the mean change in total carotid IMT in the placebo and alpha-tocopherol groups. In addition, no significant difference in cardiovascular events was observed**. CONCLUSIONS: **High-dose RRR-alpha-tocopherol supplementation in patients with CAD was safe and significantly reduced plasma biomarkers of oxidative stress and inflammation but had no significant effect on carotid IMT during 2 years**.

Multivitamins do not improve radiation therapy-related fatigue: results of a double-blind randomized crossover trial. (de Souza et al. 2007) (randomized 40 patients to either placebo or Centrum Silver)

Fatigue is a common symptom in cancer patients receiving radiation therapy. PATIENTS AND METHODS: They conducted a **double-blind randomized crossover trial** of multivitamins versus placebo in patients with breast cancer undergoing radiation therapy to evaluate fatigue and quality of life. RESULTS: We **randomized 40 patients to either placebo or Centrum Silver.** At the middle of the radiation treatments, patients were switched from placebo to multivitamins and vice versa. Patients answered the EORTC QLQ C-30 quality of life (QOL) and Chalder fatigue questionnaires at the beginning, middle, and end of radiation therapy. Both groups experienced decreases in general and physical fatigue scores at the end of the course of placebo compared with the assessment prior to this treatment. They also observed significant improvements in functional and symptoms score scales of the QOL questionnaire in the patients on placebo. **No significant changes were elicited with the use of multivitamins.** They also observed significantly lower rates of fatigue in the patients who had just finished a course of placebo as compared with patients finishing a course of multivitamins. CONCLUSION: **Multivitamins do not improve radiation-related fatigue in patients with breast cancer.**

Combined vitamin C and E supplementation during pregnancy for preeclampsia prevention: a systematic review (Polyzos et al, 2007) (#4,680 pregnant women)

The effect of combined vitamin C and E supplementation during pregnancy on the prevention of preeclampsia and major adverse infant outcomes has been reviewed. We searched MEDLINE and the Central Library of Controlled Trials of the Cochrane Library through August 2006 for relevant clinical trials. Interstudy heterogeneity was evaluated using the chi(2) statistic

322

(Q statistic) test. Pooled relative risks (RRs) and 95% confidence intervals (CIs) were calculated with a fixed or random-effects model as appropriate. Four trials that **collectively randomized 4680 pregnant women to either the combination of vitamin C and vitamin E or placebo were included in the analysis.** There were no significant differences between the vitamin and placebo groups in the risk of preeclampsia, 11% versus 11.4%, fetal or neonatal loss, 2.6% versus 2.3%, or small for gestational age (SGA) infant, 20.6% versus 20%. Although **there was a higher risk for preterm birth in the vitamin group, 19.5% versus 18%, this finding was not significant. Combined vitamin C and E supplementation during pregnancy does not reduce the risk of preeclampsia, fetal or neonatal loss, small for gestational age infant, or preterm birth. Such supplementation should be discouraged unless solid supporting data from randomized trials become available.** MEDLINE analysis of the literature questions the use of vitamin C and E supplements.

Antioxidant therapy to prevent preeclampsia: a randomized controlled trial (Spinnato et al. 2007) (#739)

Investigators studied whether antioxidant supplementation will reduce the incidence of preeclampsia among patients at increased risk. METHODS: A **randomized, placebo-controlled, double-blind clinical trial** was conducted at four Brazilian sites. Women between 12 0/7 weeks and 19 6/7 weeks of gestation and diagnosed to have chronic hypertension or a prior history of preeclampsia were randomly assigned to daily treatment with both vitamin C (1,000 mg) and vitamin E (400 International Units) or placebo. Analyses were adjusted for clinical site and risk group (prior preeclampsia, chronic hypertension, or both). A sample size of 734 would provide 80% power to detect a 40% reduction in the risk of preeclampsia, assuming a placebo group rate of 21% and alpha=.05. The alpha level for the final analysis, adjusted for interim looks, was 0.0458. RESULTS: **Outcome data for 707 of 739 randomly assigned patients revealed no significant reduction in the rate of pre-**

eclampsia compared with placebo. **There were no differences in mean gestational age at delivery or rates of perinatal mortality, abruptio placentae, preterm delivery, and small for gestational age or low birth weight infants.** *Among patients without chronic hypertension, there was a slightly higher rate of severe preeclampsia in the study group.* CONCLUSION: **This trial failed to demonstrate a benefit of antioxidant supplementation in reducing the rate of preeclampsia among patients with chronic hypertension and/or prior preeclampsia.**

The effect of vitamin E on blood pressure in individuals with type 2 diabetes: a randomized, double-blind, placebo-controlled trial (Ward et al, 2007) (#58 with type 2 diabetes)

Oxidative stress has been suggested to play a role in the development of diabetes, hypertension and vascular dysfunction. Vitamin E, a major lipid-soluble dietary antioxidant, has two major dietary forms, alpha-tocopherol and gamma-tocopherol. The potential importance of gamma-tocopherol has largely been overlooked. Our aim was to investigate the effect of alpha-tocopherol and gamma-tocopherol supplementation on 24-h ambulatory blood pressure (BP) and heart rate, vascular function and oxidative stress in individuals with type 2 diabetes. METHOD: **Fifty-eight individuals with type 2 diabetes were randomized in a double-blind, placebo-controlled trial. Participants were randomized to a daily dose of 500 mg/day RRR-alpha-tocopherol, 500 mg/day mixed tocopherols (60% gamma-tocopherol) or placebo for 6 weeks.** Primary endpoints were 24-h ambulatory BP and heart rate, endothelium-dependent and independent vasodilation and plasma and urinary F2-isoprostanes. RESULTS: Treatment with **alpha-tocopherol significantly increased systolic BP, diastolic BP, pulse pressure and heart rate versus placebo. Treatment with mixed tocopherols significantly increased systolic BP, diastolic BP,** pulse pressure and heart rate versus placebo. **Treatment with alpha-tocopherol or mixed tocopherols significantly reduced plasma F2-isoprostanes versus placebo,** but had no effect on urinary F2-isoprostanes. Endothelium-dependent and independent vasodilation was not affected by either treatment. CONCLUSION: In contrast to our initial hypothesis, *treatment with either alpha- or mixed tocopherols significantly increased BP, pulse pressure and heart rate in individuals with type 2 diabetes.*

National Institutes of Health State-of-the-Science Conference Statement: Multivitamin/Mineral Supplements and Chronic Disease Prevention (NIH State-of-the Science Panel. 2007).

At least half of American adults take a dietary supplement, the majority of which are multivitamin/multimineral (MVM) supplements. As more and more Americans seek strategies for maintaining good health and preventing disease, and as the marketplace offers an increasing number of products to fulfill that desire, **it is important that consumers have the best possible information to make their choices.** Assessing the available scientific evidence on the benefits of MVM supplement use for chronic disease prevention, identifying the gaps in the evidence, and recommending an appropriate research agenda to meet the shortfalls are subjects considered in this report.

Most people assume that the ingredients in MVM supplements are safe. There is evidence, however, that certain ingredients in MVM supplements can produce adverse effects, including **reports from RCTs that noted excess lung cancer occurring in asbestos workers and smokers consuming β-carotene.** In addition, *esophageal cancer excess was found with long-term follow-up of older Chinese patients (the Linxian study by Blot et al.) treated with selenium, β-carotene, and vitamin E supplements* (Blot et al, 1993) (NIH State-of-the Science Panel. 2007).

CIRCA 2008

High maternal plasma antioxidant (vit. C) concentrations associated with preterm delivery (Joshi et al, 2008) (#140 normotensive women)

Our earlier study has shown that **increased maternal oxidative stress and reduced antioxidants like vitamin E and C play an important role in fetal growth in preeclampsia**. However, the role of antioxidants and their effects on gestation and birth outcome in normotensive pregnancies are not conclusive. The present study examined plasma malondialdehyde as a marker of oxidative stress and antioxidant concentrations (vitamins E and C) in maternal as well as in cord blood samples in normotensive women who delivered both preterm and at term. METHODS: **140 normotensive pregnant women** were recruited at Bharati Medical Hospital, Pune, India, during the year 2007. Maternal and cord samples were examined for oxidative stress levels and vitamin C and E concentrations in women who delivered preterm (n=40) and at term (n=100). Mean values were compared with those of women delivering at term using the t test. RESULTS: Increased (p<0.05) oxidative stress was seen in preterm mothers as well as in cord samples. ***Preterm mothers had higher vitamin C concentrations (p<0.05), and these were positively associated with oxidative stress*** (p=0.02). **Vitamin E levels were comparable between groups**. CONCLUSIONS: Increased maternal circulating vitamin C concentrations and increased oxidative stress are associated with preterm delivery. **I believe that the increased vitamin C level in preterm (mothers) deliveries is significant and a cause of problems in the newborns.**

Vitamin E and age-related cataract in a randomized trial of women. (#39,876) (Christen et al. 2008).

Investigators studied whether vitamin E supplementation decreases the risk of age-related cataract in women.

DESIGN: Randomized, double-masked, placebo-controlled trial. **PARTICIPANTS: Thirty-nine thousand eight hundred seventy-six** (39,876) apparently healthy female health professionals aged 45 years or older. **INTERVENTION:** Participants were assigned randomly to receive either 600 IU natural-source vitamin E on alternate days or placebo and were followed up for presence of cataract for an average of 9.7 years.

MAIN OUTCOME MEASURE: Age-related cataract defined as an incident, age-related lens opacity, responsible for a reduction in best-corrected visual acuity to 20/30 or worse, based on self-report and confirmed by medical record review. **RESULTS:** There was no significant difference between the vitamin E and placebo groups in the incidence of cataract. In subgroup analyses of subtypes, there were no significant effects of vitamin E on the incidence of nuclear, cortical, or posterior subcapsular cataract. Results were similar for extraction of cataract and subtypes. There was no modification of the lack of effect of vitamin E on cataract by baseline categories of age, cigarette smoking, multivitamin use, or several other possible risk factors for cataract. **CONCLUSIONS: These data from a large trial of apparently healthy female health professionals with 9.7 years of treatment and follow-up indicate that 600 IU natural-source vitamin E taken every other day provides no benefit for age-related cataract or subtypes**.

Antioxidants in cardiovascular health and disease: key lessons from epidemiologic studies. (Icox et al. 2008). Interventional trials have been controversial, with some positive findings, many null findings, and some suggestion of harm in certain high-risk populations. *Because of the mismatch between the epidemiologic studies and the interventional trials, some researchers have advocated ending antioxidant work.* Others have questioned the validity of the LDL oxidative hypothesis itself.

Prof Randolph M. Howes MD, PhD

Observational studies on the effect of dietary antioxidants on asthma: a meta-analysis. (Gao et al. 2008) (#13,653) It has been suggested that the rapid increase in asthma prevalence may in part be due to a decrease in the intake of dietary antioxidants, including vitamin C, vitamin E and beta-carotene. Epidemiological studies investigating the association between dietary antioxidant intake and asthma have generated inconsistent results. A meta-analysis was undertaken to examine the association between dietary antioxidant intake and the risk of asthma.

METHODS: The MEDLINE database was searched for observational studies in English-language journals from 1966 to March 2007. Data were extracted using standardized forms. Pooled odds ratios (OR) with 95% confidence intervals (CI) were calculated using a random effects model. Ten studies were eligible for inclusion. Seven studies, comprising **13 653 subjects**, used asthma or wheeze as their outcome; three studies explored the effect of antioxidant intake on lung function. RESULTS: **A higher dietary intake of antioxidants was not associated with a lower risk of having asthma.** The pooled OR for having asthma were 1.06 for subjects with a higher dietary vitamin C intake compared with those with a lower intake; 0.88 for vitamin E; and 1.12 for beta-carotene. **There was no significant association between dietary antioxidant intake and lung function except for a positive association between vitamin C intake and an increase in FEV(1).** CONCLUSIONS: **This meta-analysis does not support the hypothesis that dietary intake of the antioxidants vitamins C and E and beta-carotene influences the risk of asthma.**

Dietary antioxidants and the long-term incidence of age-related macular degeneration: the Blue Mountains Eye Study (Tan et al. 2008) (#Of 3654 baseline (1992-1994) participants initially 49 years of older, 2454 were reexam-

328

ined after 5 years, 10 years, or both) Investigators assessed the relationship between baseline dietary and supplement intakes of antioxidants and the long-term risk of incident age-related macular degeneration (AMD). DESIGN: Australian population-based cohort study. PARTICIPANTS: Of **3654 baseline (1992-1994) participants initially 49 years of older, 2454 were reexamined after 5 years, 10 years, or both**. METHODS: Stereoscopic retinal photographs were graded using the Wisconsin Grading System. Data on potential risk factors were collected. Energy-adjusted intakes of alpha-carotene; beta-carotene; beta-cryptoxanthin; lutein and zeaxanthin; lycopene; vitamins A, C, and E; and iron and zinc were the study factors. Discrete logistic models assessed AMD risk. Risk ratios (RRs) and 95% confidence intervals (CIs) were calculated after adjusting for age, gender, smoking, and other risk factors. MAIN OUTCOME MEASURES: Incident early, late, and any AMD. RESULTS: For dietary **lutein and zeaxanthin, participants in the top tertile of intake had a reduced risk of incident neovascular AMD**, and those with above median intakes had a reduced risk of indistinct soft or reticular drusen. For total zinc intake the RR comparing the top decile intake with the remaining population was 0.56 for any AMD and 0.54 for early AMD. The highest compared with the lowest tertile of total beta-carotene intake predicted incident neovascular AMD. Similarly, beta-carotene intake from diet alone predicted neovascular AMD. This association was evident in both ever and never smokers. Higher intakes of total vitamin E predicted late AMD. CONCLUSIONS: In this population-based cohort study, higher dietary lutein and zeaxanthin intake reduced the risk of long-term incident AMD. This study confirmed the Age-Related Eye Disease Study finding of protective influences from zinc against AMD. *Higher beta-carotene intake was associated with an increased risk of age-related macular degeneration (AMD).*

CIRCA 2009

Effect of eicosapentaenoic and docosahexaenoic acid on resting and exercise-induced inflammatory

and oxidative stress biomarkers: a randomized, placebo controlled, cross-over study (Bloomer et al, 2009).

The purpose of the present investigation was to determine the effects of EPA/DHA supplementation on resting and exercise-induced inflammation and oxidative stress in exercise-trained men. **Fourteen men supplemented with 2224 mg EPA+2208 mg DHA and a placebo for 6 weeks in a random order, double blind cross-over design** (with an 8 week washout) prior to performing a 60 minute treadmill climb using a weighted pack. Blood was collected pre and post exercise and analyzed for a variety of oxidative stress and inflammatory biomarkers. Blood lactate, muscle soreness, and creatine kinase activity were also measured. RESULTS: Treatment with EPA/DHA resulted in a significant increase in blood levels of both EPA and DHA, while no differences were noted for placebo. Resting levels of CRP and TNF-alpha were lower with EPA/DHA compared to placebo. **Resting oxidative stress markers were not different. There was a mild increase in oxidative stress in response to exercise** (XO and $H2O2$). No interaction effects were noted. However, a condition effect was noted for CRP and TNF-alpha, with lower values with the EPA/DHA condition. CONCLUSION: EPA/DHA supplementation increases blood levels of these fatty acids and results in decreased resting levels of inflammatory biomarkers in exercise-trained men, but **does not appear necessary for exercise-induced attenuation in either inflammation or oxidative stress.** This may be due to the finding that trained men exhibit a minimal increase in both inflammation and oxidative stress in response to moderate duration (60 minute) aerobic exercise (Bloomer et al, 2009).

Concentrations of antioxidant vitamins in maternal and cord serum and their effect on birth outcomes. (Wang et al. 2009) (#143 mother-neonate pairs)

Emerging evidence indicates that maternal oxidative stress during pregnancy could impair fetal growth and that antioxidant vitamins (e.g. vitamins A, E and C) have a significant role in maintaining physiological processes of pregnancy and growth. AIMS: To determine the concentrations of vitamins A, E, and C in pair-matched maternal and cord serum samples of neonate, and thus to investigate the relationship between maternal serum levels of these vitamins at delivery and birth outcomes. METHODS: A total of **143 mother-neonate pairs** were recruited into the cross-sectional descriptive study. Demographic information was investigated by questionnaire. After delivery, both cord and maternal blood were collected for quantification of serum levels of vitamins A, E and C by HPLC. RESULTS: **Maternal serum levels of vitamins A and E were significantly higher than those in cord serum.** In contrast, vitamin C level in cord serum was significantly higher than that in maternal serum. Further, **we found that maternal vitamin A status was significantly correlated to both birth weight and birth height, and these were manifested by these findings:** (i) **per 250.2 g reduction in birth weight concomitant with 1 micromol/L increase in maternal serum vitamin A level;** and (ii) per 1% increase in the ratio of serum vitamin A level of neonate to mother concomitant with 0.8 cm increase in birth height. CONCLUSION: **Maternal vitamin A, but not vitamins E and C, during pregnancy had a significant effect on birth outcomes.** Further studies are necessary to investigate the role of these antioxidant vitamins in fetal growth at various gestation stages.

Does antioxidant vitamin supplementation protect against muscle damage? (McGinley et al. 2009).

The antioxidant vitamins C (ascorbic acid) and E (tocopherol) are among the most commonly used sport supplements, and are often taken in large doses by athletes and other sports persons because of their potential protective effect against muscle damage. Although there is some evidence to show that both antioxidants can reduce indices of oxidative stress, **there is little evidence to support a role for vitamin C and/or vitamin E in protecting against muscle damage.** Indeed, *antioxidant supplementation may actually interfere with the cellular signalling* *functions of ROS, thereby adversely affecting muscle performance. Since the potential for long-term harm does exist, the casual use of high doses of antioxidants by athletes and others should perhaps be curtailed.*

WHO Vitamin C and Vitamin E trial group. World Health Organisation multicentre randomised trial of supplementation with vitamins C and E among pregnant women at high risk for pre-eclampsia in populations of low nutritional status from developing countries. (Villar et al, 2009) (#687 women)

Supplementation was not associated with a reduction of pre-eclampsia, eclampsia, gestational hypertension, nor any other maternal outcome. Low birthweight (RR:, small for gestational age and perinatal deaths were also unaffected. **Vitamins C and E at the doses used did not prevent pre-eclampsia in these high-risk women.**

Vitamin and mineral use and risk of prostate cancer: the case-control surveillance study. (Zhang et al. 2009) (#1,706 prostate cancer cases and 2,404 matched controls). *Men who used zinc for ten years or more, either in a multivitamin or as a supplement, had an approximately two-fold increased risk of prostate cancer. The finding that long-term zinc intake from multivitamins or single supplements was associated with a doubling in risk of prostate cancer adds to the growing evidence for an unfavorable effect of zinc on prostate cancer carcinogenesis.*

"Is the oxidative stress theory of aging dead?" (STUDY) (Pérez et al. 2009). Because only one

(the deletion of the Sod1 gene) of the 18 genetic manipulations we studied had an effect on lifespan, our data calls into serious question the hypothesis that alterations in oxidative damage/stress play a role in the longevity of mice. **This 2009 review of experiments in mice concluded that almost all manipulations of antioxidant systems had no effect on aging.**

The oxidative stress menace to coronary vasculature: any place for antioxidants? (Briasoulis et al. 2009).

Interventional trials have been controversial, with some positive findings, many null findings, and some suggestion of harm in certain high-risk populations. Therefore, **treatment with antioxidant vitamins C and E should not be recommended for the prevention or treatment of coronary atherosclerosis.**

Oral antioxidant supplementation does not prevent acute mountain sickness: Double blind, randomized placebo-controlled trial. (Baillie et al. 2009) (#83).

daily dose of 1 g l-ascorbic acid, 400 IU of alpha-tocopherol acetate and 600 mg of alpha-lipoic acid. **There was no difference in AMS incidence or severity between the antioxidant and placebo groups using the LLS at any time at high altitude.**

Total dietary antioxidant index and survival in patients with glioblastoma multiforme. (Il'yasova et al. 2009) (#814 glioblastoma multiforme cases).

Overall, our results indicated no consistent, significant association of survival with dietary antioxidant intake or its combination with vitamin supplements.

Associations between alpha-tocopherol, beta-carotene, and retinol and prostate cancer survival (Watters et al. 2009) (#29,133)

Previous studies suggest that carotenoids and tocopherols (vitamin E compounds) may be inversely associated with prostate cancer risk, yet little is known about how they affect prostate cancer progression and survival. We investigated whether serum alpha-tocopherol, beta-carotene, and retinol concentrations, or the alpha-tocopherol and beta-carotene trial supplementation, affected survival of men diagnosed with prostate cancer during the **alpha-Tocopherol, beta-Carotene Cancer Prevention Study, a randomized, double-blind, placebo-controlled primary prevention trial** testing the effects of beta-carotene and alpha-tocopherol supplements on cancer incidence in adult male smokers in southwestern Finland (n = **29,133**). Prostate cancer survival was examined using the Kaplan-Meier method with deaths from other causes treated as censoring, and using Cox proportional hazards regression models with hazard ratios (HR) and 95% confidence intervals (CI) adjusted for family history of prostate cancer, age at randomization, benign prostatic hyperplasia, age and stage at diagnosis, height, body mass index, and serum cholesterol. As of April 2005, 1,891 men were diagnosed with prostate cancer and 395 died of their disease. **Higher serum alpha-tocopherol at baseline was associated with improved prostate cancer survival**, especially among cases who had received the alpha-tocopherol intervention of the trial and who were in the highest quintile of alpha-tocopherol at baseline or at the 3-year follow-up measurement. **Serum beta-carotene, serum retinol, and supplemental beta-carotene had no apparent effects on survival.** These findings suggest that higher alpha-tocopherol (and not beta-carotene or retinol) status increases overall prostate cancer survival. Further investigations, possibly including randomized studies, are needed to confirm this observation.

Antioxidant Supplementation and Risk of Incident Melanomas. Results of a Large Prospective Cohort Study. (Asgari et al, 2009)

(#69 671 men and women) Objective To examine whether *antioxidant supplement use is associated with melanoma risk in light of recently published data from the Supplementation in Vitamins and Mineral Antioxidants (SUVIMAX) study, which reported a 4-fold higher melanoma risk in women* randomized to receive a supplement with nutritionally appropriate doses of antioxidants. Asgari et al. did not observe increased melanoma risk with the use of supplemental beta carotene or selenium at doses comparable with those of the SUVIMAX study. Conclusion: Antioxidants taken in nutritional doses do not seem to increase melanoma risk.

Folic acid and risk of prostate cancer: results from a randomized clinical trial. (Figueiredo et al, 2009) (643 randomly assigned men).

Data regarding the association between folate status and risk of prostate cancer are sparse and conflicting. We studied prostate cancer occurrence in the Aspirin/Folate Polyp Prevention Study, a placebo-controlled randomized trial of aspirin and folic acid supplementation for the chemoprevention of colorectal adenomas conducted between July 6, 1994, and December 31, 2006. Participants were followed for up to 10.8 years and asked periodically to report all illnesses and hospitalizations. Aspirin alone had no statistically significant effect on prostate cancer incidence, but there were marked differences according to folic acid treatment. Among the **643 men who were randomly assigned** to placebo or supplementation with folic acid, *the estimated probability of being diagnosed with prostate cancer over a 10-year period was 9.7% in the folic acid group and 3.3% in the placebo group*. In contrast, baseline dietary folate intake and plasma folate in nonmultivitamin users were inversely associated with risk of prostate cancer, although these associations did not attain statistical significance in adjusted analyses. These findings highlight the potential complex role of folate in prostate cancer and the possibly different effects of folic acid-containing supplements vs natural sources of folate (Figueiredo et al, 2009).

Antioxidants do not prevent post exercise peroxidation and may delay muscle recovery (Teixeira et al. 2009) (#20)

This study aimed to determine the effects of 4 wk of antioxidants (AOX) supplementation on exercise-induced lipid peroxidation, muscle damage, and inflammation in kayakers. METHODS: **Subjects (n = 20) were randomly assigned to receive a placebo (PLA) or an AOX capsule (AOX; 272 mg of alpha-tocopherol, 400 mg of vitamin C, 30 mg of beta-carotene, 2 mg of lutein, 400 mug of selenium, 30 mg of zinc, and 600 mg of magnesium).** Blood samples were collected at rest and 15 min after a 1000-m kayak race, both before and after the supplementation period, for analysis of alpha-tocopherol, alpha-carotene, beta-carotene, lycopene, lutein plus zeaxanthin, vitamin C, uric acid, total AOX status (TAS), thiobarbituric reactive acid substances (TBARS) and interleukin-6 (IL-6) levels, and creatine kinase (CK), superoxide dismutase (SOD), glutathione reductase (Gr), and glutathione peroxidase (GPx) activities. RESULTS: With supplementation, plasma alpha-tocopherol (P = 0.003) and beta-carotene (P = 0.007) augmented significantly in the AOX group. **IL-6 (exercise, P = 0.039), TBARS (exercise, P < 0.001), and uric acid (exercise, P = 0.032) increased significantly in response to the exercise regardless of treatment group.** Cortisol level raised more from pre- to post supplementation period in the PLA group. Although TAS declined after exercise before intervention, it increased above pre-exercise values after the 4-wk period in the AOX group. CK increased after exercise in both groups and decreased from week 0 to week 4 more markedly in the PLA group. CONCLUSIONS: *AOX supplementation does not offer protection against exercise-induced lipid peroxidation and inflammation and may hinder the recovery of muscle damage* (Teixeira et al. 2009).

The response of gamma vitamin E to varying dosages of alpha vitamin E plus vitamin C (Guiterrez et al, 2009).

Vitamin E has been studied extensively in the prevention of athero-sclerosis. **Cross-sectional population studies as well as randomized controlled intervention trials have demonstrated conflicting results.** A recent meta-analysis of these trials has emphasized the ineffectiveness of vitamin E in ath-erosclerosis prevention, with a possibility of harm at higher dosages. However, vitamin E has several isomers, with **the alpha form being available via dietary supplements and the gamma form being available via dietary foodstuffs.** The gamma form of vita-min E demonstrates several superior properties (such as trapping reactive nitrogen species and detoxifying nitrogen dioxide) compared with alpha vitamin E. All clinical trials have used the alpha isomer, with little concern that this isomer of vitamin E may actually suppress the gamma isomer of vitamin E. They undertook a dose-response study in volunteers with type 2 diabetes mellitus to include all the dosages of alpha vitamin E that have been used in cardiovascular prevention trials to determine the effect of alpha vitamin E on gamma vitamin E. They also assessed the effect of alpha vitamin E on several traditional markers of atherosclerotic risk. We added vitamin C to the vitamin E because several clinical trials included this vitamin to enhance the antioxidant effects of alpha vitamin E. Volunteers received, in random-ized order for a 2-week period, one of the following vitamin dosage arms: (1) no vitamins, (2) low-dose supplemental vitamins E plus C, (3) medium-dose supplemental vitamins E plus C, and (4) high-dose supplemental vitamins E plus C. Blood levels of both alpha and gamma vitamin E were measured as well as surrogate markers of oxidative stress, hypercoagulation, and inflammation during a high-fat athero-genic meal (to increase the ambient oxidative stress level during the study). The results demonstrate that alpha vitamin E levels increased in proportion to the dose administered. However, at every dose of alpha vitamin E, gamma vitamin E concentration was significantly suppressed. **No beneficial changes in surrogate markers of atherosclerosis were observed, consistent with the negative results of prospective clinical trials using alpha vitamin E.** Their results suggest that **all prospective cardiovascular clini-cal trials that used vitamin E supplementation actually sup-pressed the beneficial antioxidant gamma isomer of vitamin**

E. No beneficial effects on several potential cardio-vascular risk factors were observed, even when the vitamin E was supplemented with vitamin C. If a standardized preparation of gamma vitamin E (without the alpha isomer) becomes available, the effects of gamma vitamin E on atherosclerotic risk will warrant additional studies (Guiterrez et al, 2009).

CIRCA 2010

Vitamin E and age-related macular degeneration in a randomized trial of women. (Christen et al. 2010) (#39,876) a large-scale randomized trial of female health professionals, long-term alternate-day use of 600 IU of natural-source vitamin E had no large beneficial or harmful effect on risk of AMD. Investigators tested whether alternate day vitamin E affects the incidence of age-related macular degeneration (AMD) in a large-scale randomized trial of women.

DESIGN: Randomized, double-masked, placebo-controlled trial. **PARTICIPANTS: Thirty-nine thousand eight hundred seventy-six (39,876)** apparently healthy female health professionals aged 45 years or older. **INTERVENTION:** Participants were assigned randomly to receive either 600 IU of natural-source vitamin E on alternate days or placebo. **MAIN OUTCOME MEASURES:** Incident AMD responsible for a reduction in best-corrected visual acuity to 20/30 or worse based on self-report confirmed by medical record review. **RESULTS:** After 10 years of treatment and follow-up, there were 117 cases of AMD in the vitamin E group and 128 cases in the placebo group.

CONCLUSIONS: In a **large-scale randomized trial of female health professionals, long-term alternate-day use of 600 IU of natural-source vitamin E had no large beneficial or harmful effect on risk of AMD.**

Vitamins C and E for prevention of pre-eclampsia in women with type I diabetes (DAPIT) (McCance et al. 2010) (#762 women)

Rates of pre-eclampsia did not differ between vitamin (15%, n=57) and placebo (19%, 70) groups. **Supplementation with vitamins C and E did not reduce risk of pre-eclampsia in women with type I diabetes.**

Daily intake of antioxidants in relation to survival among adult patients diagnosed with malignant glioma. (DeLorenze et al. 2010).

Geometric mean values for 11 fat-soluble and 6 water-soluble individual antioxidants, antioxidant index and 3 macronutrients were virtually the same when comparing all cases (n=748) to self-reported cases only (n=450). For patients diagnosed with Grade II and Grade III histology, moderate (915.8-2118.3 mcg) intake of fat-soluble lycopene was associated with poorer survival when compared to low intake (0.0-914.8 mcg), for self-reported cases only. High intake of vitamin E and moderate/high intake of secoisolariciresinol among Grade III patients indicated greater survival for all cases. In Grade IV patients, moderate/high intake of cryptoxanthin and high intake of secoisolariciresinol were associated with poorer survival among all cases. Among Grade II patients, moderate intake of water-soluble folate was associated with greater survival for all cases; high intake of vitamin C and genistein and the highest level of the antioxidant index were associated with poorer survival for all cases.

CONCLUSIONS: The associations observed in our study suggest that the influence of some antioxidants on survival following a diagnosis of malignant glioma are inconsistent and vary by histology group.

Effects of vitamin on stroke subtypes: meta-analysis of randomized controlled trials. (Schurks et al. 2010) (#118,765) Systematic review

and meta-analysis of randomized, placebo controlled trials published until January 2010. **Data sources** Electronic databases (Medline, Embase, Cochrane Central Register of Controlled Trials) and reference lists of trial reports. **Selection criteria** Randomized, placebo controlled trials with ≥1 year of follow-up investigating the effect of vitamin E on stroke. **Review methods and data extraction** Two investigators independently assessed eligibility of identified trials. Disagreements were resolved by consensus. Two different investigators independently extracted data. Risk ratios (and 95% confidence intervals) were calculated for each trial based on the number of cases and non-cases randomized to vitamin E or placebo. Pooled effect estimates were then calculated. **Results** Nine trials investigating the effect of vitamin E on incident stroke were included, **totalling 118,765 participants (59,357 randomized to vitamin E and 59,408 to placebo).** Among those, seven trials reported data for total stroke and five trials each for hemorrhagic and ischemic stroke. Vitamin E had no effect on the risk for total stroke. In contrast, the risk for hemorrhagic stroke was increased, while the risk of ischemic stroke was reduced. There was little evidence for heterogeneity among studies. Meta-regression did not identify blinding strategy, vitamin E dose, or morbidity status of participants as sources of heterogeneity. In terms of absolute risk, this translates into one additional hemorrhagic stroke for every 1,250 individuals taking vitamin E, in contrast to one ischemic stroke prevented per 476 individuals taking vitamin E. **Conclusion** In this meta-analysis, *vitamin E increased the risk for hemorrhagic stroke by 22% and reduced the risk of ischemic stroke by 10%.* This differential risk pattern is obscured when looking at total stroke. Given the relatively small risk reduction of ischemic stroke and the generally more severe outcome of hemorrhagic stroke, *indiscriminate widespread use of vitamin E should be cautioned against.*

Multivitamin/Mineral supplementation does not affect standardized assessment of academic performance in elementary school children (Perlman et al. 2010) (#students in grades three through six, approximate age

range=8 to 12 years old) Limited research suggests that micronutrient supplementation may have a positive effect on the academic performance and behavior of school-aged children. To determine the effect of multivitamin/mineral supplementation on academic performance, **students in grades three through six (approximate age range=8 to 12 years old)** were recruited from 37 parochial schools in northern New Jersey to participate in a **double-blind, placebo-controlled clinical trial** conducted during the 2004-2005 academic school year. Participants were randomized to receive either a standard children's multivitamin/mineral supplement (MVM) or a placebo. MVM or placebo was administered in school only during lunch or snack period by a teacher or study personnel who were blinded to group assignment. The main outcome measured was change in scores on **Terra Nova, a standardized achievement test administered by the State of New Jersey**, at the beginning of March 2005 compared to March 2004. **Compared with placebo, participants receiving MVM supplements showed no statistically significant improvement for Terra Nova National Percentile total scores by treatment assignment or for any of the subject area scores using repeated measures analysis of variance.** No significant improvements were observed in secondary end points: number of days absent from school, tardiness, or grade point average. In conclusion, the in-school **daily consumption of an MVM supplement by third- through sixth-grade inner-city children did not lead to improved school performance** based upon standardized testing, grade point average, and absenteeism.

Differential effects of concomitant use of vitamins C and E on trophoblast apoptosis and autophagy between normoxia and hypoxia-reoxygenation (Hung et al, 2010) *Concomitant supplementation of vitamins C and E during pregnancy has been reportedly associated with low birth weight,*

Prof Randolph M. Howes MD, PhD

the premature rupture of membranes and fetal loss or perinatal death in women at risk for preeclampsia; however, the cause is unknown. They surmise that hypoxia-reoxygenation (HR) within the intervillous space due to abnormal placentation is the mechanism and hypothesize that concomitant administration of aforementioned vitamin antioxidants detrimentally affects trophoblast cells during HR.

METHODOLOGY/PRINCIPAL FINDINGS: Using villous explants, concomitant administration of 50 microM of vitamins C and E was observed to reduce apoptotic and autophagic changes in the trophoblast layer at normoxia (8% oxygen) but to cause more prominent apoptosis and autophagy during HR. Furthermore, increased levels of Bcl-2 and Bcl-xL in association with a decrease in the autophagy-related protein LC3-II were noted in cytotrophoblastic cells treated with vitamins C and E under standard culture conditions. In contrast, vitamin treatment decreased Bcl-2 and Bcl-xL as well as increased mitochondrial Bak and cytosolic LC3-II in cytotrophoblasts subjected to HR.

CONCLUSIONS/SIGNIFICANCE: **Our results indicate that concomitant administration of vitamins C and E has differential effects on the changes of apoptosis, autophagy and the expression of Bcl-2 family of proteins in the trophoblasts between normoxia and HR.** *These changes may probably lead to the impairment of placental function and suboptimal growth of the fetus*.

Is vitamin C supplementation beneficial? Lessons learned from randomised controlled trials (Lyddesfeldt and Poulsen, 2010).

In contrast to the promised 'antioxidant miracle' of the 1980s, several randomized controlled trials have shown no effect of antioxidant supplements on hard endpoints such as morbidity and mortality. The **former over-optimistic attitude** has clearly called for a more realistic assessment of the benefit:harm ratio of antioxidant supplements. **They have examined the literature on vitamin C intervention with the inten-**

tion of drawing a conclusion on its possible benefi- cial or deleterious effect on health and the result is discouraging. One of several important issues is that vitamin C uptake is tightly controlled, resulting in a wide-ranging bioavailability depending on the current vitamin C status. Lack of proper selection criteria dominates the currently available literature. Thus, while **supplementation with vitamin C is likely to be without effect for the majority of the Western population due to satura- tion through their normal diet**, there could be a large subpopula- tion with a potential health problem that remains uninvestigated. The present review discusses the relevance of the available literature on vitamin C supplementation and proposes guidelines for future ran- domized intervention trials (Lyddesfeldt and Poulsen, 2010).

Bioactive Dietary Polyphenols Decrease Heme Iron Absorption by Decreasing Basolateral Iron Release in Human Intestinal Caco-2 cells (Ma et al. 2010).

Because **dietary polyphenolic compounds have a wide range of effects in vivo and vitro, including chelation of metals such as iron**, it is prudent to test whether the regular consumption of dietary bioactive polyphenols impair the utilization of dietary iron. **Because our previous study showed the inhibitory effect of (-) -epigal- locatechin-3-gallate (EGCG) and grape seed extract (GSE) on nonheme iron absorption,** we investigated whether EGCG and GSE also affect iron absorption from heme. The fully differentiated in- testinal Caco-2 cells grown on microporous membrane inserts were incubated with heme ^{55}Fe in uptake buffer containing EGCG or GSE in the apical compartment for 7 h. Both EGCG and GSE decreased transepithelial transport of heme-derived iron. However, apical heme iron uptake was increased by GSE. Despite the increased cellular lev- els of heme ^{55}Fe, the transfer of iron across the intestinal basolat- eral membrane was extremely low, indicating that basolateral export was impaired by GSE. In contrast, EGCG moderately decreased the cellular assimilation of heme ^{55}Fe, but the basolateral iron transfer was extremely low, suggesting that *the basolateral efflux of heme iron was also inhibited by EGCG.* Expression of heme oxygenase, ferroportin, and hephaestin protein was not changed by EGCG and GSE. The apical uptake of heme iron was temperature dependent and saturable in fully differentiated Caco-2 cells. Our data show that ***bioactive dietary polyphenols inhibit heme iron absorption*** mainly by reducing basolateral iron exit rather than decreasing apical heme iron uptake in intestinal cells (Ma et al. 2010). ***Polyphenols bind to iron in the intestinal cells, forming a non-transportable complex.*** *This iron-polyphenol complex cannot enter the blood stream. Instead, it is excreted in the feces when cells are sloughed off and replaced.*

References- 69 additional studies

(Anderssen et al. 1996) (Andersson SO, Wolk A, Bergström R, Giovannucci E, Lindgren C, Baron J, Adami HO. Energy, nutrient intake and prostate cancer risk: a population-based case-control study in Sweden. Int J Cancer. 1996 Dec 11;68(6):716-22).

(Asgari et al. 2009) (Maryam M. Asgari, Sonia S. Maruti, Lawrence H. Kushi, Emily White. Antioxidant Supplementation and Risk of Incident Melanomas. *Arch Dermatol.* 2009;145(8):879-882)

(Avenell et al. 2005) (Effect of multivitamin and multimineral supplements on morbidity from infections in older people (MAVIS trial): Pragmatic, randomized, double blind, placebo controlled trial. Avenell A. et al. BMJ 2005;331:324).

(Baillie et al. 2009) . (Baillie JK, Thompson AA, Irving JB, Bates MG, Sutherland AI, Macnee W, Maxwell SR, Webb DJ. Oral antioxidant supplementation does not prevent acute mountain sickness: double blind, randomized placebo-controlled trial. QJM. 2009 May;102(5):341-8).

(Bloomer et al, 2009) (Bloomer RJ. et al. Effect of eicosapentaenoic and docosahexaenoic acid on resting and exercise-induced inflammatory and oxidative stress biomarkers: a randomized, placebo controlled, cross-over study. Lipids Health Dis. 2009 Aug 19;8:36).

(Blot et al, 1993) (Blot WJ, Li JY, Taylor PR, Guo W, Dawsey S, Wang GQ, et al. Nutrition intervention trials in Linxian, China: supplementation with specific vitamin/mineral combinations, cancer incidence, and disease-specific mortality in the general population. J Natl Cancer Inst. 1993;85:1483–92).

(Bonnefoy et al. 2002) (Bonnefoy M, Drai J, Kostka T. Antioxidants to slow aging, facts and perspectives. Presse Med. 2002 Jul 27;31(25):1174-84).

(Briasoulis et al. 2009) (Briasoulis A, Tousoulis D, Antoniades C, Stefanadis C. The oxidative stress menace to coronary vasculature: any place for antioxidants? Curr Pharm Des. 2009;15(26):3078-90).

(Christen et al. 2004) (Christen W, Glynn R, Sperduto R, Chew E, Buring J. Age-related cataract in a randomized trial of beta-carotene in women. Ophthalmic Epidemiol. 2004 Dec;11(5):401-12).

(Christen et al. 2007) (Christen WG, Manson JE, Glynn RJ, Gaziano JM, Chew EY, Buring JE, Hennekens CH. Beta carotene supplementation and age-related maculopathy in a randomized trial of US physicians. Arch Ophthalmol. 2007 Mar;125(3):333-9).

(Christen et al. 2008) (Christen WG, Glynn RJ, Chew EY, Buring JE. Vitamin E and age-related cataract in a randomized trial of women. Ophthalmology. 2008 May;115(5):822-829.e1).

(Christen et al. 2010) (Christen WG, Glynn RJ, Chew EY, Buring JE. Vitamin E and age-related macular degeneration in a randomized trial of women. Ophthalmology. 2010 Jun;117(6):1163-8).

(DeLorenze et al. 2010) (DeLorenze GN, McCoy L, Tsai AL, Quesenberry CP Jr, Rice T, Il'yasova D, Wrensch M. Daily intake of antioxidants in relation to survival among adult patients diagnosed with malignant glioma. BMC Cancer. 2010 May 19;10:215).

(Demling et al. 2002) (Demling R, Ikegami K, Picard L, Lalonde C. Administration of large doses of vitamin C does not decrease oxidant-induced lung lipid peroxidation caused by bacterial-independent acute peritonitis Inflammation. 2002. Volume 18, Number 5, 499-510, DOI: 10.1007/BF01560697). ANIMAL STUDY

(Devaraj et al. 2007) (Devaraj S, Tang R, Adams-Huet B, Harris A, Seenivasan T, de Lemos JA, Jialal I. Effect of high-dose alpha-tocopherol supplementation on biomarkers of oxidative stress and inflammation and carotid atherosclerosis in patients with coronary artery disease. Am J Clin Nutr. 2007 Nov;86(5):1392-8).

(de Souza et al. 2007) (de Souza et al. Multivitamins do not improve radiation therapy-related fatigue: results of a double-blind randomized crossover trial. 2007. Am J Clin Oncol. 2007 Aug;30(4):432-6)

(de Waart et al. 2000) (de Waart FG, Smilde TJ, Wollersheim H, Stalenhoef AF, Kok FJ. Smoking characteristics, antioxidant vitamins, and carotid artery wall thickness among life-long smokers. J Clin Epidemiol. 2000 Jul;53(7):707-14).

(Duthie et al. 1994) (Duthie GG, Beattie JA, Arthur JR, Franklin M, Morrice PC, James WP. Blood antioxidants and indices of lipid peroxidation in subjects with angina pectoris. Nutrition. 1994 Jul-Aug;10(4):313-6).

(Evans et al. 1998) (Evans RW, Shaten BJ, Day BW, Kuller LH. Prospective association between lipid soluble antioxidants and coronary heart disease in men. The Multiple Risk Factor Intervention Trial. Am J Epidemiol. 1998; 147: 180–186).

(Fusco et al. 2007) (Fusco D, Colloca G, Lo Monaco MR, Cesari M. Effects of antioxidant supplementation on the aging process. Clin Interv Aging. 2007;2(3):377-87).

(Gao et al. 2008) (Gao J, Gao X, Li W, Zhu Y, Thompson PJ. Observational studies on the effect of dietary antioxidants on asthma: a meta-analysis. Respirology. 2008 Jun;13(4):528-36).

(Genkinger et al. 2004) (Genkinger JM, Platz EA, Hoffman SC, Comstock GW, Helzlsouer KJ. Fruit, vegetable, and antioxidant intake and all-cause, cancer, and cardiovascular disease mortality in a community-dwelling population in Washington County, Maryland. Am J Epidemiol. 2004 Dec 15;160(12):1223-33).

(Grievink et al. 1998) (Grievink L, Smit HA, Ocké MC, van 't Veer P, Kromhout D. Dietary intake of antioxidant (pro)-vitamins, respiratory symptoms and pulmonary function: the MORGEN study. Thorax. 1998 Mar;53(3):166-71).

(Guiterrez et al, 2009) (Guiterrez AD, et al, The response of gamma vitamin E to varying dosages of alpha vitamin E plus vitamin C. Metabolism. 2009 Apr;58(4):469-78).

(Hak et al. 2003) (Hak AE, Stampfer MJ, Campos H, Sesso HD, Gaziano JM, Willett W, Ma J: Plasma carotenoids and tocopherols and risk of myocardial infarction in a low-risk population of US male physicians. Circulation 108:802 :E9012 –E9013,2003).

(Hemila et al. 2004) (Hemilä H, Virtamo J, Albanes D, Kaprio J. Vitamin E and beta-carotene supplementation and hospital-treated pneumonia incidence in male smokers. Chest. 2004 Feb;125(2):557-65).

(Hense et al. 1993) (Hense HW, Stender M, Bors W, Keil U. Lack of an association between serum vitamin E and myocardial infarction in a population with high vitamin E levels. Atherosclerosis. 1993 Oct;103(1):21-8).

Prof Randolph M. Howes MD, PhD

(Herbert et al. 2006) (Herbert KE, Fletcher S, Chauhan D, Ladapo A, Nirwan J, Munson S, Mistry P. Dietary supplementation with different vitamin C doses: no effect on oxidative DNA damage in healthy people. Eur J Nutr. 2006 Mar;45(2):97-104).

(Hung et al, 2010) (Hung TH, Chen SF, Li MJ, Yeh YL, Hsieh TT. Differential effects of concomitant use of vitamins C and E on trophoblast apoptosis and autophagy between normoxia and hypoxia-reoxygenation. PLoS One. 2010 Aug 16;5(8):e12202).

(Icox et al. 2008) (Icox BJ, Curb JD, Rodriguez BL. Antioxidants in cardiovascular health and disease: key lessons from epidemiologic studies. Am J Cardiol. 2008 May 22;101(10A):75D-86D).

(Il'yasova et al. 2009) (Il'yasova D, Marcello JE, McCoy L, Rice T, Wrensch M. Total dietary antioxidant index and survival in patients with glioblastoma multiforme. Cancer Causes Control. 2009 Oct;20(8):1255-60).

(Joshi et al. 2008) (Joshi SR, Mehendale SS, Dangat KD, Kilari AS, Yadav HR, Taralekar VS. High maternal plasma antioxidant concentrations associated with preterm delivery. Ann Nutr Metab. 2008;53(3-4):276-82).

(Keith et al, 2001) (Keith ME, Jeejeebhoy KN, Langer A, Kurian R, Barr A, O'Kelly B, Sole MJ. A controlled clinical trial of vitamin E supplementation in patients with congestive heart failure. Am J Clin Nutr. 2001 Feb;73(2):219-24)

(Kinlay et al. 2004) (Kinlay S, Behrendt D, Fang JC, Delagrange D, Morrow J, Witztum JL, Rifai N, Selwyn AP, Creager MA, Ganz P. Long-term effect of combined vitamins E and C on coronary and peripheral endothelial function. J Am Coll Cardiol. 2004 Feb 18;43(4):629-34).

(Leppala et al. 2000) (Leppala JM, Virtamo J, Fogelholm R, Huttunen JK, Albanes D, Taylor PR, et al. Controlled trial of alpha-tocopherol and beta-carotene supplements on stroke incidence and mortality in male smokers. Arterioscler Thromb Vasc Biol 2000;20:230-5).

(Lyddesfeldt and Poulsen, 2010) (Lyddesfeldt J, Poulsen HE. Is vitamin C supplementation beneficial? Lessons learned from randomised controlled trials. Br J Nutr. 2010 May;103(9):1251-9).

(Ma et al. 2010) (Ma Q, Kim E-Y, Han O. Bioactive Dietary Polyphenols Decrease Heme Iron Absorption by Decreasing Basolateral Iron

348

Release in Human Intestinal Caco-e Cells. J. Nutr. June 2010. Vol 140. No. 6. pp. 1117-1121).

(Marchioli et al. 2001) (Marchioli R, Schweiger C, Levantesi G, Tavazzi L, Valagussa F. Antioxidant vitamins and prevention of cardiovascular disease: epidemiological and clinical trial data. Lipids. 2001;36 Suppl:S53-63).

(Mayer-Davis et al. 1998) (Mayer-Davis EJ, Bell RA, Reboussin BA, Rushing J, Marshall JA, Hamman RF. Antioxidant nutrient intake and diabetic retinopathy: the San Luis Valley Diabetes Study. Ophthalmology. 1998 Dec;105(12):2264-70).

(McCance et al. 2010) (McCance DR, Holmes VA, Maresh MJ, Patterson CC, Walker JD, Pearson DW, Young IS; Diabetes and Preeclampsia Intervention Trial (DAPIT) Study Group. Vitamins C and E for prevention of pre-eclampsia in women with type 1 diabetes (DAPIT): a randomised placebo-controlled trial. Lancet. 2010 Jul 24;376(9737):259-66).

(McGinley et al. 2009) (McGinley C, Shafat A, Donnelly AE. Does antioxidant vitamin supplementation protect against muscle damage? Sports Med. 2009;39(12):1011-32).

(Milner et al. 2004) (Joshua D. Milner, Daniel M. Stein, Robert McCarter, Rachel Y. Moon. Early Infant Multivitamin Supplementation Is Associated With Increased Risk for Food Allergy and Asthma. PEDIATRICS Vol. 114 No. 1 July 2004, pp. 27-32).

(Moyad et al. 2002) (Moyad MA. Selenium and vitamin E supplements for prostate cancer: evidence or embellishment? Urology. 2002 Apr;59(4 Suppl 1):9-19).

(Neunteufl et al. 2000) (Neunteufl T, Priglinger U, Heher S, Zehetgruber M, Söregi G, Lehr S, Huber K, Maurer G, Weidinger F, Kostner K. Effects of vitamin E on chronic and acute endothelial dysfunction in smokers. J Am Coll Cardiol. 2000 Feb;35(2):277-83).

(NIH State-of-the Science Panel. 2007) (National Institutes of Health State-of-the-Science Conference Statement: Multivitamin/Mineral Supplements and Chronic Disease Prevention. NIH State-of-the Science Panel. Am. J. Clin. Nutr. 2007;85:257S-264S).

(Pérez et al. 2009) (Pérez VI, Bokov A, Van Remmen H, Mele J, Ran Q, Ikeno Y, Richardson A. "Is the oxidative stress theory of aging dead?". Biochimica et Biophysica Acta (BBA) - General Subjects (2009). 1790 (10): 1005–1014).

(Perlman et al. 2010) (Perlman et al. Multivitamin/Mineral supplementation does not affect standardized assessment of academic performance in elementary school children. 2010. J Am Diet Assoc. 2010 Jul;110(7):1089-93).

(Polyzos et al, 2007) (Polyzos NP et al. Combined vitamin C and E supplementation during pregnancy for preeclampsia prevention: a systematic review. Obstet Gynecol Surv. 2007 Mar;62(3):202-6).

(Priemé et al. 1997) (Priemé H, Loft S, Nyyssönen K, Salonen JT, Poulsen HE. No effect of supplementation with vitamin E, ascorbic acid, or coenzyme Q10 on oxidative DNA damage estimated by 8-oxo-7,8-dihydro-2'-deoxyguanosine excretion in smokers. Am J Clin Nutr. 1997 Feb;65(2):503-7).

(Raitakari, et al. 2000) (Raitakari OT, Adams MR, McCredie RJ, Griffiths KA, Stocker R, Celermajer DS. Oral vitamin C and endothelial function in smokers: short-term improvement, but no sustained beneficial effect. J Am Coll Cardiol. 2000 May;35(6):1616-21).

(Rohan et al. 1995) (Rohan TE, Howe GR, Burch JD, Jain M. Cancer Causes Control. Dietary factors and risk of prostate cancer: a case-control study in Ontario, Canada. 1995 Mar;6(2):145-54).

(Rumbold et al, Apr 18, 2005. CD004072) (Rumbold A, Middleton P, Crowther CA. Vitamin supplementation for preventing miscarriage. Cochrane Database Syst Rev. 2005 Apr 18;(2):CD004069).

(Rumbold et al, Apr 18, 2005. CD004072) (Rumbold A, Crowther CA. Vitamin E supplementation in pregnancy. Cochrane Database Syst Rev. 2005 Apr 18;(2):CD004069).

(Rumbold et al, 2006) (Rumbold AR, Crowther CA, Haslam RR, Dekker GA, Robinson JS, ACTS Study Group. Vitamins C and E and the risks of preeclampsia and perinatal complications. N Engl J Med. 2006 Apr 27;354(17):1796-806).

(Schurks et al. 2010) (Effects of vitamin on stroke subtypes: meta-analysis of randomised controlled trials. Markus Schurks, Robert J

Glynn, Pamela M. Rist, Christophe Tzourio, Tobias Kurth. BMJ 2010; 341:c5702 (online 11-4-10).

(Selman et al. 2006) (Selman C, McLaren JS, Meyer C, Duncan JS, Redman P, Collins AR, Duthie GG, Speakman JR. Life-long vitamin C supplementation in combination with cold exposure does not affect oxidative damage or lifespan in mice, but decreases expression of antioxidant protection genes. Mech Ageing Dev. 2006 Dec;127(12):897-904). ANIMAL STUDY

(Sesso et al, 2008) (Sesso, HD. et al. Vitamins E and C in the prevention of cardiovascular disease in men: the Physicians' Health Study II randomized controlled trial. JAMA. 2008 Nov 12;300(18):2123-33. Epub 2008 Nov 9)

(Skrha et al. 1997) (J. Skrha, G. Sindelka and J. Hilgertova. The effect of fasting and vitamin E on insulin action in obese type 2 diabetes mellitus. Annals of the New York Academy of Sciences, Vol 827, Issue 1 556-560, 1997).

(Spinnato et al. 2007) (Spinnato JA et al. Antioxidant therapy to prevent preeclampsia: a randomized controlled trial. Obstet Gynecol. 2007 Dec;110(6):1311-8).

(Stanner et al. 2004) (Stanner SA, Hughes J, Kelly CN, Buttriss J. A review of the epidemiological evidence for the 'antioxidant hypothesis'. Public Health Nutr. 2004 May;7(3):407-22).

(Tam et al. 2005) (Tam LS, Li EK, Leung VY, Griffith JF, Benzie IF, Lim PL, Whitney B, Lee VW, Lee KK, Thomas GN, Tomlinson B. Effects of vitamins C and E on oxidative stress markers and endothelial function in patients with systemic lupus erythematosus: a double blind, placebo controlled pilot study. J Rheumatol. 2005 Feb;32(2):275-82).

(Tan et al. 2008) (Tan JS, Wang JJ, Flood V, Rochtchina E, Smith W, Mitchell P. Dietary antioxidants and the long-term incidence of age-related macular degeneration: the Blue Mountains Eye Study. Ophthalmology. 2008 Feb;115(2):334-41).

(Teixeira et al. 2009) (Teixeira VH et al. Antioxidants do not prevent post-exercise peroxidation and may delay muscle recovery. Med Sci Sports Exerc. 2009 Sep;41(9):1752-60).

(Thomson et al. 2007) (Thomson MJ, Puntmann V, Kaski JC. Atherosclerosis and oxidant stress: the end of the road for antioxidant vitamin treatment? Cardiovasc Drugs Ther. 2007 Jun;21(3):195-210).

(Villar et al, 2009) (Villar J, Purwar M, Merialdi M, Zavaleta N, Thi Nhu Ngoc N, Anthony J, De Greeff A, Poston L, Shennan A; WHO Vitamin C and Vitamin E trial group. World Health Organisation multicentre randomised trial of supplementation with vitamins C and E among pregnant women at high risk for pre-eclampsia in populations of low nutritional status from developing countries. BJOG. 2009 May;116(6):780-8).

(Voutilainen et al. 2006) (Sari Voutilainen, Tarja Nurmi, Jaakko Mursu and Tiina H Rissanen. Carotenoids and cardiovascular health American Journal of Clinical Nutrition, Vol. 83, No. 6, 1265-1271, June 2006).

(Wang et al. 2090) (Wang YZ, Ren WH, Liao WQ, Zhang GY. Concentrations of antioxidant vitamins in maternal and cord serum and their effect on birth outcomes. J Nutr Sci Vitaminol (Tokyo). 2009 Feb;55(1):1-8).

(Ward et al, 2007) (Ward NC, Wu JH, Clarke MW, Puddey IB, Burke V, Croft KD, Hodgson JM. The effect of vitamin E on blood pressure in individuals with type 2 diabetes: a randomized, double-blind, placebo-controlled trial. J Hypertens. 2007 Jan;25(1):227-34).

(Watters et al. 2009) (Watters JL, Gail MH, Weinstein SJ, Virtamo J, Albanes D. Associations between alpha-tocopherol, beta-carotene, and retinol and prostate cancer survival. Cancer Res. 2009 May 1;69(9):3833-41).

(Yuen et al. 2005) (Yuen B, Furrer L, Ballmer PE. Antioxidant vitamin supplementation in the prevention of cardiovascular disease. Ther Umsch. 2005 Sep;62(9):615-8).

(Yusoff, 2002) (Yusoff K. Vitamin E in cardiovascular disease: has the die been cast? Asia Pac J Clin Nutr. 2002;11 Suppl 7:S443-7).

(Zhang et al. 2009) (Zhang Y, Coogan P, Palmer JR, Strom BL, Rosenberg L. Vitamin and mineral use and risk of prostate cancer: the case-control surveillance study. Cancer Causes Control. 2009 Jul;20(5):691-8).

CHAPTER SIXTEEN

NAC, N-ACETYLCYSTEINE

Even the powerful antioxidant, NAC, does not alter disease course.

Thirteen (13) studies, with over 6,500 participants showed that NAC is no more effective than a placebo and 2 of these studies found harmful effects.

CIRCA 2003-2010

1) **Acetylcysteine, coronary procedure and prevention of contrast-induced worsening of renal function: which benefit for which patient? (Kefer et al. 2003) (#108)** This study was designed to determine whether acetylcysteine could provide a protective effect on renal function in a population of patients with normal renal function or mild to moderate chronic renal failure, usually referred for a coronary procedure. BACKGROUND: Contrast-induced nephropathy is a well-recognized complication of coronary angiography. Recent studies suggest that saline hydration and acetylcysteine reduce the incidence of contrast-induced worsening of renal function in patients with pre-existing chronic renal failure who are undergoing computed tomography examinations. METHODS: **One hundred eight patients were blindly and randomly assigned to receive either acetylcysteine or placebo** before and after administration of contrast agent in

association with a moderate hydration protocol. Serum creatinine and urea nitrogen were measured before and 24 hours after coronary procedure. RESULTS: The mean serum creatinine concentration remained unchanged 24 hours after contrast agent administration in both groups: from 1.04 +/- 0.26 to 1.03 +/- 0.29 mg/dl in the acetylcysteine group and from 1.16 +/- 1.1 to 1.06 +/- 0.41 mg/dl in the control group. We divided the population into 3 subgroups according to their creatinine clearance: no significant change of serum creatinine concentration was observed in patients with normal renal function nor in patients with pre-existing mild to moderate chronic renal failure in both groups. **There was no significant difference for the incidence of contrast-induced nephropathy between both groups.** CONCLUSIONS: **Our data do not support the systematic use of acetylcysteine before a coronary procedure in patients with normal renal function or mild to moderate chronic renal failure, to prevent contrast-induced nephropathy**. Division of Cardiology, University of Louvain, Brussels, Belgium.

2) Oral acetylcysteine does not protect renal function from moderate to high doses of intravenous radiographic contrast (Boccalandro et al. 2003) (#106 consecutive patients)

The use of radiographic contrast during cardiac catheterization can cause acute renal failure with an increase in morbidity and mortality. Prophylactic acetylcysteine plus intravenous hydration have been shown to prevent contrast-induced nephropathy (CIN) in patients with chronic renal failure undergoing computed tomography scan, who receive low doses of intravenous contrast. Whether the use of prophylactic acetylcysteine can decrease the incidence of CIN when larger doses of contrast are used remains to be determined. We sought to evaluate whether the prophylactic administration of acetylcysteine plus intravenous hydration is superior to intravenous hydration alone in prevention of CIN in patients with chronic renal failure undergoing cardiac catheterization and receiving moderate to high doses of intravenous contrast (> 1 cc/kg). **Seventy-three consecutive patients with renal insufficiency who received intravenous hydration and**

600 mg of acetylcysteine twice a day 24 hr before and the day of the cardiac catheterization were compared with **106 consecutive patients** who received hydration alone. Baseline and 48-hr serum creatinine concentrations were compared between the two groups before and after cardiac catheterization. **Multivariate and univariate analysis** were performed to assess the effects of acetylcysteine and other clinical variables in the change of serum creatinine after the procedure. Both groups had comparable clinical characteristics and received similar volumes of intravenous hydration. The volume of contrast used was similar for the two groups. A mean change in serum creatinine of 0.17 +/- 0.54 mg/dl for the acetylcysteine group vs. 0.19 +/- 0.40 mg/dl for the control group was observed at 48 hr. The incidence CIN was 13% in the acetylcysteine vs. 12% in the control group. **Acetylcysteine, whether analyzed with multivariate or univariate analysis, failed to demonstrate a significant effect in the change of serum creatinine after cardiac catheterization.** In patients with chronic renal insufficiency, acetylcysteine in a dose of 600 mg twice a day before and after cardiac catheterization, along with intravenous fluids, is as effective as fluids alone in the prevention of CIN when moderate to high doses of contrast are used. University of Texas Medical School and Memorial Hermann Hospital, Houston, Texas.

3) Perioperative N-acetylcysteine to prevent renal dysfunction in high-risk patients undergoing cabg surgery: a randomized controlled trial (Burns KE, et al. 2005) (#295 patients required elective or urgent CABG) Renal dysfunction is a complication of coronary artery bypass graft (CABG) surgery performed with cardiopulmonary bypass (CPB) that is associated with increased morbidity and mortality. N-acetylcysteine, an antioxidant and vasodilator, counteracts renal ischemia and hypoxia. OBJECTIVE: To determine whether perioperative intravenous (IV) N-acetylcysteine preserves renal function in high-risk patients undergoing CABG surgery with CPB compared with placebo. DESIGN, SETTING, AND PATIENTS: Randomized, quadruple blind, placebo-controlled trial (October 2003-September 2004) in operating rooms and general intensive care units (ICUs) of 2

Ontario tertiary care centers. The **295 patients required elective or urgent CABG** and had at least 1 of the following: preexisting renal dysfunction, at least 70 years old, diabetes mellitus, impaired left ventricular function, or undergoing concomitant valve or redo surgery. INTERVENTIONS: Patients received 4 (2 intraoperative and 2 postoperative) doses of IV N-acetylcysteine (600 mg) (n = 148) or placebo (n = 147) over 24 hours.

MAIN OUTCOME MEASURES: The primary outcome was the proportion of patients developing postoperative renal dysfunction, defined by an increase in serum creatinine level greater than 0.5 mg/dL (44 micromol/L) or a 25% increase from baseline within the first 5 postoperative days. Secondary outcomes included postoperative interventions and complications, the requirement for renal replacement therapy (RRT), adverse events, hospital mortality, and ICU and hospital length of stay. RESULTS: There was no difference in the proportion of patients with postoperative renal dysfunction in the N-acetylcysteine and placebo groups, respectively. We noted nonsignificant differences in postoperative interventions and complications, the need for RRT and serious adverse events, hospital mortality, and ICU and hospital length of stay between the N-acetylcysteine and placebo groups. A post hoc subgroup analysis of patients (baseline creatinine level >1.4 mg/dL [120 micromol/L]) showed a nonsignificant trend toward fewer patients experiencing postoperative renal dysfunction in the N-acetylcysteine group compared with the placebo group. CONCLUSIONS: **N-acetylcysteine did not prevent postoperative renal dysfunction, interventions, complications, or mortality in high-risk patients undergoing CABG surgery with CPB.** Further research is required to identify CABG patients at risk for postoperative renal events, valid markers of renal dysfunction, and to establish renal thresholds associated with important clinical outcomes. Division of Critical Care Medicine, University of Western Ontario, London, Ontario, Canada.

4) Phase II, randomized, controlled trial of high-dose N-acetylcysteine in high-risk cardiac surgery patients (Haase M, et al. 2007) (#60 cardiac surgery patients at higher risk of postoperative renal failure)

To assess the effect of high-dose N-acetylcysteine on renal function in cardiac surgery patients at higher risk of postoperative renal failure. DESIGN: **Multiblind, placebo-controlled, randomized, phase II clinical trial**. SETTING: Operating rooms and intensive care units of two tertiary referral hospitals. PATIENTS: A total of **60 cardiac surgery patients at higher risk of postoperative renal failure**. INTERVENTIONS: Patients were allocated to either 24 hrs of high-dose **N-acetylcysteine infusion (300 mg/kg body weight in 5% glucose, 1.7 L)** or placebo (5% glucose, 1.7 L). MEASUREMENTS AND MAIN RESULTS: The primary outcome measure was the absolute change in serum creatinine from baseline to peak value within the first five postoperative days. Secondary outcomes included the relative change in serum creatinine, peak serum creatinine level, serum cystatin C, and in urinary output. Further outcomes were needed for renal replacement therapy, length of ventilation, and length of stay in the intensive care unit and hospital. Randomization was successful and patients were well balanced for preoperative and intraoperative characteristics. There was no significant attenuation in the increase in serum creatinine from baseline to peak when comparing N-acetylcysteine with placebo. Also, there was no attenuation in the increase in serum cystatin C from baseline to peak for N-acetylcysteine compared with placebo. Likewise, there was no evidence for differences in any other clinical outcome. CONCLUSIONS: **In this phase II, randomized, controlled trial, high-dose N-acetylcysteine was no more effective than placebo in attenuating cardiopulmonary bypass-related acute renal failure in high-risk cardiac surgery patients**. Department of Intensive Care, Austin Hospital, University of Melbourne, Australia.

5) Clinical outcomes of contrast-induced nephropathy in patients undergoing percutaneous coronary intervention: a prospective, multicenter, randomized study to analyze the effect of hydration and acetylcysteine (Chen SL, et al. 2008) (#936)

The potential role of hydration in prevention of contrast-induced nephropathy (CIN) still remains to be unclear. METHODS: **Nine-hundred**

and thirty-six patients scheduled for percutaneous coronary intervention (PCI) were enrolled into the present study, and divided into normal (serum creatinine<1.5 mg/dl) and abnormal (serum creatine> or =1.5 mg/dl) groups according to their baseline serum concentration of creatinine. Each group was further randomly divided into two subgroups: hydration and nonhydration. **All patients in abnormal group took twice orally loading dose of 1200 mg acetylcysteine (ATLS)** at 12 h before scheduled time for coronary angiogram and immediately after procedure. Creatinine concentration was remeasured at the time of admission (just before catheterization), every day for the following three days. The primary end point during 6-month follow-up included clinical driven revascularization (either PCI or CABG), death from all causes, and requiring emergency renal-replacement therapy. RESULTS: **The incidence of CIN was more commonly in abnormal group that in normal group** (6.52% vs. 37.68%, p<0.001). Hydration had potentials in prevention of CIN only in patients with elevated baseline concentration of creatinine. Multivariate analysis demonstrated that the following variables remained to be significant factors correlating with CIN: age> or =70 years, contrast volume> or =320 ml, diabetes mellitus, and peripheral arterial disease. Patients with CIN in abnormal group had worse clinical outcomes, compared to patients with CIN in normal group. CONCLUSION: Hydration with 0.45% sodium *Patients with CIN and preexisting renal insufficiency had worse clinical outcomes.* chloride alone had no potential effect on the occurrence of CIN in patients with normal renal function. Combination of hydration with ATLS could reduce the incidence of CIN in patients at high risk. Nanjing First Hospital of Nanjing Medical University, Department of Cardiology, 68# Changle Road, 210006, Nanjing, China.

6) NAC had no effect on disease progression in non-diabetic kidney failure patients (Renke M. et al. 2008) (#20 non-diabetic patients with proteinuria)

Inhibition of the renin-angiotensin-aldosterone system with angiotensin-converting enzyme inhibitors (ACEI) and/or angiotensin II subtype I receptor antagonists (ARB) constitutes a strategy in the management of patients with chronic kidney disease. There is still no optimal therapy which can stop the progression of chronic kidney disease. **Antioxidants such as N-acetylcysteine (NAC) have been reported as a promising strategy** in this field. METHODS: In a **placebo-controlled, randomized**, open, 2-period cross-over study, we evaluated the influence of NAC (1,200 mg/day) added to renin-angiotensin-aldosterone system blockade on proteinuria and surrogate markers of tubular injury and renal fibrosis in **20 non-diabetic patients with proteinuria** (0.4-6.36 g/24 h) with normal or decreased kidney function (estimated glomerular filtration rate 61-163 ml/min). Subjects entered the **8-week** run-in period during which the therapy using ACEI and/or ARB was established with blood pressure below 130/80 mm Hg. Next, patients were randomly assigned to 1 of 2 treatment sequences: NAC/washout/placebo or placebo/washout/NAC. Clinical evaluation and laboratory tests were performed at the randomization point and after each period of the study. RESULTS: **No significant changes in laboratory tests were observed.** CONCLUSION: **NAC had no effect on proteinuria, surrogate markers of tubular injury or renal fibrosis in non-diabetic patients with chronic kidney disease.**

7) N-acetylcysteine to reduce renal failure after cardiac surgery: a systematic review and meta-analysis (Naughton et al. 2008) (#Seven randomized controlled trials (RCTs, n = 1000)

To assess the effect of N-acetylcysteine (NAC) on acute renal failure and important clinical outcomes after cardiac surgery. METHODS: Two reviewers performed literature searches, using EMBASE and PubMed, of randomized controlled trials investigating the renoprotective effect of N-acetylcysteine in cardiac surgery. Treatment effects were calculated as relative risks (RR) with 95% confidence intervals (CI). Heterogeneity and publication bias were assessed using the I(2) test and funnel plots, respectively. Meta regression was performed to assess the effect of baseline renal function and the use of aprotinin on renal function. RESULTS: **Seven randomized controlled trials (RCTs) (n = 1000)** were identified. No study could demonstrate, either independently or meta-analytically, an improvement in the postoperative increase in creatinine, mortality, renal failure requiring renal replacement therapy, myocardial infarction, atrial fibrillation, or stroke. *There was a small, though significant increase in post-operative blood loss among patients treated with NAC* (weighted mean difference 119 mL 95% CI 51, 187). After meta regression neither increase in postoperative creatinine nor renal replacement therapy was associated with the baseline creatinine or with NAC dose. CONCLUSION: **This analysis did not find that treatment with NAC was associated with clinical renal protection during cardiac surgery, or improvement in other clinical outcomes**. Department of Anesthesia and Pain Management, University Health Network, Toronto General Hospital, University of Toronto, Ontario, Canada.

8) N-acetylcysteine does not prevent contrast-induced nephropathy after cardiac catheterization in patients with diabetes mellitus and chronic kidney disease: a randomized clinical trial (Amini et al. 2009) (#90 patients) Patients with diabetes mellitus (DM) and chronic kidney disease (CKD) constitute to be a high-risk population for the development of contrast-induced nephropathy (CIN), in which the incidence of CIN is estimated to be as high as 50%. We performed this trial to assess the efficacy of N-acetylcysteine (NAC) in the prevention of this complication. METHODS: In a prospective, double-blind, placebo controlled, randomized clinical trial, we studied **90 patients undergoing elective diagnostic coronary angiography with DM and CKD** (serum creatinine > or = 1.5 mg/dL for men and > or = 1.4 mg/dL for women). The patients were **randomly assigned** to receive either oral NAC (600 mg BID, starting 24 h before the procedure) or placebo, in adjunct to hydration. Serum creatinine was measured prior to and 48 h after coronary angiography. The primary end-point was the occurrence of CIN, defined as an increase in serum creatinine > or = 0.5 mg/dL (44.2 micromol/L) or > or = 25% above baseline at 48 h after exposure to contrast medium. RESULTS: Complete data on the outcomes were available on 87 patients, 45 of whom had received NAC. **There were no significant differences between the NAC and**

placebo groups in baseline characteristics, amount of hydration, or type and volume of contrast used, except in gender and the use of statins. CIN occurred in 5 out of 45 (11.1%) patients in the NAC group and 6 out of 42 (14.3%) patients in the placebo group. CONCLUSION: **There was no detectable benefit for the prophylactic administration of oral NAC over an aggressive hydration protocol in patients with DM and CKD**. Department of cardiology, Tehran Heart Center, Tehran University of Medical Sciences, Tehran, Iran.

9) N-acetylcysteine in cardiovascular-surgery-associated renal failure: a meta-analysis (Nigwekar SU, Kandula P. 2009) (#Twelve studies comprising 1,324 patients)

Clinical trials with N-acetylcysteine (NAC) in perioperative cardiovascular settings have shown inconsistent effects for renal endpoints. We aimed to systematically review these trials to ascertain its role in prevention of post-cardiovascular surgery acute renal failure. METHODS: We searched MEDLINE, EMBASE, Cochrane Renal Health Library, and Google Scholar for randomized controlled studies that evaluated NAC in adult patients undergoing cardiovascular surgery. Acute renal failure, acute renal failure requiring dialysis, and mortality were the primary outcomes. Additional outcomes studied were length of intensive care unit stay, postoperative serum creatinine, creatinine clearance, renal biomarkers, and adverse effects of NAC. RESULTS: **Twelve studies comprising 1,324 patients** were found to be eligible. **Meta-analytic estimates showed that NAC was not associated with reduction in acute renal failure, acute renal failure requiring dialysis or mortality. N-acetylcysteine was well tolerated but was not associated with any reduction in the length of intensive care unit stay**. It had inconsistent effects on postoperative serum creatinine, creatinine clearance, and renal biomarkers. Subgroup analysis restricted to studies using intravenous NAC preparation showed a nonsignificant trend toward reduction in acute renal failure without any significant change in other outcomes. CONCLUSIONS: **Overall analysis of the existent literature shows that NAC is not beneficial in the prevention of post-cardiovascular surgery re-**

nal dysfunction. Routine use of NAC for this indication should be avoided. Department of Internal Medicine, Rochester General Hospital and University of Rochester School of Medicine, Rochester, New York 14621, USA.

10) Meta-analysis of N-acetylcysteine to prevent acute renal failure after major surgery (Ho M, Morgan DJ. 2009) (#10 studies involving a total of 1,193 adult patients)

Acute renal failure after major surgery is associated with significant mortality and morbidity that theoretically may be attenuated by N-acetylcysteine. DESIGN: Meta-analysis of relevant studies sourced from the Cochrane Controlled Trial Register (2007 issue 4), EMBASE, and MEDLINE databases (1966 to February 1, 2008) without language restriction. SETTING & POPULATION: Adult patients undergoing major surgery without the use of radiocontrast. SELECTION CRITERIA FOR STUDIES: **Randomized controlled studies** comparing N-acetylcysteine with a placebo perioperatively. DATA ANALYSIS: Categorical variables are reported as odds ratio (OR) with 95% confidence interval (CI), and continuous variables are reported as weighted-mean-difference (WMD) with 95% CI. OUTCOME MEASURES: Effects of N-acetylcysteine on mortality and acute renal failure requiring dialysis were the main outcomes of interest. Additional outcome measures included an incremental increase in serum creatinine concentration greater than 25% above baseline, surgical reexploration for bleeding, amount of allogeneic blood transfusion, and length of intensive care unit stay. RESULTS: **10 studies involving a total of 1,193 adult patients undergoing major surgery were considered. N-Acetylcysteine use was not associated with a decrease in mortality**, acute renal failure requiring dialysis, incremental increase in serum creatinine concentration greater than 25% above baseline, **or length of intensive care unit stay**. N-acetylcysteine did not appear to increase the risk of surgical reexploration for bleeding or amount of allogeneic blood transfusion required. LIMITATIONS: Most studied patients had cardiac surgery and normal renal function preoperatively.

CONCLUSIONS: **There is no current evidence that N-acetylcysteine used perioperatively can alter mor-**

tality or renal outcomes when radio-contrast is not used. Intensive Care Unit, Royal Perth Hospital, Perth, WA 6000, Australia.

11) Efficacy of N-acetylcysteine in preventing renal injury after heart surgery: a systematic review of randomized trials (Adabag et al. 2009) (#1163)

The aim of this study was to assess whether perioperative N-acetyl-cysteine (NAC), an antioxidant, prevents **acute renal injury (ARI)** after cardiac surgery. METHODS AND RESULTS: We performed **a systematic review** of **randomized controlled trials (RCTs) of NAC in adult cardiac surgery patients.** The RCTs were identified by searching MEDLINE (1960-2008), clinicaltrials.gov website, and hand-searching references of relevant publications. Primary outcome was ARI (absolute increase >0.5 mg/dL or relative increase >25%, in serum creatinine from baseline within 5 days after surgery). Random effects model was used to perform **a meta-analysis**. Forest plots and I(2) test were used to assess heterogeneity among studies. **Ten RCTs (n = 1163 patients)** were included. Mean age was 70 +/- 7.4 years, 71% were male, and 66% underwent coronary artery bypass surgery. **N-Acetylcysteine did not reduce ARI incidence.** Overall, 3.3% of patients required and 3% died. There was a trend towards reduced ARI incidence among patients with baseline chronic kidney disease assigned to intravenous NAC. CONCLUSION: This **meta-analysis of RCTs showed that prophylactic perioperative NAC in cardiac surgery does not reduce ARI, hemodialysis, or death.** Division of Cardiology (111 C), Minneapolis Veterans Affairs Medical Center, The Minneapolis VA Center for Chronic Disease Outcomes Research, and the University of Minnesota.

12) Impact of high-dose N-acetylcysteine versus placebo on contrast-induced nephropathy and myocardial reperfusion injury in unselected patients with ST-segment elevation myocardial infarction undergoing primary percutaneous coronary intervention. The LIPSIA-N-ACC (Prospective, Single-Blind,

Placebo-Controlled, Randomized Leipzig Imme-diate PercutaneouS Coronary Intervention Acute Myocardial Infarction N-ACC) Trial (Thiele H, et al. 2010) (#251) The aim of this **randomized, single-blind, controlled trial** was to assess N-acetylcysteine effects on contrast-induced nephropathy and reperfusion injury in ST-segment elevation myocardial infarction patients undergoing primary angioplasty with moderate contrast volumes. BACKGROUND: High-dose N-acetyl-cysteine reduced the incidence of **contrast-induced nephropathy (CIN)** in patients with high contrast volumes and reduced reperfusion injury in animal trials. METHODS: Patients undergoing primary angioplasty were **randomized to either high-dose N-acetylcysteine (2 x 1,200 mg/day for 48 h; n = 126) or placebo plus optimal hydration (n = 125).** The 2 primary end points were: 1) the occurrence of >25% increase in serum creatinine level <72 h after randomization; and 2) a reduction in reperfusion injury measured as myocardial salvage index by magnetic resonance imaging. RESULTS: The median volume of an iso-osmolar contrast agent during angiography was 180 ml in the N-acetylcysteine and 160 ml in the placebo group. The primary end point contrast-induced nephropathy occurred in 14% of the N-acetylcysteine group and in 20% of the placebo group. The myocardial salvage index was also not different between both treatment groups. **Activated oxygen protein products and oxidized low-density lipoprotein as markers for oxidative stress were reduced by as much as 20% in the N-acetylcysteine group, whereas no change was evident in the placebo group.** CONCLUSIONS: **High-dose intravenous N-acetylcysteine reduces oxidative stress.** However, **it does not provide an additional clinical benefit to placebo with respect to CIN and myocardial reperfusion injury in nonselected patients undergoing angioplasty with moderate doses of contrast medium and optimal hydration.** The LIPSIA-N-ACC. Department of Internal Medicine-Cardiology, University of Leipzig Heart Center, Leipzig, Germany.

13) NAC had no effect on blood pressure and surrogate markers of cardiovascular injury in non-

diabetic patients with CKD (Renke et al. 2010) (#20 non-diabetic patients with albuminuria) Cardiovascular complications in patients with chronic kidney disease **(CKD) are frequent.** They show increased cardiovascular mortality and morbidity attributable to accumulation of several risk factors; e.g., hypertension, oxidative stress and elevated plasma homocysteine concentration. Despite recent progress in their management, there is still no optimal therapy that can stop progression of CKD and decrease cardiovascular outcome in these patients. **Antioxidants, e.g., N-acetylcysteine (NAC), have been suggested as a promising medicament** in this field. MATERIAL/METHODS: In a **placebo-controlled, randomized,** two-period cross-over study we evaluated the influence of **eight weeks** of **NAC therapy (1200 mg/ day)** added to pharmacological renin-angiotensin system blockade on ambulatory blood pressure and surrogate markers of cardiovascular risk and injury in **20 non-diabetic patients with albuminuria** [30-915 mg per creatinine mg] and normal or slightly decreased kidney function [eGFR 61-163 ml/min]. After eight weeks run-in period during which the therapy using angiotensin converting enzyme inhibitors and/or angiotensin receptor blockers was settled, patients were randomly assigned to one of two treatment sequences: NAC/washout/placebo or placebo/washout/NAC. RESULTS: **No significant changes in blood pressure, albuminuria and homocysteine plasma level were observed.** CONCLUSIONS: **NAC had no effect on blood pressure and surrogate markers of cardiovascular injury in non-diabetic patients with CKD**.

Two studies showing harmful **NAC** effects:

- *Patients with CIN and preexisting renal insufficiency had worse clinical outcomes when taking NAC.* **(Chen SL, et al. 2008)**
- *There was a small, though significant increase in postoperative blood loss among patients treated with NAC.* **(Naughton et al. 2008)**

REFERENCES FOR NAC, N-acetylcysteine

(Adabag et al. 2009) (Adabag AS, Ishane A, bloomfield HE, Ngo AK, Wilt TJ. Efficacy of N-acetylcysteine in preventing renal injury after heart surgery: a systematic review of randomized trials. Eur Heart J. 2009 Aug;30(15):1910-7).

(Amini et al. 2009) (Amini M, Salarifar M, Amirgaigloo A, Masoudk-abir F, Esfahane F. N-acetylcysteine does not prevent contrast-induced nephropathy after cardiac catheterization in patients with diabetes mellitus and chronic kidney disease: a randomized clinical trial. Trials. 2009 Jun 29;10:45).

(Boccalandro et al. 2003) (Boccalandro F, Amhad M, Smalling RW, Sdringola S. Oral acetylcysteine does not protect renal function from moderate to high doses of intravenous radiographic contrast. Catheter Cardiovasc Interv. 2003 Mar;58(3):336-41).

(Burns KE, et al. 2005) (Burns KE, et al. Perioperative N-acetylcys-teine to prevent renal dysfunction in high-risk patients undergoing cabg surgery: a randomized controlled trial. JAMA. 2005 Jul 20;294(3): 342-50).

(Chen SL, et al. 2008) (Chen SL, et al. Clinical outcomes of contrast-induced nephropathy in patients undergoing percutaneous coronary intervention: a prospective, multicenter, randomized study to ana-lyze the effect of hydration and acetylcysteine. Int J Cardiol. 2008 Jun 6;126(3):407-13).

(Haase M, et al. 2007) (Haase M, et al. Phase II, randomized, controlled trial of high-dose N-acetylcysteine in high-risk cardiac surgery pa-tients. Crit Care Med. 2007 May;35(5):1324-31).

(Ho M, Morgan DJ. 2009) (Ho M, Morgan DJ. Meta-analysis of N-acetylcysteine to prevent acute renal failure after major surgery. Am J Kidney Dis. 2009 Jan;53(1):33-40).

(Kefer et al. 2003) (Kefer JM, Hanet CE, Boitte S, Wilmotte L, DeKock M. Acetylcysteine, coronary procedure and prevention of contrast-induced worsening of renal function: which benefit for which patient? Acta Cardiol. 2003 Dec;58(6):555-60).

(Naughton et al. 2008) (Naughton F, Wijeysundera D, Karkouti K, Tait G, Beattie WS. N-acetylcysteine to reduce renal failure after cardiac surgery: a systematic review and meta-analysis. Can J Anaesth. 2008 Dec;55(12):827-35).

(Nigwekar SU, Kandula P. 2009) (Nigwekar SU, Kandula P. N-acetylcysteine in cardiovascular-surgery-associated renal failure: a meta-analysis. Ann Thorac Surg. 2009 Jan;87(1):139-47).

(Renke M. et al. 2008) (Renke M. et al. The effect of N-acetylcysteine on proteinuria and markers of tubular injury in non-diabetic patients with chronic kidney disease. A placebo-controlled, randomized, open, cross-over study. Kidney Blood Press Res. 2008;31(6):404-10).

(Renke et al. 2010) (Renke M. et al. The effect of N-acetylcysteine on blood pressure and markers of cardiovascular risk in non-diabetic patients with chronic kidney disease: a placebo-controlled, randomized, cross-over study. Med Sci Monit. 2010;16(7):PI13-8).

(Thiele H, et al. 2010) (Thiele H, et al. Impact of high-dose N-acetylcysteine versus placebo on contrast-induced nephropathy and myocardial reperfusion injury in unselected patients with ST-segment elevation myocardial infarction undergoing primary percutaneous coronary intervention. The LIPSIA-N-ACC (Prospective, Single-Blind, Placebo-Controlled, Randomized Leipzig Immediate PercutaneouS Coronary Intervention Acute Myocardial Infarction N-ACC) Trial. J Am Coll Cardiol. 2010 May 18;55(20):2201-9).

CHAPTER SEVENTEEN

THE PLOT THICKENS

The oxidative stress menace to coronary vasculature: any place for antioxidants?

Oxidative stress was believed to be involved in the pathogenesis of atherosclerosis. However, **interventional trials have been controversial, with some positive findings, many null findings, and some suggestion of harm in certain high-risk populations.** Therefore, **treatment with antioxidant vitamins C and E should not be recommended for the prevention or treatment of coronary atherosclerosis.** New antioxidant strategies are needed to clarify the exact role of antioxidant treatment in coronary atherosclerosis (Briasoulis et al, 2009). 1st Cardiology Unit, Hippokration Hospital, Athens University Medical School, Athens, Greece.

Other popular antioxidant failures:

Glutathione and reductive stress

In 2007, Ivor Benjamin of the University of Utah, found the first bona fide example of the role that "reductive stress" can play in disease. Mice with one of the mutant genes, áB-crystallin, specifically in the heart develop the same symptoms seen in human patients, including heart enlargement, progressive heart failure, and an early death.

They further show that the animals' hearts are under reductive stress. Benjamin found the mice had "markedly reduced" oxidative stress levels due to an abundance of a natural antioxidant known as glutathione, producing excess levels of the reduced glutathione and a condition of **reductive stress**. This supports my ROSI syndrome (Reactive Oxygen Species Insufficiency) (Howes, 2008) and my Unified Theory (Howes, 2004).

Pine bark

No beneficial effects of pine bark extract on cardiovascular disease risk factors (Drieling et al. 2010) (#130 individuals with increased cardiovascular disease risk)

Although modifiable cardiovascular disease risk factors are common, some patients eschew conventional drug treatments in favor of natural alternatives. **Pine bark extract, a dietary supplement source of antioxidant oligomeric proanthocyanidin complexes**, has multiple putative cardiovascular benefits. Studies published to date about the supplement have notable methodological limitations. METHODS: They **randomized 130 individuals with increased cardiovascular disease risk** to take **200 mg of a water-based extract of pine bark** (n = 64; Toyo-FVG, Toyo Bio-Pharma, Torrance, California; Shinyaku Co, Ltd, Saga, Japan; also marketed as Flavagenol in Japan) or placebo (n = 66) **once per day**. Blood pressure, our primary outcome, and other cardiovascular disease risk factors were measured at baseline and at **6 and 12 weeks.** Statistical analyses were conducted using regression models. RESULTS: Baseline characteristics did not differ between the study groups. Over the 12-week intervention, the sum of systolic and diastolic blood pressures decreased by 1.0 mm Hg in the pine bark extract-treated group and by 1.9 mm Hg. Other outcomes were likewise not significantly different, including body mass index, lipid panel measures, liver transaminase test results, lipoprotein cholesterol particle size, and levels of insulin, lipoprotein(a), fasting glucose, and high-sensitivity C-reactive protein. **There were no subgroups for whom intake of pine bark extract affected cardiovascular disease risk factors.** CONCLUSIONS: **This pine bark extract (at a dosage of 200 mg/d) was safe but was not** associated with improvement in cardiovascular disease risk factors. Although variations among participants, dosages, and chemical preparations could contribute to different findings compared with past studies, **our results are consistent with a general failure of antioxidants to demonstrate cardiovascular benefits.**

Don't Count on Selenium to Prevent Lung Cancer Recurrence

A June 5, 2010 study shows that taking the popular mineral supplement selenium doesn't reduce the likelihood of lung cancer recurrence.

Lead author Dr. Daniel D. Karp, a professor in the department of thoracic/head and neck medical oncology at the University of Texas M.D. Anderson Cancer Center, is scheduled to present the finding Saturday 6/5/10 at the American Society of Clinical Oncology annual meeting, in Chicago.

"Several epidemiological and animal studies have long-suggested a link between deficiency of selenium and cancer development," said Karp in a news release. **"Interest and research escalated in the late 1990s after a skin cancer and selenium study, published in 1996, found no benefit against the skin cancer, but did suggest an approximate 30 percent reduction of prostate and lung cancers.** Our lung cancer research and another major study for the prevention of prostate cancer evolved from that finding."

But the new study found that **among more than 1,500 stage 1 (early) non-small cell lung cancer patients who had survived their initial bout with the disease, selenium offered no protection against recurrence or the onset of a new cancer or second primary cancer.**

The patients were tracked from 2000 to 2009, after all had undergone surgery to remove their initial tumors and remained cancer-free for a minimum of six months post-treatment. Half the patients were placed on a regimen of **200 micrograms of selenium**, while the other half took a placebo.

Those in the placebo group had better survival rates five years later than those taking the supplement (selenium)– an observation that led the research team to halt the study earlier than planned.

While 78 percent taking the placebo stayed alive over that time frame, the rate was just 72 percent among the selenium group. And while 1.4 percent of the placebo group developed a second primary tumor within a year, that figure rose to 1.9 percent among the selenium group, the researchers said.

Some benefit of selenium was observed in a small group of patients who had never smoked, but the study authors said the group was too small to render the finding meaningful.

I believe that this indicates that the antioxidant, selenium, not only does not improve the survival of lung cancer patients, it may increase their mortality or raise the incidence of developing of a second primary tumor. This is similar to and consistent with my collective study data on the antioxidant vitamins A, C and E reported in *Death In Small Doses?*.

ANIMAL STUDIES with vitamin C

Life-long vitamin C supplementation does not affect oxidative damage or lifespan in mice, but decreases expression of antioxidant protection genes. (Selman et al. 2006) (MICE study). High dietary doses of vitamin C are ineffective at prolonging lifespan in mice because any positive benefits derived as an antioxidant are offset by compensatory reductions in endogenous protection mechanisms, leading to no net reduction in accumulated oxidative damage.

Lipid peroxidation caused by bacterial-independent acute peritonitis

Administration of large doses of vitamin C does not decrease oxidant-induced lung lipid peroxidation caused by bacterial-independent acute peritonitis in-flammation. (Demling et al. 2002). Acute zymosan-induced peritonitis in rats produces lung inflammation and lipid peroxidation. The effect of this process on plasma and lung tissue ascorbic acid was determined, as was the effect of infusing 150 mg/kg of ascorbic acid immediately after zymosan on the degree of lung insult. Ascorbic acid levels were significantly decreased in plasma and lung tissue at 24 h after zymosan, and lung tissue conjugated diene and neutrophil content was also significantly increased. Vitamin C infusion increased postzymosan plasma levels by 50% over normal control levels. However, **lung tissue ascorbic acid was still decreased, and no decrease in the lung injury process was noted.** Added ascorbic acid also did not prevent a decrease in plasma vitamin E with the peritonitis. We conclude that **the amount of ascorbic acid given in this study did not diminish the lung oxidant inflammatory changes.** An insufficient dose or inadequate time for plasma ascorbic acid to equilibrate with the lung cytosol are possible explanations for the lack of attenuation of lung oxidant stress.

Quercetin and ferulic acid

The Safety Questioned Of Certain 'Healthful' Plant-Based Antioxidants (quercetin and ferulic acid) (rat study)

In September of 2010, **scientists were calling for more research on the possibility that some supposedly healthful plant-based antioxidants - including those renowned for their apparent ability to prevent cancer - may actually aggravate or even cause cancer in some individuals**.

Their recommendation followed a study in which *two such antioxidants - quercetin and ferulic acid - appeared to aggravate kidney cancer in severely diabetic laboratory rats.* **The study appears in ACS' bi-weekly *Journal of Agricultural and Food Chemistry.***

Kuan-Chou Chen, Robert Peng, and colleagues note that vegetables, fruits, and other plant-based foods are rich in antioxidants that appear to fight cancer, diabetes, heart disease, and other disorders. **Among those antioxidants is quercetin, especially abundant in onions and black tea, and ferulic acid, found in corn, tomatoes, and rice bran.** Both also are ingredients in certain herbal remedies and dietary supplements. **But questions remain about the safety and effectiveness of some antioxidants, with research suggesting that quercetin could contribute to the development of cancer,** the scientists note.

They found that **diabetic laboratory rats fed either quercetin or ferulic acid developed more advanced forms of kidney cancer, and *concluded the two antioxidants appear to aggravate or possibly cause kidney cancer.*** *"Some researchers believe that quercetin should not be used by healthy people for prevention until it can be shown that quercetin does not itself cause cancer,"* the report states. *"In this study we report that* **quercetin aggravated, at least, if not directly caused, kidney cancer in rats,"* *it adds, suggesting that health agencies like the U. S. Food and Drug Administration should re-evaluate the safety of plant-based antioxidants.* Article: "Quercetin and Ferulic Acid Aggravate Renal Carcinoma in Long-Term Diabetic Victims" Source: Michael Bernstein, American Chemical Society.

Lycopene

Are the health attributes of lycopene related to its antioxidant function?

A variety of epidemiological trials have suggested that higher intake of lycopene-containing foods (primarily tomato products) or blood lycopene concentrations are associated with decreased cardiovascular disease and prostate cancer risk. Of the carotenoids tested, **lyco-**

pene has been demonstrated to be the most potent in vitro antioxidant leading many researchers to conclude that the antioxidant properties of lycopene are responsible for disease prevention. In our review of human and animal trials with lycopene, or lycopene-containing extracts, **there is limited support for the in vivo antioxidant function for lycopene.** Moreover, **tissue levels of lycopene appear to be too low to play a meaningful antioxidant role.** We conclude that **there is an overall shortage of supportive evidence for the "antioxidant hypothesis" as lycopene's major in vivo mechanism of action.** Our laboratory has postulated that metabolic products of lycopene, the lycopenoids, may be responsible for some of lycopene's reported bioactivity (Erdman, Ford, Lindshield, 2009).

The scientific method demands that we change our beliefs or theories to fit the factual data. I believe that this applies directly to the Free Radi-Crap theory. Again, I say that the free radical theory has fallen.

ANOTHER ANTIOXIDANT TRAGEDY: CLIOQUINOL

In 1955 a mysterious disease, **resembling polio**, appeared in Japan and had symptoms of a **combination of diarrhea, internal bleeding and various signs of nerve degeneration. By 1959 the disease had become an epidemic.** The illness appeared to be **contagious**, but patients did not display the symptoms typically associated with infections. **By 1964 the epidemic had worsened and patients were exhibiting blindness, with some patients dying.**

During the 1960s thousands of Japanese users of the anti-diarrhea drug clioquinol were left crippled, blinded, or otherwise disabled (sometimes leading to death) by a nerve disease known as subacute myelo-optic neuropathy (SMON). Dozens of elderly women, and some men in their thirties, began filling the nearby hospitals, totaling almost 3 percent of the local population by 1971.

In May of 1964, the disease was given a formal name: **"Sub-acute Myelo-Optic Neuropathy" (SMON) and by 1971, the number of people hospitalized in the Okayama Province accounted for about three per cent of the province's population. SMON victims had received treatment for diarrhea with a number of drugs.** Upon investigation, **these different drugs turned out not to be different at all; they were all made of a substance called Clioquinol, an antioxidant, but marketed under different brand names and freely available.**

The antioxidant Clioquinol, a Ciba-Geigy product, was erroneously considered to be perfectly safe, because **its effects would be confined to the digestive tract where it was supposed to destroy germs associated with diarrhea without being absorbed into the bloodstream. But the evidence was irrefutable and** the SMON epidemic **lasted until just after the government finally banned the antioxidant drug in September 1970. But Ciba-Geigy nevertheless continued selling the drug worldwide.**

The Japanese government recognized about 11,000 SMON victims, 4,700 of whom had filed damage claims as of 1979 (Chapmann, 1979).

Curiously, overmedication is more common in Japan than elsewhere because doctors receive payment from the government health insurance for every drug they prescribe.

Clioquinol (5-chloro-7-iodo-8-hydroxyquinoline; CQ) belongs to the quinoline class of compounds and is structurally similar to 5,7-DiCl-8-OHQ. **This class of compounds possesses an established toxicology profile with the US Pharmacopoeia.** During the 1950s to the 1970s, CQ was used as an **antibiotic;** however, **it was withdrawn due to association with subacute myelo-optic neuropathy** possibly due to overdose and/or a reversible vitamin B_{12} deficiency. Recently, interest in CQ has reemerged due to studies involving its use, in combination with B$_{12}$, for treatment of Alzheimer's disease. **It has a very controversial history.**

Clioquinol (5-chloro-7-iodo-8-quinolinol) chelates zinc and copper and acts as an antioxidant. The main biochemical change induced in some studies by clioquinol was a marked reduction in lipid peroxidation at all time points. (Bareggi SR et al. 2009).

I believe that clioquinol is another example of dead bodies from antioxidant use.

One thousand and thirty-one longstanding patients with subacute myelo-optico-neuropathy (SMON; 275 males, 756 females) were examined in 2002, **32 years after banning of clioquinol.** About 41% of patients still had **difficulty to walking** independently, including 15.8% of completely loss of locomotion. One point six percent of patients were in **complete blindness** and 5.8% had severe visual impairment. As complication, **high incidence was revealed with cataract (56.2%), hypertension (40.2%),** vertebral disease (35.5%), and limb articular disease (31.5%).

These results indicate the serious sequelae of clioquinol intoxication, SMON. (Konogaya et al. 2004). **I believe that this supports my view that an EMOD insufficiency is, in part, causative of cataract formation. This is the effect of the antioxidant clioquinol.**

Blow to vitamins as antidote to aging

As of 2008,

- Antioxidants failed to protect body, study concludes.
- Theory (free radical theory) cited by health food industry is wrong.

The notion that antioxidant supplements such as vitamins C and E could slow aging has been dealt a blow by a scientific study showing that the theory behind the advice is wrong. Beloved health food shops and glossy magazines alike, antioxidants have long been peddled as preventative pills that have the ability to slow ageing and protect against diseases such as cancer. But the research has shown that the molecular mechanism proposed to explain how they work is mistaken.

David Gems, at University College London, who led the study, said: "It really demonstrates finally that trying to boost your antioxidant levels is very unlikely to have any effect on ageing."

The dominant theory for aging has been around since the 1950s; it blames glitches in cells caused by the damaging byproducts of our metabolism. As cells break down sugars to release energy, they also unleash reactive forms of oxygen such as superoxide. These supposedly cause the damage which is the hallmark of ageing.

Gems' team set about testing the theory that raising or lowering the body's natural defences against superoxide could affect an individual's lifespan: make the defenses stronger, and lifespan should increase; make them weaker, and it should decrease.

As it would be unethical to experiment on humans, his team used the nematode worm, Caenorhabditis elegans. By tweaking its genes, the scientists were able to "tune" the worms' natural defenses - enzymes it produces to tackle superoxide. However, this made no difference to the worms' lifespan.

"You can drastically change the natural defense levels and there's just no effect on ageing," said Gems, who published his results yesterday in the journal Genes and Development. He added that molecular damage was probably caused by numerous different chemicals within the cell. "With increasing lifespan comes greater exposure and vulnerability to the aging process," said Alan Schafer, head of molecular and physiological sciences at the Wellcome Trust. "Research such as this points to how much we have to learn about ageing, and the importance of understanding the mechanisms behind this process. This new study will encourage researchers to explore new avenues in ageing research."

Gems's findings coincide with a recent US study on the effectiveness of antioxidants against cancer. The clinical trial on nearly 15,000 men tested whether vitamin C and E supplements were effective against the disease. After following the subjects for several years, **researchers found no statistical difference in the number of cancers between the groups taking the vitamins and those on a placebo**.

References for chapter seventeen

(Bareggi SR et al. 2009) (Bareggi SR et al. Effects of clioquinol on memory impairment and the neurochemical modifications induced by scrapie infection in golden hamsters. Brain Res. 2009 Jul 14;1280:195-200). Department of Pharmacology, Chemotherapy and Medical Toxicology, School of Medicine, Milano, Italy.

(Briasoulis et al, 2009) (Briasoulis A, et al, The oxidative stress menace to coronary vasculature: any place for antioxidants? Curr Pharm Des. 2009;15(26):3078-90).

(Chapmann, 1979) (William Chapmann, "A Japanese Tragedy, Dirodo-hydroxyquinoline," *Washington Post* 18 March 1979.).

(Demling et al. 2002) (Robert Demling, Keiichi Ikegami, Lisa Picard and Cheryl Lalonde. Administration of large doses of vitamin C does not decrease oxidant-induced lung lipid peroxidation caused by bacterial-independent acute peritonitis Inflammation. 2002. Volume 18, Number 5, 499-510, DOI: 10.1007/BF01560697).

(Drieling et al. 2010) (Drieling RL, Gardner CD, Ma J, Ahn DK, Stafford RS. No beneficial effects of pine bark extract on cardiovascular disease risk factors. Arch Intern Med. 2010 Sep 27;170(17):1541-7). Program on Prevention Outcomes and Practices, Stanford Prevention Research Center, Stanford University School of Medicine, Stanford, California.

(Erdman, Ford, Lindshield, 2009) (Erdman JW Jr, Ford NA, Lindshield BL. Are the health attributes of lycopene related to its antioxidant function? Arch Biochem Biophys. 2009 Mar 15;483(2):229-35).

(Howes, 2004) (Howes, R. M. U.T.O.P.I.A. - Unified Theory of Oxygen Participation in Aerobiosis. © 2004. Free Radical Publishing Co. Kentwood, LA, available at www.iwillfindthecure.org.)

(Howes, 2008) (R. M. Howes. Reactive Oxygen Species Insufficiency (ROSI) as the Basis for Disease Allowance and Coexistence: Extraordinary Support for an Extraordinary Theory. Free Radical Publishing. Vol I, II & III. © 2008; 1564 pages. available at: www.iwillfindthecure. org)

(Konogaya et al.) (Konogaya M, et al. Clinical analysis of longstanding subacute myelo-optico-neuropathy: sequelae of clioquinol at 32 years after its ban. Journal of the Neurological Sciences. Volume 218, Issue 1 , Pages 85-90, 15 March 2004).

(Selman et al. 2006) (Selman C, McLaren JS, Meyer C, Duncan JS, Redman P, Collins AR, Duthie GG, Speakman JR. Life-long vitamin C supplementation in combination with cold exposure does not affect oxidative damage or lifespan in mice, but decreases expression of antioxidant protection genes. Mech Ageing Dev. 2006 Dec;127(12): 897-904).

SECTION THREE

181 STUDIES FROM "DEATH IN SMALL DOSES?"

AN EPIC CHRONOLOGY OF ANTIOXIDANT VITAMIN STUDIES

I have included this section from my prior book to make the referenced material complete, such that both this new book and the prior book total 250 studies showing marginal or negligible effects. A total of eighty (80) of these 250 studies have shown harmful effects.

ANTIOXIDANT VITAMIN FAILURES

I have 181 reports, on over 8 million subjects, showing "disappointing" results with antioxidants in preventing or reversing disease. Thus, prudent questions are, "Why take them in the absence of a deficiency state?" "Why waste money for marginally effective or harmful pills?"

181 Antioxidant Intervention Trial & Analysis Studies:
Failures & Nullification of the Free Radical Theory
R.M. Howes M.D., Ph.D.

This is a selective systematic over view of 181 **interventional initial or follow up studies,** showing either marginal effect, negligible effect or no effect at all. Fifty seven of these studies/reports showed harmful effects of the antioxidant vitamins **A** (beta carotene), **C** (ascorbic acid) or **E** (alpha tocopherol) or combinations thereof. Total number of participants for all of the above studies is in excess of **8,600,000 subjects,** some of which may have been repeats in follow up or parallel studies. Studies with multi-vitamins, which contain the antioxidant vitamins, were also included.

The list of studies or reports is arranged as follows: Paper (study) number; Title of Study or Paper; Author reference; and Chronological Year; and Number of participants or trials in the respective study.

1. **Failure of High-dose Vitamin C (ascorbic acid) Therapy to Benefit Patients with Advanced Cancer. A Controlled Trial.** (Creagan et al, 1979) (#159 patients with advanced cancer)

2. **High-dose Vitamin C versus Placebo in the Treatment of Patients with Advanced Cancer Who Have had no Prior Chemotherapy.** (Moertel et al, 1985) (#100 patients with advanced colorectal cancer)

3. **Skin Cancer Prevention Study** (Greenberg et al, 1990) (#1,805 men and women with recent nonmelanoma skin cancer)

4. **Diet in the Epidemiology of Postmenopausal Breast Cancer in the New York State Cohort** (Graham et al, 1992) (#18,586 postmenopausal women)

5. **Women's Health Study (WHS) (Buring and Hennekens, 1992); (#39,876 healthy women)**

6. **Isotretinoin-Basal Cell Carcinoma Study Group** (Tangrea et al, 1992, 1993) (#981 patients with two or more previously treated basal cell carcinomas)

7. **Prospective Study of the Intake of Vitamins C, E, and A and the Risk of Breast Cancer** (Hunter et al, 1993) (#89,494 women)

8. **Serum micronutrients and the subsequent risk of cervical cancer in a population-based nested case-control study.** (Batieha, 1993) (#15,161 women)

9. **A randomized trial of vitamin A and vitamin E supplementation for retinitis pigmentosa.** (Berson, 1993) (#601 patients aged 18 through 49 years with retinitis pigmentosa)

10. **Alpha-Tocopherol, beta-Carotene Cancer Prevention Study (ATBC study)** (Heinonen et al, **1994) (#29,133 men)**

11. **Polyp Prevention Study** (Greenberg et al, 1994) (#864)

12. **Effect of vitamin C supplementation on lipoprotein cholesterol, apolipoprotein, and triglyceride concentrations** (Jaques et al, 1995) (#139)

13. **The effect of high-dose ascorbate supplementation on plasma lipoprotein(a) levels in patients with premature coronary heart disease** (Bostom et al, 1995) (#44 patients with premature CHD)

14. **Cholesterol Lowering Atherosclerosis Study (CLAS) (1995)** (Hodis et al, 1995) (#156 men)

15. **Effects of Vitamin E on susceptibility of low-density lipoprotein and low-density lipoprotein subfractions to oxidation and on protein glycation in NIDDM.** (Reaven, 1995) (#21 men with NIDDM)

16. **Excretion of alpha-tocopherol into human seminal plasma after oral administration** (Moilanen and Hovatta, 1995) (#15 unselected male volunteers)

17. **The beta-Carotene and Retinol Efficacy Trial (CARET)** (Omenn et al, 1996) (#14,254 heavy smokers and 4,060 asbestos workers) (total #18,314)

18. **Cambridge Heart Antioxidant Study (CHAOS)** (Stephens et al., 1996) (#2,002 patients with coronary atherosclerosis)

19. **Physicians' Health Study (PHSI)** (Hennekens et al, 1996) (#22,071 US Physicians and Malignant Neoplasms or CVD)

20. **Dietary Antioxidant Vitamins and Death from Coronary Heart Disease in Postmenopausal Women** (Kushi et al, 1996) (#34,486 postmenopausal women with no cardiovascular disease)

21. **Mortality associated with low plasma concentration of beta carotene and the effect of oral supplementation** (Greenberg et al, 1996) (#1,720 men and women)

22. **The effect of antioxidant treatment on human spermatozoa and fertilization rate in an in vitro fertilization program** (Geva et al, 1996) (#Fifteen fertile normospermic males)

23. **Antioxidant Vitamin Effect on Traditional CVD Risk Factors** (Miller et al, 1997) (#297 retired teachers)

24. **ATBC Sub-Study Shows Increased CVD Deaths** (Rapola et al, 1997) (#1,862 men, with prior myocardial infarction)

25. **Effect of preoperative supplementation with alpha-tocopherol and ascorbic acid on myocardial injury in patients undergoing cardiac operations** (Westhuyzen et al, 1997) (#77 undergoing elective coronary artery bypass grafting)

26. **The influence of antioxidant nutrients on platelet function in healthy volunteers** (Calzada et al, 1997) (#40 healthy volunteers)

27. **The Multivitamins and Probucol Study** (Tardif et al, 1997) (#317 participants)

28. **Vitamin C intake and cardiovascular disease risk factors in persons with non-insulin-dependent diabetes mellitus** (Mayer-Davis et al, 1997) (#Insulin Resistance Atherosclerosis Study (IRAS, n = 520) **and from the San Luis Valley Diabetes Study (SLVDS, n = 422)** (total #942)

29. **Preformed Vitamin A Study Showed No Trend to Reduce Breast Cancer Risk.** (Longnecker, 1997) (#3,543 cases and 9,406 controls)

30. **Effect of Vitamin E and Beta Carotene on the Incidence of Primary Nonfatal Myocardial Infarction and Fatal Coronary Heart Disease** (Virtamo et al, 1998) (#27,271 Finnish male smokers)

31. **SU.VI.MAX** (Vasquez et al., 1998) (#13,017 French adults)

32. **A Sub-Study of SU.VI.MAX** (#1,162 subjects aged older than 50 years)

33. **The Nurses' Health Study and Folic Acid and Colon Cancer** (Giovannucci, 1998) (#88,756 women taking vitamin C and B-carotene, for 8 years)

34. **Effect of B-group vitamins and antioxidant vitamins on hyperhomocysteinemia** (Woodside, et al. 1998) (#101 men)

35. **Relationships of serum carotenoids, retinol, alpha-to-copherol, and selenium with breast cancer risk: results from a prospective study in Columbia, Missouri (United States).** (Dorgan, 1998) (#105 cases of histologically confirmed breast cancer)

36. **Incidence of cataract operations in Finnish male smokers unaffected by alpha tocopherol or beta carotene supplements.** (Teikari, 1998) (#28,934 male smokers)

37. **Effects of alpha tocopherol and beta carotene supplements on symptoms, progression, and prognosis of angina pectoris.** (Rapola et al, 1998) (#1,795 male smokers aged 50–69 years who had angina pectoris)

38. **The effects of antioxidant supplementation during Percoll preparation on human sperm DNA integrity** (Hughes et al, 1998) (#150 patients)

39. **GISSI-Prevention Trial** (GISSI-Prevenzione Investigators;1999) (#11,324 patients with recent MI)

40. **Women's Health Study** (Lee et al., 1999) (#39,876 healthy women); 50 mg beta-carotene (alternate days)

41. **The Health Professionals Follow-Up Study** (Ascherio et al. 1999) (#43,738 men)

42. **Familial hypercholesterolemia, intima-to-media thickness (FH IMT study)** (Raal et al, 1999) (#15 with homozygous familial hypercholesterolemia)

43. **Beta carotene supplementation in prevention of basal-cell and squamous-cell carcinomas of the skin** (Green et al, 1999) (#1,383 participants)

44. **Vitamins A, C and E and the risk of breast cancer: results from a case-control study in Greece,** (Bohlke, 1999) (#830 patients with breast cancer plus 1,548 controls)

45. **Dietary antioxidants and risk of myocardial infarction in the elderly: the Rotterdam Study.** (Klipstein-Grobusch et al, 1999) (#4,802 participants of the Rotterdam Study aged 55–95 y who were free of MI)

46. **A prospective study of vitamin supplement intake and cataract extraction among US women.** (Chasan-Taber et al, 1999) (#47,152 female nurses)

47. **Antioxidant treatment of patients with asthenozoospermia or moderate oligoasthenozoospermia with high-dose vitamin C and vitamin E: a randomized, placebo-controlled, double-blind study** (Rolf et al, 1999) (#31 without genital infection but with asthenozoospermia)

48. **Antioxidant supplementation in vitro does not improve human sperm motility** (Donnelly et al, Fertil Steril. 1999) (#60 patients)

49. **The effect of ascorbate and alpha-tocopherol supplementation in vitro on DNA integrity and hydrogen peroxide-induced DNA damage in human spermatozoa** (Donnelly et al, Mutagenesis. 1999) (#Semen samples with normozoospermic and asthenozoospermic profiles (n = 15 for each control and antioxidant group)

50. **Heart Outcome Prevention Evaluation Study (HOPE) (Yusuf et al, 2000)** (#9,541 patients at high risk for cardiovascular events or diabetes)

51. **Meta-Analysis of Vitamin E in CVD, Ischemic Heart Disease (IHD) and Mortality** (Dagenais et al. 2000) (#51,000 participants)

52. **Vitamin C and the risk of acute myocardial infarction.** (Riemersma et al, 2000) (#180 males with a first AMI and 177 healthy volunteers)

53. **The effects of combined conventional treatment, oral antioxidants and essential fatty acids on sperm biology in subfertile men** (Comhaire et al, 2000) (#27 infertile men)

54. **Dietary antioxidant vitamins, retinol, and breast cancer incidence in a cohort of Swedish women.** (Michels, 2001) (#59,036 women free of cancer)

55. **The secondary prevention HDL Atherosclerosis Treatment study (HATS)** (Brown et al., 2001) (#160 patients with coronary disease)

56. **The Perth Carotid Ultrasound Disease Assessment Study (CUDAS)** (McQuillan et al 2001) (#1,111 subjects)

57. **Randomized Trial of Supplemental beta-Carotene to Prevent Second Head and Neck Cancer** (Mayne et al, 2001) (#264 patients who had been curatively treated for a recent early-stage squamous cell carcinoma of the oral cavity, pharynx, or larynx.)

58. **Age-Related Eye Disease Study Research Group (AREDS)** (AREDS, 2001) (#4,757 participants)

59. **HDL Atherosclerosis Treatment study (HATS)** (Brown et al, 2001) (#160 participants)

60. **Vitamin C and Vitamin E Supplement Use and Colorectal Cancer Mortality in a Large American Cancer Society cohort. (Cancr Prevention Study II cohort - CPS-II)** (Jacobs, 2001) (#711,891 men and women in U.S.A.)

61. **Risk of Ovarian Carcinoma and Consumption of Vitamins A, C and E and Specific Carotenoids: a prospective analysis.** (Fairfield, 2001) (#80,326 women)

62. **Carotenoids, Alpha-tocopherols, and Retinol in Plasma and Breast Cancer Risk in Northern Sweden.** (Hulten, 2001) (#201 cases and 290 referents)

63. **The Vitamin E Atherosclerosis Prevention Study (VEAPS)** (Hodis et al, 2002) **(#353 were randomized (176 placebo, 177 vitamin E)**

64. **MRC/BHF** (MRC/BHF, 2002) (#20,536); (600 mg vitamin E, 250 mg vitamin C and 20 mg beta-carotene daily)

65. **Antioxidant Vitamins and US Physician CVD Mortality** (Muntwyler et al. 2002) (#83,639 male U.S.A. physicians)

66. **Women's Angiographic Vitamin and Estrogen (WAVE) Trial** (Waters et al, 2002) (#423 postmenopausal women, with at least one 15% to 75% coronary stenosis)

67. **Mega-dose vitamins and minerals in the treatment of non-metastatic breast cancer: an historical cohort study** (Lesperance et al, 2002) (#90 patients with non-metastatic breast cancer who received conventional treatment)

68. **The Roche European American Cataract Trial (REACT)** (Chylack et al. 2002) **(#445** patients)

69. **Vitamin E supplementation and macular degeneration** (Taylor et al, 2002) (#1,193 subjects)

70. **Vitamin E on Cardiovascular and Microvascular Outcomes in High-Risk Patients With Diabetes. Results of the HOPE Study and MICRO-HOPE Substudy** (Lonn et al. 2002) (#3,654 with diabetes)

71. **Vitamin C and Vitamin E Supplement Use and Bladder Cancer Mortality in a Large Cohort of US Men and Women** (Cancer Prevention Study II (CPS-II) (Jacobs et al., 2002) (#991,522 US adults in the Cancer Prevention Study II (CPS-II) cohort.)

72. **Supplemental Vitamin C & E and Multivitamin use and Stomach cancer Mortality in U.S.A.** (Jacobs et al. Jan. 2002) (#1,045,923)

73. **Vitamin E and C Supplements and Risk of Dementia** (Laurin et al, 2002) (#3,734 Japanese men)

74. **Retinol intake and bone mineral density in the elderly: the Rancho Bernardo Study.** (Promislow et al, 2002) (#570 women and 388 men)

75. **Vitamin A intake and hip fractures among postmenopausal women.** (Feskanich et al, 2002) (#72,337 postmenopausal women)

76. **A prospective study on supplemental vitamin E intake and risk of colon cancer in women and men.** (Wu et al, 2002) (#87,998 females from the Nurses' Health Study and 47, 344 males from the Health Professionals Follow-up Study) (#135,332 total participants)

77. **The Collaborative Primary Prevention Project (PPP)** (Chiabrando et al., 2002) (#144 participants with CHD risk factors)

78. **Vitamins E & A fail to reduce incidence or mortality of lung cancer: Cochrane Database Syst Rev. 2003.** (Caraballoso et al., 2003) (#109,394 participants)

79. **Use of antioxidant vitamins for the prevention of cardiovascular disease: meta-analysis of randomized trials.** (Vivekananthan et al., 2003) (The vitamin E trials involved a total of #81,788 patients, and the beta-carotene trials involved #138,113)

80. **Antioxidant Vitamins Effect on Alzheimer's Disease: Washington Heights-Inwood Columbia Aging Project** (Luchsinger et al, 2003) (#980 elderly subjects)

81. **Neoplastic and Antineoplastic Effects of Beta Carotene on Colorectal Adenoma Recurrence: Results of a Randomized Trial** (Baron et al, 2003) (#864 subjects who had had an adenoma removed and were polyp-free)

82. **Routine Vitamin Supplementation To Prevent Cardiovascular Disease: A Summary of the Evidence for the U.S. Preventive Services Task Force** (Morris and Carson, 2003)

83. **Midlife Dietary Intake of Antioxidants and Risk of Late-Life Incident Dementia: The Honolulu-Asia Aging Study** (Laurin et al, 2003) (#2,459 men)

84. **Serum retinol levels and the risk of fracture.** (Michealsson, 2003) (#2,322 men)

85. **Impact of simvastatin, niacin, and/or antioxidants on cholesterol metabolism in CAD patients with low HDL.** (Matthan et al, 2003) (#123 HATS participants)

86. **A randomized trial of beta carotene and age-related cataract in US physicians.** (Christen et al, 2003) (#22,071 Male US physicians aged 40 to 84 years)

87. **Supplemental vitamin C increase cardiovascular disease risk in women with diabetes** (Lee et al, 2004) (#1,923 postmenopausal women who reported being diabetic)

88. **Cochrane Database Syst Rev. 2004: Vitamins E & A fail to reduce incidence or mortality of gastrointestinal cancer.** (Cochrane Database Syst Rev. G. Bjelakovic et al, 2004) (#170,525 participants)

89. **ATBC 6-year followup study (2004)** (Thornwall et al., 2004) (#29,133 male smokers)

90. **HOPE study of vitamin E on renal insufficiency (2004)** (Mann et al, 2004) (#993 people with a serum creatinine > or = 1.4 to 2.3 mg/dL. And renal insufficiency)

91. **Randomized trials of vitamin E in the treatment and prevention of cardiovascular disease (2004)** (Eidelman et al., 2004) (7 large-scale randomized trials)

92. **Effect of supplemental vitamin E for the prevention and treatment of cardiovascular disease** (Shekelle et al, 2004) (#Eighty-four eligible trials)

93. **SU.VI.MAX Study (2004)** (Hercberg et al, 2004) (#A total of 13,017 French adults)

94. **Meta-analysis: high-dosage vitamin E supplementation may increase all-cause mortality** (Miller et al., 2004) (#135,967 subjects)

95. **The role of vitamin E in the prevention of coronary events and stroke. Meta-analysis of randomized controlled trials** (Alkhenizan and Al-Omran, 2004) (#80,645 subjects)

96. **Oats, Antioxidants and Endothelial Function in Overweight, Dyslipidemic Adults** (Katz et al, 2004) (#30) (16 males ≥age 35; 14 postmenopausal females)

97. **Vitamin C Worsens Coronary Atherosclerosis in Those with Two Copies of the Haptoglobin 2 Gene.** (Levy, 2004) (#299 postmenopausal women)

98. **Vitamin C for preventing and treating the common cold. Cochrane Database Syst Rev. 2004;(4):CD000980.** (Douglas, 2004) (#11,350 study participants)

99. **Vitamin E supplementation and cataract: randomized controlled trial.** (McNeil, 2004) (#1,193 eligible subjects with early or no cataract)

100. **Antioxidant vitamins and coronary heart disease risk: a pooled analysis of 9 cohorts.** (Knekt et al, 2004) (#293,172 subjects free of CHD at baseline)

101. **A review of the epidemiological evidence for the 'antioxidant hypothesis' by the British Nutrition Foundation (the Food Standards Agency).** (Stanner et al, 2004) (British Nutrition Foundation independent review)

102. **Impact of antioxidants, zinc, and copper on cognition in the elderly: a randomized, controlled trial.** (Yaffe et al, 2004) (#2,166 elderly persons)

103. **Use of multivitamins and prostate cancer mortality in a large cohort of US men.** (Stevens et al, 2005) (#475,726 men who were cancer-free)

104. **Vitamin A Supplementation for Reducing the Risk of Mother-to-child Transmission of HIV Infection.** (Wiysonge et al, 2005) (#3,033 females)

105. **The Alzheimer's Disease Cooperative Study (ADCS) Group** (Petersen et al, 2005) (#769 subjects)

106. **Vitamin E Supplementation in Alzheimer's Disease, Parkinson's Disease, Tardive Dyskinesia, and Cataract: Part 2** (Pham et al, 2005)

107. **Dementia and Alzheimer's Disease in Community-Dwelling Elders Taking Vitamin C and/or Vitamin E:** (Fillenbaum et al, 2005) (#626 elderly)

108. **HOPE-TOO Extension** (Lonn et al, 2005) (#3,994 original study enrollees)

109. **Women's Health Study (WHS)** (Lee et al, 2005) (#39,876 apparently healthy US women)

110. **A randomized trial of antioxidant vitamins to prevent second primary cancers in head and neck cancer patients** (Bairati et al, 2005 Apr 6) (#540 patients with stage I or II head and neck cancer treated by radiation therapy)

111. **Randomized trial of antioxidant vitamins to prevent acute adverse effects of radiation therapy in head and neck cancer patients** (Bairati et al, 2005 Aug 20) (#540 patients with stage I or II head and neck cancer treated by radiation therapy)

112. **Effect of intensive lipid lowering, with or without antioxidant vitamins, compared with moderate lipid lowering on myocardial ischemia** (Stone et al, 2005) (#300 patients with stable coronary disease)

113. **Vitamin C and vitamin E for Alzheimer's disease.** (Boothby and Doering, 2005)

114. **Vitamin-mineral supplementation and the progression of atherosclerosis** (Bleys et al, 2006) (searched the MEDLINE, EMBASE, and CENTRAL databases)

115. **Multivitamin/mineral supplements and prevention of chronic disease.** (Huang et al, 2006 May)

116. **The Efficacy and Safety of Multivitamin and Mineral Supplement Use To Prevent Cancer and Chronic Disease in Adults: A Systematic Review for a National**

Institutes of Health State-of-the-Science Conference. (Huang et al, 2006 Sept)

117. **Antioxidants Vitamin C and Vitamin E for the Prevention and Treatment of Cancer** (Coulter et al, 2006) (Thirty-eight studies; participant # not available)

118. **Vitamin C levels in Type 2 diabetes and low vitamin C levels does not improve endothelial dysfunction or insulin resistance** (Chen et al, 2006) (#32 type 2 diabetics)

119. **Meta-analysis: antioxidant supplements for primary and secondary prevention of colorectal adenoma (2006)** (Bjelakovic et al., 2006) (#17,620 participants)

120. **Australian Collaborative Trial of Supplements (ACTS)** (Rumbold et al, 2006) (#1,877 subjects)

121. **The Antioxidants in Prevention of Cataracts Study (APC Study): effects of antioxidant supplements on cataract progression in South India.** (Gritz, 2006) (#798)

122. **Vitamins in Pre-eclampsia (VIP) Trial Consortium** (Poston et al., 2006) (#2,410 women at increased risk for pre-eclampsia, analayzed 2,395)

123. **SU.VI.MAX (2006) Antioxidants do not affect fasting blood glucose** (Czernichow et al, 2006) (#3,146 subjects)

124. **Vitamin E and Risk of Type 2 Diabetes in the Women's Health Study** (Liu et al., 2006) (#38,716 apparently healthy U.S. women)

125. **Vitamin E supplementation and cognitive function in women: The Women's Health Study (2006)** (Kang et al., 2006) (#39,876 healthy US women)

126. **Supplemental and dietary vitamin E, beta-carotene, and vitamin C intakes and prostate cancer risk (PLCO Trial)** (Kirsh et al, 2006) (#29,361 men during up to 8 years of follow-up)

127. **Intakes of Vitamins A, C and E and Folate and Multivitamins and Lung Cancer: a pooled analysis of 8**

prospective studies. (Cho et al, 2006) (#430,281 persons over a maximum of 6-16 years in the studies)

128. **The Melbourne Atherosclerosis Vitamin E Trial (MA-VET): a study of high dose vitamin E in smokers.** (Magliano et al, 2006) (#409 male and female smokers)

129. **Mortality in Randomized Trials of Antioxidant Supplements for Primary and Secondary Prevention; Systematic Review and Meta-analysis** (Bjelakovic et al, 2007) (#232,606 participants)

130. **Multivitamin Use and Risk of Prostate Cancer in the National Institutes of Health–AARP Diet and Health Study** (Lawson et al, 2007) (#295,344 men)

131. **A Randomized Factorial Trial of Vitamins C and E and Beta Carotene in the Secondary Prevention of Cardiovascular Events in Women: Results From the Women's Antioxidant Cardiovascular Study** (Cook et al. 2007) (#8,171 female health professionals at increased risk)

132. **Use of Supplements of Multivitamins, Vitamin C, and Vitamin E in Relation to Mortality** (Pocobelli et al, 2007) (#77,719 subjects aged 50–76 years)

133. **Health Professionals Follow-up Study (2007): Effect of vitamins C, E, A and carotenoids and the occurrence of oral pre-malignant lesions** (Maserejian et al, 2007) (#42,340 men enrolled in the Health Professionals Follow-up Study) (#207 found with oral premalignant lesions)

134. **Antioxidant meta-analysis for the treatment of macular degeneration (2007)** (Chong et al, 2007) (#149,203 subjects)

135. **Effect of *RRR*-alpha-tocopherol supplementation on carotid atherosclerosis in patients with stable coronary artery disease (CAD)** (Devaraj et al, 2007) (#90 patients with CAD)

136. **Overview of the Women's Antioxidant Cardiovascular Study (WACS) (2007)** (Zaharris et al, 2007) (#8,171 women)

137. **Serum alpha-tocopherol, concurrent and past vitamin E intake, and mild cognitive impairment** (Dunn et al, 2007) (#526 subjects)

138. **The role of vitamin E in the prevention of cancer: a meta-analysis of randomized controlled trials.** (Alkhenizan and Hafez, 2007) (#167,025 subjects)

139. **Chemoprevention of Primary Liver Cancer: A Randomized, Double-Blind Trial in Linxian, China.** (Qu et al, 2007) (29,450 subjects)

140. **Risk of Mortality with Vitamin E Supplements: The Cache County Study.** (Hayden et al, 2007)

141. **Multivitamin-multimineral supplements and eye disease: age-related macular degeneration and cataract.** (Seddon, 2007) The Dietary Ancillary Study of the Eye Disease Case-Control Study (EDCCS)

142. **Antioxidant Supplementation Increases the Risk of Skin Cancers in Women but Not in Men.** (Hercberg et al, 2007) (#French adults, 7,876 women and 5,141 men. Total # = 13,017)

143. **Antioxidant Vitamin Supplement Use and Risk of Dementia or Alzheimer's Disease in Older Adults** (Gray et al, 2007) (#2,969)

144. **Antioxidant supplements for prevention of mortality in healthy participants and patients with various diseases.** (Bjelakovic, Nikolova, Gludd, Simonetti and Gludd, 2008 Apr) (#232,550 Cochrane Database Syst Rev.)

145. **Systematic review: primary and secondary prevention of gastrointestinal cancers with antioxidant supplements.** (Bjelakovic, Nikolova, Simonette and Gludd, 2008 Sept) (#211,818 participants)

146. **Vitamins E and C in the prevention of cardiovascular disease in men: the Physicians' Health Study II randomized controlled trial** (Sesso et al, 2008) (#14,641 US male physicians)

147. **Both {alpha}- and beta-Carotene, but Not Tocopherols and Vitamin C, Are Inversely Related to 15-Year Cardiovascular Mortality in Dutch Elderly Men** (Buijsse et al, 2008) (**#559** men (mean age ~72 y) free of chronic diseases)

148. **Vitamin E and selenium supplementation and risk of prostate cancer in the Vitamins and lifestyle (VITAL) study cohort** (Peters et al, 2008) (#35,242 men)

149. **VITAL (VITamins And Lifestyle) study 2008** (Slatore et al, 2008) (#77,721 men and women)

150. **Vitamin E for Alzheimer's and mild cognitive impairment. Cochrane Database Syst Rev. (2008)** (Isaac et al, 2008) (#769 participants)

151. **Efficacy of Antioxidant Supplementation in Reducing Primary Cancer Incidence and Mortality: Systematic Review and Meta-analysis** (Bardia et al, 2008) (#104,196 participants)

152. **Carotenoids and the risk of developing lung cancer: a systematic review.** (Gallicchio et al, 2008) (Six randomized clinical trials)

153. **Antioxidant enriched enteral nutrition and oxidative stress after major gastrointestinal tract surgery.** (van Stijn et al, 2008) (#21 undergoing major upper gastrointestinal tract surgery)

154. **Vitamin E supplementation may transiently increase tuberculosis risk in males who smoke heavily and have high dietary vitamin C intake.** (Hemila and Kaprio, 2008 Oct) (#29,023 males aged 50-69 years, smoking at baseline, with no tuberculosis)

155. **Vitamin E supplementation and pneumonia risk in males who initiated smoking at an early age: effect modification by body weight and dietary vitamin C.** (Hemila and Kaprio, 2008 Nov) (#21,657 ATBC Study participants who initiated smoking by the age of 20 years)

156. **Oral administration of vitamin C decreases muscle mitochondrial biogenesis and hampers training-induced adaptations in endurance performance.** (Gomez-Cabrera et al, 2008) (#14)

157. **Antioxidant vitamin and mineral supplements for preventing age-related macular degeneration.** (Evans and Henshaw, 2008) (#23,099 participants)

158. **Dietary antioxidants and the long-term incidence of age-related macular degeneration: the Blue Mountains Eye Study.** (Tan et al, 2008) (#2,454 Australian population-based cohort study)

159. **Multivitamin-multimineral supplement use and mammographic breast density.** (Berube et al, 2008) (#Premenopausal (777) and postmenopausal (783) women, total 1,560)

160. **Antioxidant supplements to prevent or slow down the progression of AMD: a systematic review and meta-analysis.** (Evans, 2008) (#23,099 people were randomized in three trials)

161. **Is there a role for supplemented antioxidants in the prevention of atherosclerosis?** (Katsiki and Manes, 2009)

162. **Plasma Carotenoids, Retinol, and Tocopherols and Postmenopausal Breast Cancer Risk in theMultiethnic Cohort Study: a nested case-control study.** (Epplein, 2009) (#286 incident postmenopausal breast cancer cases were matched to 535 controls)

163. **Vitamins E and C in the prevention of prostate and total cancer in men: the Physicians' Health Study II randomized controlled trial (2009)** (Gaziano et al, 2009) (#14,641 male physicians)

164. **Vitamin E, vitamin C, beta carotene, and cognitive function among women with or at risk of cardiovascular disease: The Women's Antioxidant and Cardiovascular Study (2009)** (Kang et al, 2009) (#2,824 participants)

165. **Effects of vitamins C and E and beta-carotene on the risk of type 2 diabetes in women at high risk of cardiovascular disease: Women's Antioxidant Cardiovascular Study (2009)** (Song et al, 2009) (#8,171 female health professionals)

166. **Vitamins C and E and Beta Carotene Supplementation and Cancer Risk: Women's Antioxidant Cardiovascular Study (2009)** (Lin et al, 2009) (#7,627 female health professionals)

167. **Effect of selenium and vitamin E on risk of prostate cancer and other cancers: the Selenium and Vitamin E Cancer Prevention Trial (SELECT) (2009)** (Lippman, 2009) (#35,533 men)

168. **Multivitamin Use and Risk of Cancer and Cardiovascular Disease in the Women's Health Initiative Cohorts** (Neuhouser et al, 2009) (#161,808 participants)

169. **Effects of antioxidant supplements on cancer prevention: meta-analysis of randomized controlled trials** (Myung et al, 2009) (#161,045 total subjects)

170. **Decision Analysis Supports the Paradigm That Indiscriminate Supplementation of Vitamin E Does More Harm than Good** (Dotan et al, 2009) (over 300,000 participants)

171. **Effects of long-term antioxidant supplementation and association of serum antioxidant concentrations with risk of metabolic syndrome in adults (SU.VI.MAX)** (Czernichow et al, 2009) (#5,220 adults)

172. **Total and Cancer Mortality After Supplementation With Vitamins and Minerals: 10 year Follow-up of the Linxian General Population Nutrition Intervention Trial.** (Qiao et al, 2009) **(#29,584 adults)**

173. **Vitamin A and retinol intakes and the risk of fractures among participants of the Women's Health Initiative Observational Study.** (Caire-Juvera et al. 2009) (#75,747

women from the Women's Health Initiative Observational Study)

174. **Modification of the effect of vitamin E supplementation on the mortality of male smokers by age and dietary vitamin C.** (Hemila and Kaprio, 2009 Apr) (#29,023 males aged 50-69 years, smoking at baseline, with no tuberculosis)

175. **Vitamin E supplement use and the incidence of cardiovascular disease and all-cause mortality in the Framingham Heart Study: Does the underlying health status play a role?** (Dietrich et al, 2009) (#4,270 Framingham study participants)

176. **Antioxidants prevent health-promoting effects of physical exercise in humans.** (Ristow et al, 2009) (#39 healthy adults)

177. **Long-term use of beta-carotene, retinol, lycopene, and lutein supplements and lung cancer risk: results from the VITamins And Lifestyle (VITAL) study.** (Satia et al, 2009) (#77,126 (VITAL) cohort Study in Washington State)

178. **Vitamin C supplements and the risk of age-related cataract: a population-based prospective cohort study in women.** (Rautiainen et al, 2010) (#24,593 women)

179. **Micronutrient concentrations and subclinical atherosclerosis in adults with HIV.** (Falcone et al, 2010) (#298 Nutrition for Healthy Living participants)

180. **Multivitamin use and breast cancer incidence in a prospective cohort of Swedish women.** (Larsson et al, 2010) (#35,329 cancer-free women)

181. **Vitamins C and E to prevent complications of pregnancy-associated hypertension** (Roberts et al, 2010) (#10,154)

Total of 181 studies with over 8,600,000 participants

REFERENCES for section three

(Alkhenizan and Al-Omran, 2004) (Alkhenizan AH, Al-Omran MA. The role of vitamin E in the prevention of coronary events and stroke. Meta-analysis of randomized controlled trials. Saudi Med J. 2004 Dec;25(12):1808-14)

(Alkhenizan and Hafez, 2007) (Alkhenizan A, Hafez K. The role of vitamin E in the prevention of cancer: a meta-analysis of randomized controlled trials. Ann Saudi Med. 2007 Nov-Dec;27(6):409-14)

(AREDS, 2001) (A randomized, placebo-controlled, clinical trial of high-dose supplementation with vitamins C and E and beta carotene for age-related cataract and vision loss: AREDS report no. 9. Age-Related Eye Disease Study Research Group. Arch Ophthalmol. 2001 Oct;119(10):1439-5)

(Ascherio et al. 1999) (Ascherio A, Rimm EB, Hernan MA, Giovannucci E, Kawachi I, Stampfer MJ, Willett WC. Relation of consumption of vitamin E, vitamin C, and carotenoids to risk for stroke among men in the United States. Ann Intern Med. 1999 Jun 15;130(12):963-70)

(Bairati et al, 2005 Apr 6) (Bairati I, Meyer F, Gélinas M, Fortin A, Nabid A, Brochet F, Mercier JP, Têtu B, Harel F, Mâsse B, Vigneault E, Vass S, del Vecchio P, Roy J. A randomized trial of antioxidant vitamins to prevent second primary cancers in head and neck cancer patients. J Natl Cancer Inst. 2005 Apr 6;97(7):481-8)

(Bairati et al, 2005 Aug 20) (Bairati I, Meyer F, Gélinas M, Fortin A, Nabid A, Brochet F, Mercier JP, Têtu B, Harel F, Abdous B, Vigneault E, Vass S, Del Vecchio P, Roy J. Randomized trial of antioxidant vitamins to prevent acute adverse effects of radiation therapy in head and neck cancer patients. J Clin Oncol. 2005 Aug 20;23(24):5805-13)

(Bardia et al, 2008) (Aditya Bardia, Imad M. Tleyjeh, James R. Cerhan, Amit K. Sood, Paul J. Limburg, Patricia J. Erwin and Victor M. Montori. Efficacy of Antioxidant Supplementation in Reducing Primary Cancer Incidence and Mortality: Systematic Review and Meta-analysis. January 2008 vol. 83 no. 1 23-34)

(Baron et al, 2003) (John A. Baron, Bernard F. Cole, Leila Mott, Robert Haile, Maria Grau, Timothy R. Church, Gerald J. Beck, E. Robert Greenberg. Neoplastic and Antineoplastic Effects of Beta Carotene on Colorectal Adenoma Recurrence: Results of a Randomized Trial. JNCI Journal of the National Cancer Institute 2003 95(10):717-722)

(Batieha et al, 1993) (Batieha AM, Armenian HK, Norkus EP, Morris JS, Spate VE, Comstock GW. Serum micronutrients and the subsequent risk of cervical cancer in a population-based nested case-control study. Cancer Epidemiol Biomarkers Prev. 1993 Jul-Aug;2(4):335-9)

(Berson et al, 1993) (Berson EL, Rosner B, Sandberg MA, et al. A randomized trial of vitamin A and vitamin E supplementation for retinitis pigmentosa. Arch Ophthalmol. 1993;111(6):761-772)

(Berube et al, 2008) (Sylvie Bérubé, Caroline Diorio and Jacques Brisson. Multivitamin-multimineral supplement use and mammographic breast density. American Journal of Clinical Nutrition, Vol. 87, No. 5, 1400-1404, May 2008)

(Bjelakovic et al, Lancet. 2004) (Bjelakovic G, Nikolova D, Simonetti RG, Gluud C. Antioxidant supplements for prevention of gastrointestinal cancers: a systematic review and meta-analysis. Lancet (2004) 364:1219–28)

(Bjelakovic et al., 2006) (Bjelakovic G, Nagorni A, Nikolova D, et al. Meta-analysis: antioxidant supplements for primary and secondary prevention of colorectal adenoma. Aliment Pharmacol Ther. 2006;24:281-91)

(Bjelakovic et al, 2007) (Goran Bjelakovic, Dimitrinka Nikolova, Lise Lotte Gluud, Rosa G. Simonetti, and Christian Gluud. "Mortality in Randomized Trials of Antioxidant Supplements for Primary and Secondary Prevention; Systematic Review and Meta-analysis." JAMA 2007;297:842-857. Vol. 297 No. 8, February 28, 2007)

(Bjelakovic, Nikolova, Gludd, Simonetti and Gludd, 2008 Apr) (Bjelakovic G, Nikolova D, Gluud LL, Simonetti RG, Gluud C.. Antioxidant supplements for prevention of mortality in healthy participants and patients with various diseases. Cochrane Database Syst Rev. 2008 Apr 16;(2):CD007176)

(Bjelakovic, Nikolova, Simonette and Gludd, 2008 Sept) (Bjelakovic G, Nikolova D, Simonetti RG, Gluud C. Systematic review: primary and secondary prevention of gastrointestinal cancers with antioxidant supplements. Aliment Pharmacol Ther. 2008 Sep 15;28(6):689-703)

(Bleys et al, 2006) (Vitamin-mineral supplementation and the progression of atherosclerosis: a meta-analysis of randomized controlled trials. Joachim Bleys, Edgar R Miller, III, Roberto Pastor-Barriuso, Lawrence J Appel and Eliseo Guallar. American Journal of Clinical Nutrition, Vol. 84, No. 4, 880-887, October 2006)

(Bohlke et al, 1999) (K Bohlke, D Spiegelman, A Trichopoulou, K Katsouyanni and D Trichopoulos. Vitamins A, C and E and the risk of breast cancer: results from a case-control study in Greece. British Journal of Cancer (1999) 79, 23–29)

(Boothby and Doering, 2005) (Boothby LA, Doering PL. Vitamin C and vitamin E for Alzheimer's disease. Ann Pharmacother. 2005 Dec;39(12):2073-80)

(Bostom et al, 1995) (Bostom AG, Hume AL, Eaton CB, Laurino JP, Yanek LR, Regan MS, McQuade WH, Craig WY, Perrone G, Jacques PF. The effect of high-dose ascorbate supplementation on plasma lipoprotein(a) levels in patients with premature coronary heart disease. Pharmacotherapy 1995 Jul-Aug;15(4):458-64)

(Brown et al, 2001) (Brown BG, Zhao XQ, Chait A, Fisher LD, Cheung MC, Morse JS, Dowdy AA, Marino EK, Bolson EL, Alaupovic P, Frohlich J, Albers JJ. Simvastatin and niacin, antioxidant vitamins, or the combination for the prevention of coronary disease. N Engl J Med. 2001 Nov 29;345(22):1583-92)

(Brown et al, 2001) (Brown BG, Zhao XQ, Chait A, et al. Simvastatin and niacin, antioxidant vitamins, or the combination for the prevention of coronary disease. N Engl J Med 2001;345:1583-1592)

(Buijsse et al, 2008) (B. Buijsse, E. J. M. Feskens, L. Kwape, F. J. Kok, and D. Kromhout. Both {alpha}- and -Carotene, but Not Tocopherols and Vitamin C, Are Inversely Related to 15-Year Cardiovascular Mortality in Dutch Elderly Men. J. Nutr., February 1, 2008; 138(2): 344 – 350)

(Buring and Hennekens, 1992) (Buring JE, Hennekens CH. The women's health study: summary of the design. J Myocardial Ischemia 1992;4:27-9)

(Caire-Juvera et al, 2009) (Caire-Juvera G,, Ritenbaugh C, Wactawski-Wende J, Snetselaar LG, Chen Z. Vitamin A and retinol intakes and the risk of fractures among participants of the Women's Health Initiative Observational Study. Am J Clin Nutr. 2009 Jan;89(1):323-30)

(Calzada et al, 1997) (Calzada C, Bruckdorfer KR, Rice-Evans CA. The influence of antioxidant nutrients on platelet function in healthy volunteers. Atherosclerosis 1997 Jan 3;128(1):97-105)

(Caraballoso et al., 2003) (Drugs for preventing lung cancer in healthy people. M. Caraballoso et al. Cochrane Database Syst Rev. 2003;(2):CD002141)

(Chasan-Taber et al, 1999) (Chasan-Taber L, Willett W C, Seddon J M. et al A prospective study of vitamin supplement intake and cataract extraction among US women. Epidemiology 1999. 10679–684)

(Chen et al, 2006) (Chen et al. High-dose oral vitamin C partially replenishes vitamin C levels in patients with Type 2 diabetes and low vitamin C levels but does not improve endothelial dysfunction or insulin resistance. Am. J. Physiol. Heart Circ. Physiol. 2006;290:H137-H145)

(Chiabrando et al., 2002) (Long-term vitamin E supplementation fails to reduce lipid peroxidation in people at cardiovascular risk: analysis of underlying factors. Chiabrando C, Avanzini F, Rivalta C, Colombo F, Fanelli R, Palumbo G, Roncaglioni MC; PPP Collaborative Group on the antioxidant effect of vitamin E. Curr Control Trials Cardiovasc Med. 2002 Mar 19;3(1):5)

(Cho et al, 2006) (Cho E. et al. Intakes of vitamins A, C and E and folate and multivitamins and lung cancer: a pooled analysis of 8 prospective studies. Int J Cancer. 2006 Feb 15;118(4):970-8)

(Chong et al, 2007) ("Dietary antioxidants and primary prevention of age related macular degeneration: systematic review and meta-analysis" Elaine W-T Chong, Tien Y Wong, Andreas J Kreis, Julie A Simpson, Robyn H Guymer. British Medical Journal (BMJ)., doi:10.1136/bmj.39350.500428.47 (published 8 October 2007)

(Christen et al, 2003) (Christen WG; Manson JE; Glynn RJ; Gaziano JM; Sperduto RD; Buring JE; Hennekens CH. A randomized trial of beta carotene and age-related cataract in US physicians. Arch Ophthalmol. 2003; 121(3):372-8)

(Chylack et al. 2002) (Chylack LT Jr, Brown NP, Bron A, Hurst M, Kopcke W, Thien U, Schalch W. The Roche European American Cataract Trial (REACT): a randomized clinical trial to investigate the efficacy of an oral antioxidant micronutrient mixture to slow progression of age-related cataract. Ophthalmic Epidemiol. 2002 Feb;9(1):49-80)

(Comhaire et al, 2000) (Comhaire FH, Christophe AB, Zalata AA, Dhooge WS, Mahmoud AM, Depuydt CE. The effects of combined conventional treatment, oral antioxidants and essential fatty acids on sperm biology in subfertile men. Prostaglandins Leukot Essent Fatty Acids. 2000 Sep;63(3):159-65)

(Cook et al, 2007) (A Randomized Factorial Trial of Vitamins C and E and Beta Carotene in the Secondary Prevention of Cardiovascular Events in Women: Results From the Women's Antioxidant Cardiovascular Study. Nancy R. Cook, ScD; Christine M. Albert, MD; J. Michael Gaziano, MD; Elaine Zaharris, BA; Jean MacFadyen, BA; Eleanor Danielson, MIA; Julie E. Buring, ScD; JoAnn E. Manson, MD, DrPH. Arch Intern Med. 2007;167(15):1610-1618)

(Coulter et al, 2006) (Antioxidants Vitamin C and Vitamin E for the Prevention and Treatment of Cancer. Coulter, Ian D.; Hardy, Mary L.; Morton, Sally C.; Hilton, Lara G.; Tu, Wenli; Valentine, Di; Shekelle, Paul G. Journal of General Internal Medicine, Volume 21, Number 7, July 2006, pp. 735-744(10))

(Creagan et al, 1979) (Creagan ET, Moertel CG, O'Fallon JR, Schutt AJ, O'Connell MJ, Rubin J, Frytak S. Failure of high-dose vitamin C (ascorbic acid) therapy to benefit patients with advanced cancer. A controlled trial. N Engl J Med. 1979 Sep 27;301(13):687-90)

(Czernichow et al, 2006) (Antioxidant supplementation does not affect fasting plasma glucose in the Supplementation with Antioxidant Vitamins and Minerals (SU.VI.MAX) study in France: association with dietary intake and plasma concentrations. S. Czernichow, A. Couthouis, S. Bertrais, A.-C. Vergnaud, L. Dauchet, P. Galan, and S. Hercberg. Am. J. Clinical Nutrition, August 1, 2006; 84(2): 395 - 399)

(Czernichow et al, 2009) (Czernichow, S. et al. Effects of long-term antioxidant supplementation and association of serum antioxidant concentrations with risk of metabolic syndrome in adults. Am. J. Clinical Nutrition, Vol. 90, No. 2, 329-335, August 2009)

(Dagenais et al, 2000) (Dagenais GR, Marchioli R, Yusuf S, Tognoni G. Beta-carotene, vitamin C, and vitamin E and cardiovascular diseases. Curr Cardiol Rep. 2000 Jul;2(4):293-9)

(Devaraj et al, 2007) (S. Devaraj, R. Tang, B. Adams-Huet, A. Harris, T. Seenivasan, J. A de Lemos, and I. Jialal. Effect of high-dose {alpha}-tocopherol supplementation on biomarkers of oxidative stress and inflammation and carotid atherosclerosis in patients with coronary artery disease. Am. J. Clinical Nutrition, November 1, 2007; 86(5): 1392 – 1398)

(Dietrich et al, 2009) (M. Dietrich, P. Jacques, M. Pencina, K. Lanier, M. Keyes, G. Kaur, P. Wolf, R. D'Agostino, R. Vasan. Vitamin E supplement use and the incidence of cardiovascular disease and all-cause mortality in the Framingham Heart Study: Does the underlying health status play a role? Atherosclerosis, 2009. Volume 205, Issue 2, Pages 549-553)

(Donnelly et al, Fertil Steril. 1999) (Donnelly ET, McClure N, Lewis SE. Antioxidant supplementation in vitro does not improve human sperm motility. Fertil Steril. 1999 Sep;72(3):484-95)

(Donnelly et al, Mutagenesis. 1999) (Donnelly ET, McClure N, Lewis SE. The effect of ascorbate and alpha-tocopherol supplementation in vitro on DNA integrity and hydrogen peroxide-induced DNA damage in human spermatozoa. Mutagenesis. 1999 Sep;14(5):505-12)

(Dorgan et al, 1998) (Dorgan JF, Sowell A, Swanson CA, et al. Relationships of serum carotenoids, retinol, alpha-tocopherol, and selenium with breast cancer risk: results from a prospective study in Columbia, Missouri (United States). Cancer Causes Control. 1998;9(1):89-97)

(Dotan, Lichtenberg and Pinchuk, 2009) (Dotan Y, Lichtenberg D, Pinchuk I. No evidence supports vitamin E indiscriminate supplementation. Biofactors. 2009 Nov-Dec;35(6):469-73)

(Douglas et al, 2004) (Douglas RM, Hemila H, D'Souza R, Chalker EB, Treacy B. Vitamin C for preventing and treating the common cold. Cochrane Database Syst Rev. 2004(4):CD000980)

(Dunn et al, 2007) (Julie E. Dunn, Sandra Weintraub, Anne M. Stoddard and Sarah Banks. Serum alpha-tocopherol, concurrent and past vitamin E intake, and mild cognitive impairment. Neurology. 200768: 670-676)

(Eidelman et al., 2004) (Eidelman RS, Hollar D, Hebert PR, Lamas GA, Hennekens CH. Randomized trials of vitamin E in the treatment and prevention of cardiovascular disease. Arch Intern Med. 2004;164:1552-1556)

(Epplein, 2009) (Meira Epplein et al. Plasma carotenoids, retinol, and tocopherols and postmenopausal breast cancer risk in the Multiethnic Cohort Study: a nested case-control study. Breast Cancer Research. 2009, 11:R49)

(Evans, 2008) (Evans J. Antioxidant supplements to prevent or slow down the progression of AMD: a systematic review and meta-analysis. Eye (Lond). 2008 Jun;22(6):751-60)

(Evans and Henshaw, 2008) (Evans JR, Henshaw K. Antioxidant vitamin and mineral supplements for preventing age-related macular degeneration. Cochrane Database Syst Rev. 2008 Jan 23;(1):CD000253)

(Fairfield et al, 2001) (Fairfield KM, Hankinson SE, Rosner BA, Hunter DJ, Colditz GA, Willett WC. Risk of ovarian carcinoma and consumption of vitamins A, C, and E and specific carotenoids: a prospective analysis. Cancer. 2001 Nov 1;92(9):2318-26)

(Falcone et al, 2010) (E Liana Falcone, Alexandra Mangili, Alice M Tang, Clara Y Jones, Margo N Coods, Joseph F Polak and Christine A Wanke . Micronutrient concentrations and subclinical atherosclerosis in adults with HIV. Am J Clin Nutr 91: 1213-1219, 2010. Vol. 91, No. 5, 1213-1219, May 2010)

(Feskanich et al, 2002) (Feskanich D, Singh F, Willett WC, Colditz GA. Vitamin A intake and hip fractures among postmenopausal women. J Am Med Assoc 2002;287:47-54)

(Fillenbaum et al, 2005) (Fillenbaum et al. Dementia and Alzheimer's Disease in Community-Dwelling Elders Taking Vitamin C and/or

Vitamin E. The Annals of Pharmacotherapy: Vol. 39, No. 12, pp. 2009-2014)

(Gallicchio et al, 2008) (Gallicchio L. et al. Carotenoids and the risk of developing lung cancer: a systematic review. Am J Clin Nutr. 2008 Aug;88(2):372-83

(Gaziano et al, 2009) (Vitamins E and C in the prevention of prostate and total cancer in men: the Physicians' Health Study II randomized controlled trial. Gaziano, JM., JAMA. 2009 Jan 7;301(1):52-62. Epub 2008 Dec 9)

(Geva et al, 1996) (Geva E, Bartoov B, Zabludovsky N, Lessing JB, Lerner-Geva L, Amit A. The effect of antioxidant treatment on human spermatozoa and fertilization rate in an in vitro fertilization program. Fertil Steril. 1996 Sep;66(3):430-4)

(Giovannucci, et al., 1998) (Giovannucci, E., M.J. Stampfer, G.A. Colditz, D.J. Hunter, C. Fuchs, B.A. Rosner, F.E. Speizer & W.C. Willett. 1998. Multivitamin use, folate, and colon cancer in women in the Nurses' Health Study. Ann. Intern. Med. 129(7):517-524)

(GISSI-Prevenzione Investigators;1999) (Dietary supplement with n-3 polyunsaturated acids and vitamin E after myocardial infarction: results of the GISSI-Prevention trial. Gruppo, Italiano per lo Studio Sopravvivenza nell'Infarto miocardico. Lancet, 1999; 354: 447-455)

(Gomez-Cabrera et al, 2008) (Gomez-Cabrera MC, Domenech E, Romagnoli M, Arduini A, Borras C, Pallardo FV, Sastre J, Viña J. Oral administration of vitamin C decreases muscle mitochondrial biogenesis and hampers training-induced adaptations in endurance performance. Am J Clin Nutr. 2008 Jan;87(1):142-9)

(Graham et al, 1992) (Graham S, Sielezny M, Marshall J, Priore R, Freudenheim J, Brasure J, Haughey B, Nasca P, Zdeb M. Diet in the epidemiology of Postmenopausal Breast Cancer in the New York State Cohort. Am J Epidemiol 1992;136:3127-37)

(Gray et al, 2007) (Gray SL et al. Antioxidant Vitamin Supplement Use and Risk of Dementia or Alzheimer's Disease in Older Adults. Journal of the American Geriatric Society. 2007. Volume 56 Issue 2, Pages 291 - 295)

(Greenberg et al, 1994) (Greenberg ER, Baron JA, Tosteson TD, Freeman DH Jr, Beck GJ, Bond JH, Colacchio TA, Coller JA, Frankl HD, Haile RW, et al. A clinical trial of antioxidant vitamins to prevent colorectal adenoma. Polyp Prevention Study Group. N Engl J Med. 1994 Jul 21;331(3):141-7)

(Greenberg et al, 1996) (Greenberg ER, Baron JA, Karagas MR, Stukel TA, Nierenberg DW, Stevens MM, Mandel JS, Haile RW. Mortality associated with low plasma concentration of beta carotene and the effect of oral supplementation. JAMA. 1996; 275: 699-703)

(Green et al, 1999) (Green A, Williams G, Neale R, et al.: Daily sunscreen application and beta carotene supplementation in prevention of basal-cell and squamous-cell carcinomas of the skin: a randomised controlled trial. Lancet 354 (9180): 723-9, 1999)

(Gritz, 2006) (Gritz DC, Srinivasan M, Smith SD, et al. The Antioxidants in Prevention of Cataracts Study: effects of antioxidant supplements on cataract progression in South India. Br J Ophthalmol. 2006;90(7):847-851)

(Hayden et al, 2007) (K. Hayden, K. Welsh-Bohmer, H. Wengreen, P. Zandi, C. Lyketsos, J. Breitner. Risk of Mortality with Vitamin E Supplements: The Cache County Study. Am J Med. 2007 Feb;120(2):180-4)

(Heinonen et al, 1994) (Heinonen, O.P., J.K. Huttunen, D. Albanes & ATBC cancer prevention study group. 1994. The effect of vitamin E and beta carotene on the incidence of lung cancer and other cancers in male smokers. N. Engl. J. Med. 330:1029-1035)

(Hemila and Kaprio, 2008 Oct) (Hemilä H, Kaprio J. Vitamin E supplementation may transiently increase tuberculosis risk in males who smoke heavily and have high dietary vitamin C intake. Br J Nutr. 2008 Oct;100(4):896-902)

(Hemila and Kaprio, 2008 Nov) (Hemilä H, Kaprio J. Vitamin E supplementation and pneumonia risk in males who initiated smoking at an early age: effect modification by body weight and dietary vitamin C. Nutr J. 2008 Nov 19;7:33)

(Hemila and Kaprio, 2009 Apr) (Hemilä H, Kaprio J. Modification of the effect of vitamin E supplementation on the mortality of male smokers by age and dietary vitamin C. Am J Epidemiol. 2009 Apr 15;169(8):946-53)

(Hennekens et al, 1996) (Hennekens CH, Buring JE, Manson JE, et al. Lack of effect of long-term supplementation with beta carotene on the incidence of malignant neoplasms and cardiovascular disease. N Engl J Med. 1996;334:1145-1149)

(Hercberg et al,2004) (Hercberg S,Galan P,Preziosi P,Bertrais S,Mennen L, Malvy D, Roussel A-M, Favier A, Briançon S. SU.VI.MAX Study. Arch Intern Med 2004;164:2335–42)

(Hercberg et al, 2007) (Serge Hercberg et al.Antioxidant Supplementation Increases the Risk of Skin Cancers in Women but Not in Men. American Society for Nutrition J. Nutr. 137:2098-2105, September 2007)

(Hodis et al, 1995) (Hodis HN, Mack WJ, LaBree L, et al. Serial coronary angiographic evidence that antioxidant vitamin intake reduces progression of coronary artery atherosclerosis. JAMA 1995;273(23):1849-54)

(Hodis et al, 2002) (Hodis HN, Mack WJ, LaBree L, Mahrer PR, Sevanian A, Liu CR, Liu CH, Hwang J, Selzer RH,Azen SP;VEAPS Research Group. Alpha-tocopherol supplementation in healthy individuals reduces low-density lipoprotein oxidation but not atherosclerosis: the Vitamin E Atherosclerosis Prevention Study (VEAPS). Circulation. 2002; 106: 1453–1459)

(Huang et al, 2006 May) (Huang HY, Caballero B, Chang S, Alberg A, Semba R, Schneyer C,Wilson RF, Cheng TY, Prokopowicz G, Barnes GJ 2nd,Vassy J, Bass EB. Multivitamin/mineral supplements and prevention of chronic disease. Evid Rep Technol Assess (Full Rep). 2006 May;(139):1-117)

(Huang et al, 2006 Sept) (H. Huang et al. The Efficacy and Safety of Multivitamin and Mineral Supplement Use To Prevent Cancer and Chronic Disease in Adults: A Systematic Review for a National Institutes of Health State-of-the-Science Conference. September 5, 2006, Vol. 145. Issue 5. Pages 372-385)

(Hughes et al, 1998) (Hughes CM, Lewis SE, McKelvey-Martin VJ, Thompson W. The effects of antioxidant supplementation during

Percoll preparation on human sperm DNA integrity. Hum Reprod. 1998 May;13(5):1240-7)

(Hulten, 2001) (Hulten K, Van Kappel AL, Winkvist A, et al. Carotenoids, alpha-tocopherols, and retinol in plasma and breast cancer risk in northern Sweden. Cancer Causes Control. 2001;12(6):529-537)

(Hunter et al, 1993) (A Prospective Study of the Intake of Vitamins C, E, and A and the Risk of Breast Cancer. David J. Hunter, JoAnn E. Manson, Graham A. Colditz, Meir J. Stampfer, Bernard Rosner, Charles H. Hennekens, Frank E. Speizer, and Walter C. Willett. The New England Journal of Medicine. Vol. 329:234-240. No. 4. July 22, 1993)

(Isaac et al, 2008) (Vitamin E for Alzheimers and mild cognitive impairment. Isaac MG, Quinn R, Tabet N. .Cochrane Database Syst Rev. 2008 Jul 16;(3):CD002854)

(Jacobs, 2001) (Jacobs EJ, Connell CJ, Patel AV, Chao A, Rodriguez C, Seymour J, McCullough ML, Calle EE, Thun MJ. Vitamin C and vitamin E supplement use and colorectal cancer mortality in a large American Cancer Society cohort. Cancer Epidemiol Biomarkers Prev. 2001 Jan;10(1):17-23)

(Jacobs et al., 2002) (Jacobs EJ, Henion AK, Briggs PJ, Connell CJ, McCullough ML, Jonas CR, Rodriguez C, Calle EE, Thun MJ. Vitamin C and vitamin E supplement use and bladder cancer mortality in a large cohort of US men and women. American Journal of Epidemiology 2002;156: 1002-10)

(Jacobs et al. Jan. 2002) (Jacobs EJ, Connell CJ, McCullough ML, Chao A, Jonas CR, Rodriguez C, Calle EE, Thun MJ. Vitamin C, vitamin E, and multivitamin supplement use and stomach cancer mortality in the Cancer Prevention Study II cohort. Cancer Epidemiol Biomarkers Prev. 2002 Jan;11(1):35-41)

(Jaques et al, 1995) (Jacques PF, Sulsky SI, Perrone GE, Jenner J, Schaefer EJ Epidemiology Program, US Department of Agriculture Human Nutrition Research Center on Aging, Tufts University, Boston, MA 02111, USA. (Jacques PF, Sulsky SI, Perrone GE, Jenner J, Schaefer EJ. Effect of vitamin C supplementation on lipoprotein cholesterol, apolipoprotein, and triglyceride concentrations. Ann Epidemiol 1995 Jan;5(1):52-9)

(Kang et al., 2006) (A randomized trial of vitamin E supplementation and cognitive function in women. Kang JH, Cook N, Manson J, Buring JE, Grodstein F. Arch Intern Med. 2006 Dec 11-25;166(22):2462-8)

(Kang et al, 2009) (Vitamin E, vitamin C, beta carotene, and cognitive function among women with or at risk of cardiovascular disease: The Women's Antioxidant and Cardiovascular Study. Kang JH, Cook NR, Manson JE, Buring JE, Albert CM, Grodstein F. Circulation. 2009 Jun 2;119(21):2772-80. Epub 2009 May 18)

(Katsiki and Manes, 2009) (Katsiki N, Manes C. Is there a role for supplemented antioxidants in the prevention of atherosclerosis? Clin Nutr. 2009 Feb;28(1):3-9)

(Katz et al, 2004) (D. L. Katz, M. A. Evans, W. Chan, H. Nawaz, B. P. Comerford, M. L. Hoxley, V. Y. Njike, and P. M. Sarrel. Oats, Antioxidants and Endothelial Function in Overweight, Dyslipidemic Adults. J. Am. Coll. Nutr., October 1, 2004; 23(5): 397 – 403)

(Kirsh et al, 2006) (Kirsh VA, Hayes RB, Mayne ST, Chatterjee N, Subar AF, Dixon LB, et al. Supplemental and Dietary Vitamin E, Beta-Carotene, and Vitamin C Intakes and Prostate Cancer Risk. PCLO. J Natl Cancer Inst 2006;98:245-254)

(Klipstein-Grobusch et al, 1999) (K. Klipstein-Grobusch, J. M Geleijnse, J. H den Breeijen, H. Boeing, A. Hofman, D. E Grobbee, and J. C. Witteman. Dietary antioxidants and risk of myocardial infarction in the elderly: the Rotterdam Study. Am. J. Clinical Nutrition, February 1, 1999; 69(2): 261 - 266)

(Knekt et al, 2004) (P. Knekt, J. Ritz, M. A Pereira, E. J O'Reilly, K. Augustsson, G. E Fraser, U. Goldbourt, B. L Heitmann, G. Hallmans, S. Liu, et al. Antioxidant vitamins and coronary heart disease risk: a pooled analysis of 9 cohorts. Am. J. Clinical Nutrition, December 1, 2004; 80(6): 1508 - 1520)

(Kushi et al, 1996) (L. H. Kushi et al. Dietary Antioxidant Vitamins and Death from Coronary Heart Disease in Postmenopausal Women. New England Journal of Medicine. Vol. 334. No. 18. May 2, 1996. pp. 1156-1162)

(Larsson et al, 2010) (Susanna C Larsson, Agneta Åkesson, Leif Bergkvist, and Alicja Wolk. Multivitamin use and breast cancer incidence in a prospective cohort of Swedish women. Am J Clin Nutr Published online 24 March 2010. Am J Clin Nutr Vol. 91, No. 5, 1268-1272, May 2010)

(Laurin et al, 2002) (Laurin D, Foley DJ, Masaki KH, et al. Vitamin E and C supplements and risk of dementia. JAMA 2002;288:2266–8)

(Laurin et al, 2003)(Midlife Dietary Intake of Antioxidants and Risk of Late-Life Incident Dementia: The Honolulu-Asia Aging Study)

(Lawson et al, 2007) (Lawson KA, Wright ME, Subar A, Mouw T, Schatzkin A, Leitzmann MF. Multivitamin use and risk of prostate cancer in the National Institutes of Health–AARP Diet and Health Study. J Natl Cancer Inst (2007) 99:754–64)

(Lee et al., 1999) (Lee IM, Cook NR, Manson JE, Buring JE, Hennekens CH. Beta-carotene supplementation and incidence of cancer and cardiovascular disease: the Women's Health Study. J Natl Cancer Inst. 1999 Dec 15;91(24):2102-6)

(Lee et al, 2004) (Duk-Hee Lee, Aaron R Folsom, Lisa Harnack, Barry Halliwell and David R Jacobs, Jr. Does supplemental vitamin C increase cardiovascular disease risk in women with diabetes? American Journal of Clinical Nutrition, Vol. 80, No. 5, 1194-1200, November 2004)

(Lee et al, 2005) (Vitamin E in the primary prevention of cardiovascular disease and cancer: the Women's Health Study: a randomized controlled trial. Lee IM, Cook NR, Gaziano JM, Gordon D, Ridker PM, Manson JE, et al. JAMA. 2005;294:56–65)

(Lesperance et al, 2002) (Lesperance ML, Olivotto IA, Forde N, et al. Mega-dose vitamins and minerals in the treatment of non-metastatic breast cancer: an historical cohort study. Breast Cancer Res Treat (2002) 76(2):137–143)

(Levy et al, 2004) (Levy AP, Friedenberg P, Lotan R, et al. The effect of vitamin therapy on the progression of coronary artery atherosclerosis varies by haptoglobin type in postmenopausal women. Diabetes Care. 2004;27(4):925-930)

(Lin et al, 2009) (Vitamins C and E and Beta Carotene Supplementation and Cancer Risk: A Randomized Controlled Trial. Jennifer Lin, Nancy R. Cook, Christine Albert, Elaine Zaharris, J. Michael Gaziano,

Martin Van Denburgh, Julie E. Buring, JoAnn E. Manson. JNCI Journal of the National Cancer Institute 2009 101(1):14-23)

(Lippman et al, 2009) (Effect of selenium and vitamin E on risk of prostate cancer and other cancers: the Selenium and Vitamin E Cancer Prevention Trial (SELECT). Lippman, SM. JAMA. 2009 Jan 7;301(1):39-51. Epub 2008 Dec 9)

(Liu et al., 2006) (S. Liu, I-M. Lee, Y. Song, M. Van Denburgh, N. R. Cook, J. E. Manson, and J. E. Buring. Vitamin E and Risk of Type 2 Diabetes in the Women's Health Study Randomized Controlled Trial. Diabetes, October 1, 2006; 55(10): 2856 – 2862)

(Longnecker, 1997) (Longnecker MP, Newcomb PA, Mittendorf R, Greenberg ER, Willett WC. Intake of carrots, spinach, and supplements containing vitamin A in relation to risk of breast cancer. Cancer Epidemiol Biomarkers Prev. 1997;6(11):887-892)

(Lonn et al. 2002) (Eva Lonn et al. Effects of Vitamin E on Cardiovascular and Microvascular Outcomes in High-Risk Patients With Diabetes. Results of the HOPE Study and MICRO-HOPE Substudy. Diabetes Care 25:1919-1927, 2002)

(Lonn et al, 2005) (Effects of long-term vitamin E supplementation on cardiovascular events and cancer: a randomized controlled trial. E. Lonn et al. JAMA. 2005 Mar 16;293(11):1338-47)

(Luchsinger et al, 2003) (Luchsinger et al. Antioxidant Vitamin Intake and Risk of Alzheimer Disease. Arch Neurol 2003;60: 203-208)

(Magliano et al, 2006) (Magliano, Dianna; McNeil, John; Branley, Pauline; Shiel, Louise; Demos, Lisa; Wolfe, Rory; Kotsopoulos, Dimitra; McGrath, Barry. The Melbourne Atherosclerosis Vitamin E Trial (MAVET): a study of high dose vitamin E in smokers. European Journal of Cardiovascular Prevention & Rehabilitation. June 2006 - Volume 13 - Issue 3 - pp 341-347)

(Mann et al, 2004) (Effects of vitamin E on cardiovascular outcomes in people with mild-to-moderate renal insufficiency: results of the HOPE study. J.F. Mann et al. Kidney Int. 2004 Apr;65(4):1375-80)

(Matthan et al, 2003) (Matthan N.R. et al. Impact of simvastatin, niacin, and/or antioxidants on cholesterol metabolism in CAD patients with low HDL. Journal of Lipid Research, Vol. 44, 800-806, April 2003)

(Maserejian et al, 2007) (Maserejian NW, Giovanncci E, Rosner B, Joshipura K. Prospective Study of Vitamins C, E, A, and Carotenoids and Risk of Oral Premalignant Lesions in Men. International J of Cancer. 120(5):970-7; 2006)

(Mayer-Davis et al, 1997) (Mayer-Davis EJ, Monaco JH, Marshall JA, Rushing J, Juhaeri. Vitamin c intake and cardiovascular disease risk factors in persons with non-insulin-dependent diabetes mellitus. From the Insulin Resistance Atherosclerosis Study and the San Luis Valley Diabetes Study. Prev Med 1997 May-Jun;26(3):277-83)

(Mayne et al, 2001) (Susan T. Mayne et al. Randomized Trial of Supplemental beta-Carotene to Prevent Second Head and Neck Cancer. Cancer Research 61, 1457-1463, February 15, 2001)

(McNeil et al, 2004) (McNeil JJ, Robman L, Tikellis G, Sinclair MI, McCarty CA, Taylor HR. Vitamin E supplementation and cataract: randomized controlled trial. Ophthalmology. 2004;111(1):75-84)

(McQuillan et al. 2001) (McQuillan BM, Hung J, Beilby JP, Nidorf M, Thompson PL. Antioxidant vitamins and the risk of carotid atherosclerosis. The Perth Carotid Ultrasound Disease Assessment study (CUDAS). J Am Coll Cardiol. 2001 Dec;38(7):1788-94)

(Miller et al., 1997) (Miller, E.R. 3rd, L.J. Appel, O.A. Levander & D.M. Levine. 1997. The effect of antioxidant vitamin supplementation on traditional cardiovascular risk factors. J. Cardiovasc. Risk. 4(1):19-24)

(Miller et al., 2004) (Miller ER 3d, Pastor-Barriuso R, Dalal D, Riemersma RA, Appel LJ, Guallar E. Meta-analysis: high-dosage vitamin E supplementation may increase all-cause mortality. Ann Intern Med 2005;142:37-46)

(Moertel et al, 1985) (Moertel CG, Fleming TR, Creagan ET, Rubin J, O'Connell MJ, Ames MM. High-dose vitamin C versus placebo in the treatment of patients with advanced cancer who have had no prior chemotherapy. A randomized double-blind comparison. N Engl J Med. 1985 Jan 17;312(3):137-41)

(Moilanen and Hovatta, 1995) (Moilanen J, Hovatta O. Excretion of alpha-tocopherol into human seminal plasma after oral administration. Andrologia. 1995 May-Jun;27(3):133-6)

(Morris and Carson, 2003) (Routine Vitamin Supplementation To Prevent Cardiovascular Disease: A Summary of the Evidence for the U.S. Preventive Services Task Force. Morris and Carson. ANN INTERN MED 2003;139:56-70. Review)

(MRC/BHF, 2002) (MRC/BHF Heart Protection Study of antioxidant vitamin supplementation in 20,536 high-risk individuals: a randomized placebo-controlled trial. Lancet. 2002 Jul 6;360(9326):23-33)

(Muntwyler et al. 2002) (Muntwyler J, Hennekens CH, Manson JE, Buring JE, Gaziano JM. Vitamin supplement use in a low-risk population of US male physicians and subsequent cardiovascular mortality. Arch Intern Med. 2002 Jul 8;162(13):1472-6)

(Myung et al, 2009) (S.-K. Myung et al. Effects of antioxidant supplements on cancer prevention: meta-analysis of randomized controlled trials. Annals of Oncology Advance Access published online on July 21, 2009) (Myung, S.-K., Kim, Y., Ju, W., Choi, H. J., Bae, W. K. (2010). Effects of antioxidant supplements on cancer prevention: meta-analysis of randomized controlled trials. Ann Oncol 21: 166-179)

(Neuhouser et al, 2009) (Multivitamin Use and Risk of Cancer and Cardiovascular Disease in the Women's Health Initiative Cohorts. Marian L. Neuhouser et al. Arch Intern Med. 2009;169(3):294-304)

(Omenn et al., 1996) (Risk factors for lung cancer and for intervention effects in CARET, the Beta-Carotene and Retinol Efficacy Trial. G.S. Omenn et al. J Natl Cancer Inst. 1996 Nov 6;88(21):1550-9)

(Omenn et al, NEJM. 1996) (Omenn GS, Goodman GE, Thornquist MD, et al. Effects of a combination of beta carotene and vitamin A on lung cancer and cardiovascular disease. N Engl J Med. 1996;334:1150-1155)

(Peters et al, 2008) (U. Peters et al. Vitamin E and selenium supplementation and risk of prostate cancer in the Vitamins and lifestyle (VITAL) study cohort. Cancer Causes Control. 2008 Feb;19(1):75-87)

(Pham et al, 2005) (Pham DQ, Plakogiannis R. Vitamin E supplementation in Alzheimer's disease, Parkinson's disease, tardive dyskinesia, and cataract: Part 2. Ann Pharmacother. 2005 Dec;39(12):2065-72)

(Pocobelli et al, 2007) (Gaia Pocobelli, Ulrike Peters, Alan R. Kristal and Emily White. Use of Supplements of Multivitamins, Vitamin C, and Vitamin E in Relation to Mortality. American Journal of Epidemiology 2009 170(4):472-483)

(Poston et al., 2006) (L. Poston et al. Vitamin C and vitamin E in pregnant women at risk for pre-eclampsia (VIP trial): randomised placebo-controlled trial. The Lancet, Volume 367, Issue 9517, Pages 1145 - 1154, 8 April 2006)

(Promislow et al, 2002) (Promislow JH, Goodman-Gruen D, Slymen DJ, Barrett-Connor E. Retinol intake and bone mineral density in the elderly: the Rancho Bernardo Study. J Bone Miner Res. 2002;17(8):1349-1358)

(Qiao et al, 2009) (Y.-L. Qiao, S. M. Dawsey, F. Kamangar, J.-H. Fan, C. C. Abnet, X.-D. Sun, L. L. Johnson, M. H. Gail, Z.-W. Dong, B. Yu, et al. Total and Cancer Mortality After Supplementation With Vitamins and Minerals: Follow-up of the Linxian General Population Nutrition Intervention Trial. J Natl Cancer Inst, April 1, 2009; 101(7): 507 - 518)

(Qu et al, 2007) (Chen-Xu Qu et al, Chemoprevention of Primary Liver Cancer: A Randomized, Double-Blind Trial in Linxian, China. Journal of the National Cancer Institute. Vol 99, Issue 16. August 15, 2007. pp. 1240-1247)

(Raal et al, 1999) (Efficacy of vitamin E compared with either simvastatin or atorvastatin in preventing the progression of atherosclerosis in homozygous familial hypercholesterolemia. Raal FJ, Pilcher GJ, Veller MG, Kotze MJ, Joffe BI. Am J Cardiol. 1999 Dec 1;84(11):1344-6, A7)

(Rapola et al, 1997) (Rapola, J.M., J. Virtamo, S. Ripatti, J.K. Huttunen, D. Albanes, P.R. Taylor & O. P. Heinonen. 1997. Randomized trial of alpha-tocopherol and beta-carotene supplements on incidence of major coronary events in men with previous myocardial infarction. Lancet. 349(9067):1715-1720)

(Rapola et al, 1998) (J M Rapola, J Virtamo, S Ripatti, J K Haukka, J K Huttunen, D Albanes, P R Taylor, and O P Heinonen. Effects of alpha tocopherol and beta carotene supplements on symptoms, progression, and prognosis of angina pectoris

Heart, May 1, 1998; 79(5): 454 - 458)

(Rautiainen et al, 2010) (Susanne Rautiainen, Birgitta Ejdervik Lindblad, Ralf Morgenstern and Alicja Wolk. Vitamin C supplements and the risk of age-related cataract: a population-based prospective cohort study in women. Am J Clin Nutr 91: 487-493, 2010)

(Reaven, 1995) (Reaven PD, Herold DA, Barnett J, Edelman S. Effects of Vitamin E on susceptibility of low-density lipoprotein and low-density lipoprotein subfractions to oxidation and on protein glycation in NIDDM. Diabetes Care. 1995;18(6):807-816)

(Riemersma et al, 2000) (R. A Riemersma, K. F Carruthers, R. A Elton, and K. A. Fox. Vitamin C and the risk of acute myocardial infarction. Am. J. Clinical Nutrition, May 1, 2000; 71(5): 1181 - 1186)

(Ristow et al, 2009) (Ristow M, Zarse K, Oberbach A, Klöting N, Birringer M, Kiehntopf M, Stumvoll M, Kahn CR, Blüher M. Antioxidants prevent health-promoting effects of physical exercise in humans. Proc Natl Acad Sci U S A. 2009 May 26;106(21):8665-70)

(Roberts et al, 2010) (Roberts JM et al, Vitamins C and E to prevent complications of pregnancy-associated hypertension. N Engl J Med (2010) 362: 1282-91)

(Rolf et al, 1999) (Rolf C, Cooper TG, Yeung CH, Nieschlag E. Antioxidant treatment of patients with asthenozoospermia or moderate oligoasthenozoospermia with high-dose vitamin C and vitamin E: a randomized, placebo-controlled, double-blind study. Hum Reprod. 1999 Apr;14(4):1028-33)

(Rumbold et al, 2006) (Vitamins C and E and the Risks of Preeclampsia and Perinatal Complications Alice R. Rumbold, Ph.D., Caroline A. Crowther, Ross R. Haslam, Gustaaf A. Dekker, and Jeffrey S. Robinson, for the ACTS Study Group. N Engl J Med. 2006 Apr 27;354(17): 1796-806)

(Satia et al, 2009) (Satia JA, Littman A, Slatore CG, Galanko JA, White E. Long-term use of beta-carotene, retinol, lycopene, and lutein supplements and lung cancer risk: results from the VITamins And Lifestyle (VITAL) study. Am J Epidemiol. 2009 Apr 1;169(7):815-28)

(Seddon, 2007) (Johanna M Seddon. Multivitamin-multimineral supplements and eye disease: age-related macular degeneration and cataract. American Journal of Clinical Nutrition, Vol. 85, No. 1, 304S-307S, January 2007)

(Seifried et al, 2003) (Seifried HE, McDonald SS, Anderson DE, Greenwald P, Milner JA. The antioxidant conundrum in cancer. Cancer Res (2003) 63:4295–8)

(Sesso et al, 2008) (Vitamins E and C in the prevention of cardiovascular disease in men: the Physicians' Health Study II randomized controlled trial. Sesso, HD. et al. JAMA. 2008 Nov 12;300(18):2123-33. Epub 2008 Nov 9)

(Shekelle et al, 2004) (Shekelle PG, Morton SC, Jungvig LK, et al. Effect of supplemental vitamin E for the prevention and treatment of cardiovascular disease. J Gen Intern Med 2004;19:380-389)

(Slatore et al, 2008) (Christopher G. Slatore, Alyson J. Littman, David H. Au, Jessie A. Satia, and Emily White Long-Term Use of Supplemental Multivitamins, Vitamin C, Vitamin E, and Folate Does Not Reduce the Risk of Lung Cancer. Am. J. Respir. Crit. Care Med. 177: 524-530. First published online Nov. 7, 2007 as doi:10.1164/rccm.200709-1398OC. Published in print March 1, 2008)

(Song et al. 2009) (Song Y, Cook NR, Albert CM, Van Denburgh M, Manson JE. Effects of vitamins C and E and beta-carotene on the risk of type 2 diabetes in women at high risk of cardiovascular disease: a randomized controlled trial. Am J Clin Nutr 2009 Aug;90(2):429-37)

(Stanner et al, 2004) (Stanner SA, Hughes J, Kelly CN, Buttriss J (2004). "A review of the epidemiological evidence for the 'antioxidant hypothesis'". Public Health Nutr 7 (3): 407–22)

(Stephens et al., 1996) (Stephens, NG et al. Randomized controlled trial of vitamin E in patients with coronary artery disease: Cambridge Heart Antioxidant Study (CHAOS)," Lancet, March 23, 1996; 347: 781-786.)

(Stevens et al, 2005) (Stevens VL, McCullough MI, Diver WR, Rodriguez C, Jacobs EJ, thun MJ, Calle EE. Use of multivitamins and prostate cancer mortality in a large cohort of US men. Cancer Causes Control. 2005 Aug; 16(6):643-50)

(Stone et al, 2005) (P.H. Stone et al. Effect of intensive lipid lowering, with or without antioxidant vitamins, compared with moderate lipid lowering on myocardial ischemia in patients with stable coronary artery disease: the Vascular Basis for the Treatment of Myocardial Ischemia Study. Circulation. 2005 Apr 12;111(14):1747-55)

(Tan et al, 2008) (Tan JS, Wang JJ, Flood V, Rochtchina E, Smith W, Mitchell P. Dietary antioxidants and the long-term incidence of age-related macular degeneration: the Blue Mountains Eye Study. Ophthalmology. 2008 Feb;115(2):334-41)

(Tangrea et al, 1992) (Tangrea JA, Edwards BK, Taylor PR, et al.: Long-term therapy with low-dose isotretinoin for prevention of basal cell carcinoma: a multicenter clinical trial. Isotretinoin-Basal Cell Carcinoma Study Group. J Natl Cancer Inst 84 (5): 328-32, 1992)

(Tangrea et al, 1993) (Tangrea JA, Adrianza E, Helsel WE, et al.: Clinical and laboratory adverse effects associated with long-term, low-dose isotretinoin: incidence and risk factors. The Isotretinoin-Basal Cell Carcinomas Study Group. Cancer Epidemiol Biomarkers Prev 2 (4): 375-80, 1993 Jul-Aug)

(Tardif et al, 1997) (Tardif, J.C., Cote, G and Lesperance, J., et al. Probucol and multivitamins in the prevention of restenosis after coronary angioplasty. Multivitamins and Probucol Study Group. N Engl J Med 1997; 337(6): 365-372)

(Teikari et al, 1998) (Teikari JM, Rautalahti M, Haukka J, et al. Incidence of cataract operations in Finnish male smokers unaffected by alpha tocopherol or beta carotene supplements. J Epidemiol Community Health. 1998;52(7):468-472)

(Taylor et al, 2002) (Taylor HR, Tikellis G, Robman LD, McCarty CA, McNeil JJ. Vitamin E supplementation and macular degeneration: randomised controlled trial. BMJ. 2002 Jul 6;325(7354):11)

(Thörnwall et al., 2004) (Effect of alpha-tocopherol and beta-carotene supplementation on coronary heart disease during the 6-year post-trial follow-up in the ATBC study. Markareetta E. Törnwall et al. European Heart Journal 2004 25(13):1171-1178)

(van Stijn et al, 2008) (van Stijn MF, Ligthart-Melis GC, Boelens PG, Scheffer PG, Teerlink T, Twisk JW, Houdijk AP, van Leeuwen PA. Antioxidant enriched enteral nutrition and oxidative stress after major gastrointestinal tract surgery. World J Gastroenterol. 2008 Dec 7;14(45):6960-9)

(Vasquez et al., 1998) (The SUVIMAX (France) study: the role of antioxidants in the prevention of cancer and cardiovascular disease. Vasquez, Martínez C, Galán P, Preziosi P, Ribas L, Serra LL, Hercberg S. Rev Esp Salud Publica. 1998 May-Jun;72(3):173-83.)

(Virtamo et al, 1998) (Virtamo J, Rapola JM, Ripatti S, et al. Effect of vitamin E and beta carotene on the incidence of primary nonfatal myocardial infarction and fatal coronary heart disease. Arch Intern Med. 1998;158:668-675)

(Vivekananthan et al., 2003) (Vivekananthan DP, Penn MS, Sapp SK, Hsu A, Topol EJ. Use of antioxidant vitamins for the prevention of cardiovascular disease: meta-analysis of randomised trials 2003 Lancet 2003 June 14; 361: 2017–23)

(Waters et al, 2002) (Waters DD, Alderman EL, Hsia J, Howard BV, Cobb FR, Rogers WJ, Ouyang P, Thompson P, Tardif JC, Higginson L, Bittner V, Steffes M, Gordon DJ, Proschan M, Younes N, Verter JI. Effects of hormone replacement therapy and antioxidant vitamin supplements on coronary atherosclerosis in postmenopausal women: a randomized controlled trial. JAMA. 2002; 288: 2432–40)

(Westhuyzen et al, 1997) (Westhuyzen J, Cochrane AD, Tesar PJ, Mau T, Cross DB, Frenneaux MP, Khafagi FA, Fleming SJ. Effect of preoperative supplementation with alpha-tocopherol and ascorbic acid on myocardial injury in patients undergoing cardiac operations. J Thorac Cardiovasc Surg 1997 May;113(5):942-8)

(Wiysonge et al, 2005) (Wiysonge CS, Shey MS, Sterne JA, Brockehurst P. Vitamin A supplementation for reducing the risk of mother-to-child transmission of HIV infection. Cochrane Database Syst Rev. 2005;(4):CD003648)

(Woodside, et al. 1998) (Woodside JV, Yarnell JW, McMaster D, Young IS, Harmon DL, McCrum EE, Patterson CC, Gey KF, Whitehead AS, Evans A. Effect of B-group vitamins and antioxidant vitamins on hyper-homocysteinemia: a double-blind, randomized, factorial-design, controlled trial. Am J Clin Nutr. 1998 May;67(5):858-66)

(Wu et al, 2002) (Wu K, Willett WC, Chan JM, Fuchs CS, Colditz GA, Rimm EB, Giovannucci EL. A prospective study on supplemental vitamin E intake and risk of colon cancer in women and men. Cancer Epidemiol Biomarkers Prev 2002;11:1298-304)

(Yaffe et al, 2004) (Yaffe K, Clemons TE, McBee WL, Lindblad AS; Age-Related Eye Disease Study Research Group. Impact of antioxidants, zinc, and copper on cognition in the elderly: a randomized, controlled trial. Neurology. 2004 Nov 9;63(9):1705-7)

(Yusuf et al. 2000) (Yusuf, S., Dagenais, G., Progue, J. et al. Vitamin E supplementation and cardiovascular evens, in high-risk patients the Heart Outcomes Prevention Evaluation Study Investigators. N Engl J Med. 2000; 342; 154-160)

(Zaharris et al, 2007) (A Randomized Factorial Trial of Vitamins C and E and Beta Carotene in the Secondary Prevention of Cardiovascular Events in Women: Results From the Women's Antioxidant Cardiovascular Study. Zaharris, J. MacFadyen, E. Danielson, J. E. Buring, and J. E. Manson. Arch Intern Med, August 13, 2007; 167(15): 1610 – 1618)

www.ingramcontent.com/pod-product-compliance
Lightning Source LLC
Chambersburg PA
CBHW071353170526
45165CB00001B/27